THE ECONOMICS OF HEALTH AND MEDICAL CARE

Second Edition

Philip Jacobs, Ph.D.
University of Massachusetts
at Amherst

AN ASPEN PUBLICATION®
Aspen Publishers, Inc.

1987

Rockville, Maryland
Royal Tunbridge Wells

Library of Congress Cataloging in Publication Data

Jacobs, Philip.
The economics of health and medical care.

Bibliography: p.
Includes index.
1. Medical economics. 2. Medical economics — United States. I. Title.
RA410.J32   1986   338.4'73621   86–25908
ISBN: 0–87189–607–9

Editorial Services: Lisa J. McCullough

Library of Congress Catalog Card Number: 86–25908
ISBN: 0–87189–607–9

Printed in the United States of America

1   2   3   4   5

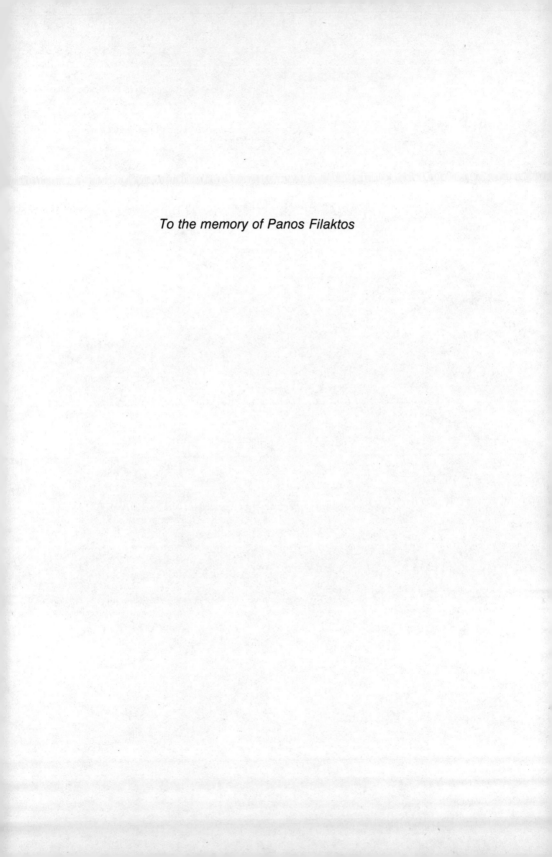

To the memory of Panos Filaktos

Table of Contents

Preface

The second edition of *The Economics of Health and Medical Care* follows closely the first in terms of its design. It is a textbook whose purpose is to provide the reader with the elements necessary to apply basic economic principles to the health care field. It is assumed that the reader has no prior background in economics. Only high school level mathematics is required to follow the presentation of the text. The concepts presented in this book are at a level of exposition similar to those in introductory economics principles texts. Emphasis is placed on those tools of particular relevance to health care as well as on the degree to which these concepts are appropriate to deal with problems in this field. The reader will find that, even at this introductory level, economic analysis can provide pertinent and systematic insights into the workings of the health care system and the evaluation of health care policies. The presentation is designed for use in undergraduate or graduate level health economics classes in public health, health care administration, and other health related disciplines.

The approach of the book is to develop usable economic tools. The orientation is designed to give the reader a task focus so that he or she is aware of the questions being answered by the analysis. As a consequence of this approach, the subject matter has been divided into three parts, each of which corresponds to one of the major tasks of economics. These tasks are description, explanation or prediction, and evaluation or prescription. The book is organized in a progressive manner; the concepts developed in Part II (explanation) and Part III (evaluation) build on those of Part I (description).

It should also be pointed out that *The Economics of Health and Medical Care* is not a critique of the health economics literature, although it should help students in further study of specific topics in the area. Although institutional and policy aspects of health economics are covered, the book is not intended as a survey of current policy in the health care field. Such information is best obtained from current periodicals and recent policy-oriented books. It is hoped, however, that in studying this book the reader will be better prepared to make up his or her mind on many current policy issues.

In recent years health policy in the United States has undergone major changes. These include a growing emphasis on competition from alternative delivery and transacting systems (for instance, health maintenance organizations and preferred provider organizations); the introduction by Medicare of a diagnosis-based prospective payment system for hospitals; the growth of for-profit providers and multihospital chains; and a deemphasis on some forms of regulation. I have incorporated these and other new subjects into this edition where the appropriate principles apply. As a result, many chapters are substantially revised from the first edition. I also felt that it was necessary to add two new chapters, one on the economic principles relating to market power and one on competition policy.

In addition to these changes, Part III, dealing with evaluative economics and health care policy, has been substantially rewritten. I have tried to provide a unified policy framework for this portion. I have also tried to develop a closer link between Part II and Part III by relating each policy analysis to the relevant explanatory model. This technique will better enable the reader to apply basic economic models to specific policy problems.

Acknowledgments

I would like to acknowledge the help of a number of people, currently or formerly connected with the University of South Carolina, in the preparation of this edition. I found the advice of Dave Adcock, Marty Bridges, John Chilton, Alan Chovil, Todd Sandler, and Cindy Woods to be of considerable help. Jin-hua Chen, Ron Wilder, and Glyn Williams provided friendship, encouragement, and advice. Joan Altekruse of the Department of Preventive Medicine gave me invaluable support, personal as well as institutional, including the help of Jamie McCullough and Rosemarie Gunter. Everose Alexander was a writer's dream-come-true with her work on the word processor. And as with the first edition, my wife Frosso was instrumental in my undertaking this rewriting and in helping me keep my momentum; in addition, she had to take over a disproportionate share of Louis, Alex, and Jo's time. Without her help, I wouldn't have started or completed this book.

Introduction

This book is an introduction to the economic approach to understanding health care problems. Our approach is based on the identification of scarcity as a fundamental cause of many of these problems. *Scarcity* can be defined as a deficiency in the quantity or quality of goods and services that are available in relation to those amounts that people desire. For example, most parents would welcome a greater availability of obstetricians and pediatricians. Many children of elderly and disabled parents would like their parents to have increased access to nursing home care. Many who suffer accidents would benefit from additional emergency medical services. The list of deficiencies could go on almost indefinitely.

Yet the fundamental problem is not merely one of "not enough" to go around. Side by side with the "not enough" problems are instances where there seems to be "too much." In 1984, total expenditures on health care in the United States reached $376 billion, over 10 percent of the Gross National Product (GNP), which is the dollar sum of all final goods and services produced. In 1965, health care expenditures were only 5.6 percent of the GNP. Included in these expenditures are services with high costs whose impact on health has been questioned. Among these services are the large-volume "little ticket" items, such as x-rays and lab tests, which make up about a quarter of all hospital costs; high-cost procedures, such as coronary artery bypass grafting, whose effectiveness is unproved; and some hospital services for the terminally ill, which consume a disproportionate share of the health care dollar (Angell, 1985). A number of commentators have asserted that a considerable amount of ineffective or what is termed "flat of the curve" medicine is being practiced (Enthoven, 1980). Issues of "too much," when raised side by side with those of "not enough," point to the importance of studying the entire resource-allocation process in health care.

Economics is the science that deals with the consequences of resource scarcity, and health economics deals with the specific portion of the economic problem that is concerned with health and health care. Because of its very broad scope, economics does not provide a body of rigid doctrines about scarce resources. Rather, economics offers an overall viewpoint toward understanding many problems, all of which relate to scarcity in one form or another. Within the context of the economic viewpoint, specific approaches can be taken to illuminate issues in health care. The common thread running through all of them is that some aspect of scarcity lies at the root of the problem.

As an introductory text, this book focuses on how to "do" economics. The organization of the book divides the discipline into three separate areas, which can be regarded as the tasks of economics. The exposition of these tasks in a health context is the objective of the book; the performance of these tasks should be regarded as the objective of the reader. These tasks include asking specific questions and searching for answers to these questions. Both of these activities, asking and answering, are performed when practicing economics. It should be stressed that the search for relevant questions is as critical a part of the process of analyzing economic problems as is the provision of answers. By formulating a problem in the context of scarcity, a deeper understanding of many problems is obtained, which may ultimately lead the way to the discovery of a solution or a means of accommodation.

Three major categories of economics tasks are presented: description, explanation, and evaluation. The next portion of this chapter is devoted to a discussion of what comprises these tasks. The section that follows describes the tools used in the book, that is, graphs and models. The final section presents an outline of the book.

THREE MAJOR TASKS OF ECONOMICS

The three major tasks of economics covered in this book, description, explanation, and evaluation, will usually not be performed in isolation from one another. Rather, descriptive economics will be used to complement an explanation or evaluation of an event whose occurrence has been explained. Nevertheless, even though these tasks may be intermingled in economic analysis, the specific task being performed should be kept clearly in mind.

Descriptive Economics

Description refers to the identification, definition, and measurement of phenomena. This task is concerned with determining the nature of the phenomena and obtaining estimates of their magnitudes. Having performed this task, we obtain some notion of the existing facts. It should be pointed out that this task only amounts to fact finding. There is, at this stage, no explanation of why the facts are what they are and no pronouncement or judgment evaluating the phenomena.

Examples of descriptions are the statistics that, in 1974, Americans 65 years and older visited physicians' offices on the average of 4.7 times per year while those in the 25 to 44 year old age group paid 2.6 visits per year (*Health United States* 1976-7, p. 257).

Explanatory Economics

The second task of economics is explaining and predicting certain phenomena. This task involves conducting an analysis of a cause–effect format. In undertaking such a task, we are moving one step beyond description. We are now explaining the causes of certain events that have occurred. This task is performed with the aid of models that classify various causal factors (assuming there is more than one) in a systematic framework. Based on this framework, hypotheses are developed about the net effect of each causal factor on the phenomena we want to explain. We do not go any further at this stage. That is, we do not pass judgment on whether the phenomena we have observed are present in the desired amounts. As an example of an explanation, let us say we want to determine why those in the 65-year-old and above age group mentioned previously utilized more medical care than those in the 25- ro 44-year-old age group. First, we would develop a framework that incorporated the major causal factors relevant to this phenomenon; usually there will be several. In this case let us say that our framework contains two essential causal factors: (1) the health status of each group, and (2) the price paid by the members of each group for their medical care. Using these causal factors, we could then hypothesize that quantity of medical care demanded will increase when health status is lowered and when consumers pay less for their medical care. These causal factors relate to our example because (1) the health status of the older group is lower, and (2) because of government-sponsored health insurance for the elderly, the older group might pay considerably less for medical care. If these facts were true, our hypothesis would predict that the older group will demand medical care in greater quantities. Should these increased quantities also be available, then the older group will utilize more.

The essential point in this example is the type of task we are performing when we develop our hypothesis; we are attempting to explain an event that has occurred or will occur.

Evaluation

The third task of economics is evaluation. This task involves judging or ranking alternative phenomena according to some standard. In other words, an acceptable standard must be obtained, and, based on this standard, alternative ways of using scarce resources are then ranked. In choosing the standard, one major criterion is *acceptability*. Standards by themselves are easy to come by; however, standards are often controversial concepts, and some degree of acceptability must usually be attached to the choice of standard. In light of this standard, alternative economic phenomena, that is, alternative uses of scarce resources, can be evaluated. For example, if we choose a standard that says that the more medical care one has the better off one is, then according to this standard the older group in our previous example is better off than the younger group. Furthermore, any measure that raises the utilization of the younger group (by lowering the price paid by this group and by increasing the available resources for use by this group) would, according to our standard, lead to a better allocation of resources (Hemenway, 1982).

TOOLS USED IN ECONOMIC ANALYSIS

Several tools are used in economic analysis. The first is graphic analysis. The purpose of graphic analysis is to illustrate relations between economic variables. The second tool is a model, which allows us to draw inferences about the relations we might expect to occur when specific underlying conditions are present. Such a tool forces us to be explicit about the underlying factors that are present in the workings of the resource-allocation process.

Economic Variables

An economic variable is an economically relevant phenomenon whose value or magnitude may vary. Examples of economic variables include prices, costs, incomes, and quantities of commodities. Economic variables can be measured along a scale, once appropriate units of measurement have been chosen. For example, price can be measured in cents or dollars per unit or quantities can be expressed in terms of numbers of visits, numbers of hospital days, numbers of hospital beds, and so forth. Two examples of units of measurement are shown along the axis in Figure 1. Along the vertical axis, values of the price of medical care are shown. We have shown the price per visit to a physician, which is the economic variable that we are examining, in terms of cents. Along this axis the price can be, alternatively, 0, 100, 200, 300, and so on. Along the horizontal axis we measure alternative values of the quantity of visits to a physician's office. These are measured in terms of number of visits.

Relations between Economic Variables

The next step after the identification and measurement of economic variables involves determining relations among these variables. Relations show how one variable changes with respect to another variable. These relations can be specified in a causal or noncausal manner. For example, we can state that one variable, total health care costs, has increased, while another variable, time, has also increased.

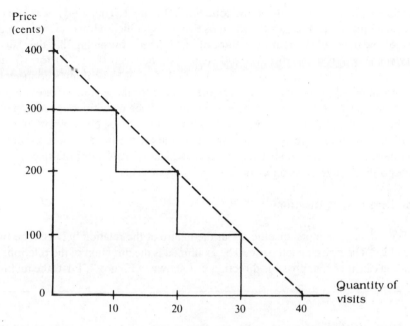

Figure 1 Relations between price and quantity of visits. The dashed line shows continuous values, and the solid line shows discrete values.

This is an example of a noncausal relation because it is not the time itself that has caused these costs to increase. As time has passed, other influencing variables have changed, and these have caused the health care costs to increase.

In a causal relation, when the value of one economic variable changes, the value of a second economic variable also changes as a result of the change in the first. For example, if the price falls for a visit to the doctor, more visits would be demanded at the lower price than at the higher price. Causal relations are usually expressed in the form of hypothetical statements, such as, if price falls, then quantity demanded will increase.

Graphic Representation of Relation

Let us start with a simple relation between price and quantity of visits such that, when the price is at a level of 400 cents, the quantity of visits is 0; when the price is 300, the quantity of visits is 10; when the price is 200, the quantity of visits is 20; and when the price is 100, the quantity of visits is 30. Associated with each price is a specific quantity: 0 visits with 400 cents, 10 visits with 300 cents, and so forth. Each of these associations can be represented by a point, as shown in Figure 1. All these points together form the relation. If we know only these values, we can draw this relation diagrammatically as the solid line in Figure 1. This solid line is known as a step function and relates to only those values specified. However, we can go further and generalize about the nature of our function by saying that the values between 0 and 100, or 100 and 200 cents, and between 0 and 10, or 10 and 20 visits, can also be specified as part of the relation. We can draw a continuous curve joining all the points specified in the relation for those values not explicitly expressed, such as 155 cents, 5 visits, and so on. Such a continuous relation can be shown as the dashed line in Figure 1, which joins all the points specified in the relation. Once we have drawn a continuous curve, we have a more complete specification of the relation between price and quantity. Any value of price, within our specified ranges, has an associated quantity of visits.

The Direction of Relations

We can now be more specific about the nature of the relation between the two variables. The first characteristic to be examined is the direction of the relation. A relation can have four possible directions, as shown in Figure 2. First, the relation

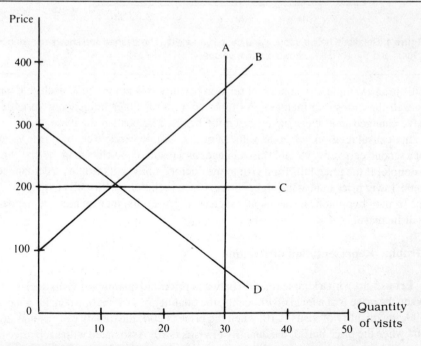

Figure 2 Direction of relations: curve *A*, constant quantity for all prices; curve *B*, price and quantity positively related; curve *C*, a constant price; and curve *D*, price and quantity negatively related.

may be positive, as shown by curve *B*. Here higher values of price are associated with higher values of quantity of visits. If there were a causal relation between them, and if the direction of causation ran from price to quantity, we would hypothesize that, as price increases, so does quantity. The opposite type of relation is shown by curve *D*, which indicates a negative relation and states that the greater the price, the smaller the quantity. Thus higher values of price are associated with lower values of quantity of visits. The third type of relation is shown by curve *C*. This relation (or, to be more precise, nonrelation) shows that, whatever the quantity of visits, the price will stay the same. In this illustration the price will remain at a value of 200 cents. The final type of relation, shown by curve *A*, is also a nonrelation. Curve *A* shows that, whatever the price may be, the quantity of visits will remain the same (in Figure 2, at a level of 30).

The Slope of Relations

The slope of a geometric relation shows how much of a change in one variable is associated with a given change in a related variable. In causal terms, slope can be expressed as the magnitude of response. Several examples are shown in Figure 3.

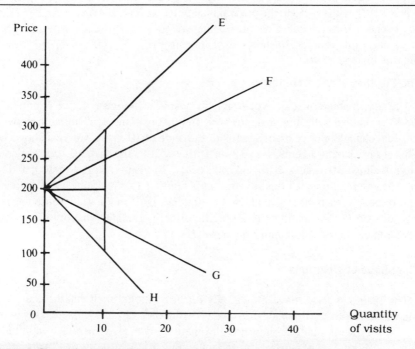

Figure 3 Slope of relations. With *E*, price increases by more than *F* for a given increase in quantity. With *H*, price decreases by more than *G* for a given increase in quantity.

Let us first look at the slope of relation, or curve, *F*. Curve *F* touches the price axis where the price equals 200 cents. This price is associated with a quantity of visits of 0. If we raise the price by 50 cents to a level of 250 cents, the associated new quantity of visits as shown by curve *F* is 10. An increase in the price by 50 cents is associated with an increase in quantity by 10 visits. The slope of curve *F* is thus 50/10, with regard to the quantity axis, or 10/50, with regard to the price axis. Because relation *F* is a straight line, the slope remains constant at every point on the line. (Some nonlinear relationships are presented later.) A second positive slope relationship is *E*. As can be seen in Figure 3, relation *E* shows a greater change in price associated with a given change in quantity as compared to relation *F*. From the initial price of 200 cents and 0 visits, a quantity change of 10 is associated with a price change from 200 to 300. The slope is 100/10 with regard to the quantity axis or 10/100 with regard to the price axis. Comparing relations *E* and *F*, we can say that, for the same quantity change, the price change in relation *E* must be double that in relation *F*.

Relations *G* and *H* can be regarded in a similar manner, but now the direction of the relation is such that a higher price is associated with a lower quantity. Relation *G* has a slope such that a fall in price of 50 cents is associated with an increase in quantity of 10 visits. The slope of the curve with regard to the quantity axis is 50/10; with regard to the price axis, it is 10/50. This shows a change in price of 50 cents associated with a quantity change of 10 visits in the opposite direction. In comparison, relation *H* shows a change in price of 100 associated with a quantity change of 10.

The Position of the Relation

The next characteristic of a relation is its position. In Figure 4, two relations, *J* and *K*, are shown with similar slopes but different positions. Each relation shows a 100-cent change in price associated with a change of 10 visits. Curve *J* shows no visits at a price of 300 cents, 10 visits at a price of 200, and so on. By comparison, curve *K* shows 10 visits at a price of 300 cents, 20 visits at a price of 200, and so on. The essential point of this illustration is how the two relations are positioned with respect to each other. Relation *K* is greater than *J* in the same sense that, at any point on *K* corresponding to a specific price, the related quantity of visits is greater than the related quantity on curve *J*.

The Shape of Relations

The examples so far have shown only linear relations, such that the change in one variable with regard to a given change in another variable is fixed. This is not the only type of relation, however. Sometimes we also encounter nonlinear relations. For this type of relation, the magnitude of the response will vary along the curve. Relations *L* and *M* in Figure 5 are two such examples.

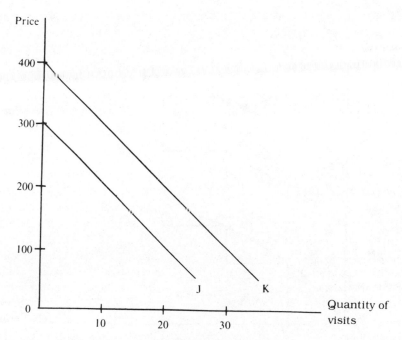

Figure 4 Position of relations. *K* shows a greater quantity than *J* for any given price.

Curve *M* shows the relation between the total cost of production of lab tests and the number of tests produced. At a quantity of 0, there is a total cost of $10; at a quantity of 1, there is a total cost of $11; at a quantity of 2, there is a total cost $14; and at a quantity of 3, the total cost is $19. The slope of the relationship changes as more lab tests are produced. For the first test, the slope is such that a $1 change in cost is associated with a change of one lab test. The next change of one lab test is associated with a $3 change in cost, and later with a $5 change in cost. The slope with reference to the lab test axis is increasing as the number of lab tests increases. Curve *M* is a smoothed out version of this relation. The relation shape is such that *M* curves as production increases.

Curve *L* shows declining slopes with increasing production. A total cost of 0 is associated with a 0 level of output. An output level of 1 is associated with a cost of $5, an output level of 2 is associated with a cost of $8, and an output level of 3 is associated with a cost of $9. The slope of the relation between 0 and 1 units of production, with regard to the production axis, is 5/1; for the next unit of production, it is 3/1; and for the next it is 1/1. The smoothed out relation is shown by curve *L*, with its tendency to level off.

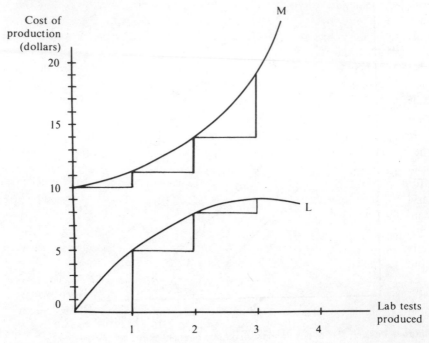

Figure 5 Shape of relations. *M* shows additional higher costs at successively higher levels of lab tests produced. *L* shows lower additional costs at successively higher levels of tests.

The Nature of Economic Propositions

Many statements made in this book regarding the resource-allocation process in the health care field will be propositions that attempt to spell out the consequences of certain conditions. The propositions are hypothetical statements of the form "if . . . then. . . ." That is, if certain conditions $x, y,$ and z hold, then, as a consequence, phenomenon q will occur. Having made this statement, we have made a prediction of what will cause the phenomenon we want to explain. The "if" portions of these statements are called *conditions* or *assumptions*; the "if/ then" statement in its entirety is the *conclusion, implication,* or *prediction*.

As an example, let us form a model to explain how much medical care an individual will demand. Our model contains initial assumptions. The first, A1, is that the price of medical care to an individual is $5 per visit; this $5 includes all services provided by the doctor, including transfusions, intravenous feedings (should they be needed), and so on. The second assumption in our model, A2, states that the individual has a weekly income of $100 that can be spent on any of a number of commodities. This assumption about the constraint on the individual brings the example within the realm of economics since scarcity is now introduced. The third assumption, A3, is about the behavior of the individual: the individual has an objective, or an end, of consuming only medical care; he or she does not want to consume any other commodity. Our assumptions are such that this is entirely feasible. If an individual does not consume food, for example, he or she would begin to starve and have to visit a physician. For a fee of $5, the individual would receive an intravenous solution. Note that all deficiencies in our example can be effectively met by obtaining medical care.

What consequences do these assumptions have for the consumer's behavior? The implications of the model are that the individual will consume 20 visits of medical care. Given his or her economic situation, this is all the individual can afford to consume, and given that he or she wants only medical care and can survive by consuming only this commodity, then he or she will not consume less than 20 visits. The resulting implication is a prediction of our model; the prediction is based on the initial conditions or assumptions of the model. Predictions are derivatives of the assumptions and can be regarded as the consequences of what would happen if the assumptions were to hold.

Let us now change one of our initial assumptions, A1. In its place let us propose assumption A1a, which states that the price of medical care is $1 per visit. Now the implications of our model are that the quantity demanded of medical care will be 100 visits. With a fall in price, the quantity demanded has increased. This is a prediction of our model when we consider all the assumptions and draw a comparative analysis.

Another comparative analysis would be to predict the consequences of what happens if the individual's income increases. In this instance, assumption A2 changes to A2a, which states that weekly income is now $110. This new assumption, coupled with the original assumptions A1 and A3, yields the conclusion that quantity demanded will increase. By performing a comparative analysis of the initial conditions with the new conditions, we can conclude that an increase in income will lead to an increase in the quantity of medical care demanded.

The mere predicting, or deriving, of conclusions about the resource-allocation process is not the end of our task, however. Our conclusions are hypotheses or propositions. They are suggestions about how the world might behave if the assumptions we have posited in the model are adequate approximations to those conditions that exist in reality. In explanatory economics, we will test these implications against actual circumstances to see if what we predicted actually does occur. The true test of an explanatory model is how well it explains or predicts actual data movements or phenomena. In evaluative economics, our task is somewhat different in that we are comparing actual against ideal sets of events. Nevertheless, whether we are deriving explanatory or evaluative principles, we place our proposition in a logical form that allows us to simultaneously incorporate a number of variables into our analysis.

OUTLINE OF THE BOOK

This book introduces the analysis of the economics of health care in the context of the three tasks just outlined. Part I, which consists of Chapters 1 and 2, introduces the description of economic dimensions of the health care field. Part II, consisting of Chapters 3 through 9, presents explanatory analyses of a number of health-related events. Part III (Chapters 10 through 14) develops evaluative analyses of several important aspects of health care resource use.

Chapter 1 presents a discussion of the output of the health care sector. Two stages of output are identified: (1) health care, which is an activity designed to improve health, and (2) health itself. Measurements of both types of output are presented. In Chapter 2, economic dimensions of the health care sector are identified and some measures of these dimensions are presented. In this chapter some of the basic problems of the health care sector are described for explanation and evaluation in subsequent sections of the book.

Chapter 3, the first explanatory chapter, develops a model to explain the demand for medical care by consumers. A number of separate factors are identified as influences on the demand for medical care. These are welded together into a single model that allows us to predict the effects of each factor when all other relevant factors are held constant. In Chapter 3 the demand for medical care is presented as if medical care were an ordinary commodity in the consumer's budget. However, medical care has characteristics that, although not totally unique to this commodity, combine to warrant special treatment. In Chapter 4 a number of these characteristics are introduced and analyzed in light of the standard model developed in Chapter 3.

In Chapters 5 and 6 we turn our attention to the behavior of health care suppliers, such as doctors, hospitals, and laboratories. Chapter 5 develops the relationships between resource use and output produced and between the cost and the scale of output produced. Both relationships are examined with regard to the individual supplying organizations. Chapter 6 presents the analysis of the supply behavior of individual producers and of groups of suppliers (i.e., market supply). The behavior of for-profit and nonprofit supply units is treated separately, since nonprofit and governmental suppliers are of particular importance in the health care field.

In Chapter 7 we examine a standard textbook explanation of how the market resource-allocation process works. This is the competitive market model, which has drawn a good deal of attention recently. However, not all market behavior is competitive. In Chapter 8 we examine the concept of market power: how it is acquired by suppliers and demanders and, when they acquire it, how this affects market outcomes, that is, prices, quantities, and qualities of output.

Some observers have stated that, because of some specific characteristics, medical care markets are special, and so they have developed models tailor-made to medical care. In Chapter 9 we examine several such models, including those where supplier-induced demand predominates and where insurance and service markets interact.

Chapter 10 introduces the topic of evaluation by identifying several alternative standards that have been used in evaluating resource use in the health care field. These standards include efficiency and equity. Based on efficiency analysis, a series of specific public policy goals is identified; using the basic models of Part II, we show how public programs and policies can be evaluated in light of these goals in Chapters 11 and 12.

In Chapter 11, public and private health insurance is discussed. Two major public programs, Medicare and Medicaid, are introduced. Specific policy problems are presented and, using the explanatory economic models developed in Chapters 3 to 9, the effects of specific policy measures are evaluated in light of the specific policy goals identified in Chapter 10.

The role of government policy in influencing the performance of the health care market is discussed in Chapter 12. Two views of regulation are presented. In the first, the public-interest view, the government establishes regulations to ensure that providers behave in the public (consumer's) interest. Evidence relating to this view has not been very convincing. A second view of regulation is based on a wider picture of the market: according to this interpretation, the government is a participant in the wider marketplace that incorporates both the suppliers and demanders of the traded product, as well as politicians and regulators. In this wider marketplace, various regulations and laws that have an impact on the supply–demand situation are "traded." The market outcome is thus influenced by regulation. Faced with discontent over the results of traditional market regulation, some observers have proposed that the medical market *can* be reshaped in the competitive mold. Two types of policies aimed in this direction, antitrust policy and tax reform, are presented in Chapter 13.

Finally, Chapter 14 presents the overall design of evaluation in the form of cost–benefit and cost-effectiveness analyses. Some basic principles of cost–benefit and cost-effectiveness analysis are set forth, and several of the tougher measurement problems are addressed.

REFERENCES

Aaron, H.J., & Schwartz, W.B. (1984). *The painful prescription*. Washington, DC: Brookings Institution.

Angell, M. (1985). Cost containment and the physician. *Journal of the American Medical Association*, *253*, 1203–1207.

Arrow, K.J. (1972). Problems of resource allocation in United States medical care. In R.M. Kunz & H. Fehr (Eds.), *The challenge of life* (pp. 392–410). Basel: Birkhauser-Verlag.

Enthoven, A.C. (1980). *Health plan*. Reading, Mass: Addison-Wesley Publishing Co., Inc.

Fuchs, V. (1974). *Who shall live?* New York: Basic Books, Inc.

Hemenway, D. The optimal location of doctors. *New England Journal of Medicine, 306,* 397–401.

Littenberg, B., & Neuhauser, D. (1981). To hell with economics? *American Journal of Public Health, 71,* 363–365.

Reinhardt, U. (1985). Future trends in the economics of medical practice and care. *American Journal of Cardiology, 56,* 50C–58C.

U.S. Department of Health, Education, and Welfare (1976/1977). *Health United States.*

Part I

Descriptive Economics

Chapter 1

Output of the Health Care Sector

1.1 INTRODUCTION

In this chapter we begin the first task of our study of the health care system, the task of description. This involves identifying the phenomena with which we are concerned, defining them so we can be precise about their nature, and measuring them so we can obtain an understanding of their magnitude. At this stage, we only wish to discover what phenomena exist, not what causes them (the task of explanation) or in what quantities they *should* exist (the task of evaluation).

The processes generated within the health care system can be looked at in two ways. The first approach is to regard them as consisting of the components of *health care* that are part of the process of influencing health. These health-influencing factors can be classified as life-style factors, such as diet, sleep, and other individual behaviors; environmental factors, such as air and water purification; genetic factors; and medical care, such as physicians' examinations and treatments. Thus health care is composed of the activities that are intended to influence health. Section 1.2 focuses on the definition and measurement of medical care. It identifies and defines the phenomena associated with medical care and discusses measures that indicate how much medical care is provided.

The second approach stems from the assertion that medical care is not the true output of the medical care sector, and that the true end of medical care is health. When measuring this output, the rationale continues, we should therefore be measuring how much health is being produced. In some cases we simply may be satisfied with knowing how much medical care is being utilized. If, however, we feel that changes in the quantity of medical care may not necessarily be beneficial, a more logical approach would be to measure what medical care is ideally supposed to produce, that is, health. Section 1.3 examines issues of definition and measurement associated with health. In Section 1.4 actual measurements are discussed.

3

1.2 MEDICAL CARE

Medical care is a process or activity in which certain inputs or factors of production (such as doctors' and nurses' services, services of medical instruments and equipment, and pharmaceuticals) are combined in varying quantities to yield an output. The process itself is the output and thus is the concept we wish to measure. An individual visiting a doctor's office receives an examination involving the services of the doctor, nurse, or paramedic and the use of some equipment. The services provided by these inputs vary from one visit to another. One patient may receive more friendly treatment than another. Physicians vary in thoroughness, knowledge, and technique. Thus the *quality* of the visit varies considerably among patients for the same doctor and among doctors.

The difficulty in measuring the medical care process stems from this quality factor. If we measure doctor care by the number of patient visits to a doctor's office, two cursory examinations count as two visits. But one visit by a patient who receives a cursory examination followed by one visit with a more thorough set of tests also counts as two visits, even though more medical care was provided.

It should be stressed that *quality* is a very broad and elusive term. The gist of the term relates to a state of being good or better. Medical care units can vary in terms of their degree of desirability in many ways. One set of desirable characteristics relates to the amount of personal attention received by the consumer in the process of acquiring medical care. Another is associated with the accuracy of diagnoses and the effectiveness of treatments in producing health. A third set relates to the amounts and types of training of the care providers and the types of medical equipment used. Associated with these are different techniques used in the provision of care. For example, a CT scan machine that takes cross-sectional x-ray pictures is generally considered to provide a higher-quality product than a standard x-ray. All these characteristics, as well as others, have been identified under the rubric of "quality." The problem with quality measurement, then, is that there are many ways of viewing quality; the fact that the term has so many potential meanings has hindered agreement on identifying the quality of care. For this reason, the use of visits as a measure of physician care should be used guardedly.

Hospital care requires the same consideration. Hospital output has frequently been measured by bed days or by the number of cases admitted to the hospital. Over time, however, a single admitted patient receives a greater intensity of services as technology advances. To count an admission in 1965 as having the same output as an admission in 1986 (given the type of case) would understate the amount of output in 1986 as opposed to 1965.

Despite these objections, physician visits to measure the output of medical care and hospital admission or bed days to measure the output of hospital care have been frequently used because of their immediate availability. Recently, in the hospital area, efforts have been made to develop additional measures that incorporate the changing quality of inputs per admission or per bed day. These measures are discussed in Section 1.4.1 on medical care output.

Using changes or differences in the number of physician visits or the number of days of in-hospital treatment as measures of movements or differences in the output of the medical care industry gives rise to another issue, which is concerned with the actual nature of the industry's output. People seek medical care, not in and of itself, but to maintain and improve their health. Thus the output of the medical care sector should perhaps be regarded as the health produced by medical care, rather than the medical care itself. If this is the case, we should try to identify and measure health and use the measure of changed health status caused by the medical care as a measure of the change in the industry's output. The next section discusses this topic.

1.3 HEALTH STATUS

The concept of health seems so familiar to us that we can almost reach out and touch it. It seems easy to distinguish the 97-pound weakling from the body-builder who kicks sand in his face at the beach or to recognize a healthy complexion when we see one. More precise measures, however, are harder to obtain; the two categories of *healthy* and *unhealthy* are not exact. The main reason for this is that we have not defined health precisely; lacking such a definition, two observers can have different opinions as to whether one person is healthier than another. The essence of the scientific procedure is to obtain some form of universal agreement about the nature of the phenomena. If we lack an implementable definition, we can hardly expect two independent observers to reach agreement concerning the status of the phenomena. A definition is useful if it helps pinpoint the characteristics of the phenomena we are trying to describe and eventually measure.

Health is not an easy concept to define with any degree of precision. As the English epidemiologist Sir Richard Doll remarked concerning the concept of health, "Positive health seems to be as elusive to measure as love, beauty, and happiness" (Doll, 1974). Yet in an effort to give some recognizable form to the concept, the World Health Organization has defined health as, "a complete state of physical, mental and social well-being, and not merely the absence of illness or disease." This is a very broad definition, and the characteristics of health based on this definition are not easy to pinpoint and measure. Yet one thing that is conspicuous in the definition is the positive orientation it gives to health. One individual with a well-functioning body can be healthier than another individual, also with a well-functioning body. Still, if we wish to measure health in this way, we must be able to pinpoint and measure these differences.

For many years health was measured by illness (morbidity) or death (mortality) rates in the community: the lower the death rate (adjusting for differences in age levels, sex ratios, or races), the healthier the community. In recent years we have been searching for other measures of health; because the death rate has fallen, it has become increasingly recognized that a community with a low death rate is not necessarily a healthy community. To arrive at what *is* a healthy community, the concept of positive health has become the point of focus.

Attempts at identifying and measuring health have focused on certain characteristics we would expect in a healthy person. These characteristics include the physical functioning of the individual's body in relation to some norm; the physical capabilities of an individual to perform certain acts, such as getting up or dressing; the social capabilities of an individual, that is, how well he or she interacts with others; and how an individual feels. These characteristics are by no means distinct from one another, a fact that has led to much disagreement among researchers who have tried to invent a unique measurement of health status. Different research efforts have focused on individual capabilities (Culyer, 1976; Boyle and Torrance, 1984), on the physical functioning of peoples' bodies in relation to some norm (Williamson, 1971; Kass, 1975), and on a mixture of physical, mental, and social characteristics (Breslow, 1972).

Despite the considerable difficulties in arriving at widely acceptable indexes of health status, the importance of the topic ensures that investigators will keep trying. To appreciate some of the difficulties in this task, let us construct a simple health-status indicator with two dimensions or attributes, physical mobility (called M) and pain (called P). First, we need an index scaling each dimension. Our mobility index might be as follows: 6 = "able to leap tall buildings in a single bound," 5 = normal mobility, 4 = mildly incapacitated, 3 = severely incapacitated, 2 = fully incapacitated, but alive, and 1 = dead. Our pain index might be 6 = no pain (but alive), 5 = slight pain, 4 = moderate pain, 3 = severe pain, 2 = excruciating pain, and 1 = dead.

For these scales to be operable, we must have very specific information as to the correspondence of each number on the scale to readily identifiable patient conditions. Assuming that we have this and that there is a good degree of correspondence among ratings across raters, we must then develop a formula to combine M and P to obtain our overall Health Status Index, HS. A number of mathematical formulas are usable; two of the more popular are $HS = M + P$ and $HS = M \times P$ (Boyle and Torrance, 1984). Using the multiplicative formula, the healthiest individual would have an index value of 36, whereas a dead individual would have a value of 1. Most individuals would fall somewhere along the scale. So the use of such an index, when aggregated, would allow a more refined estimate of group health status.

At a more specific level, a single-dimension index for specific diseases has been developed (Gonnella, Hornbrook, and Louis, 1984). This index classifies cases of a disease according to stages, ranging from extremely mild to fatal. Such an index would permit us to track the development of a case through the various stages. Its use in the measurement of output is discussed in more detail later.

1.4 MEASURING OUTPUT

Output measurements are usually conducted to make comparisons, either against other output measures or against some standard. There are two types of output comparisons: time-series and cross-sectional. A time-series comparison measures the output of the same commodity and phenomena at different times. Cross-sectional comparisons measure the output of the commodity as consumed and/or produced by different groups at the same time. For example, the output of medical care can be compared among consumers in different age groups or different races or geographic areas, according to diagnoses or according to similar comparative bases. The output of medical-care-supplying groups can be compared by size of institution, geographic region, and so on.

1.4.1 Medical Care Output

Medical care output can be measured at three sources:

1. The suppliers of medical care can be surveyed to measure how much medical care they have produced.
2. The payors for medical care can be surveyed to measure how much medical care they have paid for.
3. The consumers of medical care can be surveyed to determine the quantity of consumption.

With perfect measurement, all measures will be equal; however, because of measurement difficulties, considerable differences will arise. A continuing source of data for medical care received by consumers is the information obtained from the National Health Survey, an annual nationwide sample survey of households on health-related matters compiled for the U.S. Public Health Service. Much of the information from this survey is summarized in the Public Health Service's annual compendium of health-related data, *Health United States*.

The National Health Survey is the major source of data on medical care administered by physicians outside the hospital; this care is measured by the number of visits to physicians. As an illustration of the use of time-series data, comparisons were made of (noninpatient) physician visits per year for individuals in the 45 to 64 and 65 and over age groups. For the 45 to 64 age group, visits per person were 5.0 for 1964, 5.7 in 1976, and 5.1 in 1981; the numbers of visits for the over-65 group were 6.7, 6.9, and 6.3 for the respective years. These data do not indicate that there was increase in the output of ambulatory care for these groups (see U.S. Department of Health and Human Services, *Health United States,* 1984). Also, one visit in 1964 was counted as the equivalent of one visit in 1982 since quality-difference adjustments were not made. It is very likely that quality did increase in this period because of new technology, better equipment, and better training; such information should be collected from supply sources (i.e., physicians). Unfortunately, there are few national data to measure this aspect of output (Freiman, 1985).

An alternative measure of physician output is by procedure. A procedure (such as an appendectomy) can be measured in a number of dimensions (e.g., average time of performance, complexity, overhead expenses) and, based on these, comparable weights can be developed for each procedure (Hsiao and Stason, 1979). This approach better captures the differences among various physician tasks.

Hospital data show a very different picture. The numbers of discharges from short-stay hospitals per 1,000 population in the 45 to 64 age group were 146.4 in 1964, 166 in 1977, and 176.3 in 1982. Comparable data for the over-65 group were 190.1, 274.6, and 299.6 (U.S. Department of Health and Human Services, *Health United States,* 1984). These data can be translated into total output by multiplying them by the number of individuals in their respective populations. The picture for number of patients in the over-45 groups receiving hospital care, then, shows a rapid increase through the early 1980s. When comparable data become available for the middle 1980s, they will show a turning point and a decline in hospital admissions. (See Section 2.4.3 for a discussion of early indications of this change in trend.)

To gather a picture of product *quality,* we must look at data collected from hospitals. Hospital output data are available from the *Vital and Health Statistics* (Series 13) of the Public Health Service, the American Hospital Association's annual compendium of hospital data (*Hospital Statistics*), and various issues of *Hospitals: Journal of the American Hospital Association.*

The AHA formerly published a series of indexes that extensively covered the concept of measuring quality changes in hospital care over time (Phillip, 1977). This index attempted to measure the quality change of a day of care by changes in service intensity, defined as the quantity of real services that go into one typical day of hospitalization. The AHA's *Hospital Intensity Index (HII)* incorporated 46 services, including number of dialysis treatments, obstetric unit worker hours, and pharmacy worker hours. A weighted average of these 46 services was calculated annually for data from a sample of hospitals to derive an average number of services per patient day offered during the year. Compared with 1969 (whose value equaled 100), these annual averages formed an index that measured changes in the service-intensity component of output over time. Although these data are no longer published, they provide an excellent illustration of how important a component of medical care output service intensity is.

In Table 1–1, national data are shown for three components of hospital care: services per day, average length of hospital stay, and number of admissions. Services per day are presented in index form with 1969 = 100, which is the HII. Average length of stay is presented in average days per stay and as an index (with 1969 = 100) in parentheses beside the average-length figure. Admissions are shown in millions; the figures in parentheses are admissions transformed into an index with 1969 = 100. As can be seen from the three indexes, service intensity was by far the largest growth component of hospital output, increasing by 68 percent in 7 years. Admissions rose by 18 percent, while the length of stay fell slightly. This is an indicator of the importance of intensity of output in medical care. However, although we often equate intensity with quality, this presupposition has been questioned as discussed later.

1.4.2 Measuring Health Output

The final output of the health care sector is health. *If* there is a close relationship between health and medical care, then indicators of medical care output can be used as indicators of the true output of the medical care sector. It has been contended that there is not necessarily such a correspondence, and so medical care should not be used as a positive indicator of the medical care sector.

The true output of the health care sector is measured by the *net change* in health that was produced by the health care or medical care provided. That is, output is not measured by the level of the health index (e.g., by the infant mortality rate),

---

Table 1–1 Components of Output in Short-term Hospital Care in the United States

Year	Index of services per day (1969 = 100)[1]	Average length of stay in days (and as index, 1969 = 100)[2]	Total admissions in millions (and as index, 1969 = 100)
1969	100.0	8.2 (100)	20.3 (100)
1970	108.7	8.2 (100)	20.9 (102)
1971	115.6	8.1 (98)	21.5 (106)
1972	119.5	8.0 (97)	21.8 (107)
1973	125.4	7.9 (96)	22.4 (110)
1974	136.9	7.9 (96)	23.3 (114)
1975	153.5	7.8 (95)	23.7 (116)
1976	168.6	7.9 (96)	24.1 (118)

Sources: Data compiled from *Hospital Intensity Index*, American Hospital Association[1] and from *Hospital Statistics: 1978 Edition*, American Hospital Association.[2]

but rather by the change in the index that was due to the medical care. For example, if the infant mortality rate fell from 12 per 1,000 births to 10 per 1,000 births subsequent to the introduction of an intensive maternity program, the output of the program would be that proportion of the reduction in infant mortality that was due to the program. It may be that other factors as well, such as the mothers' diets, could have contributed to the change in infant mortality. The presence of such confounding factors creates difficulties in finding an accurate measure of output; medical care is seldom the only factor contributing to *changes* in health status. Other factors may be difficult to identify (e.g., changes in personal behaviors) and equally difficult to measure.

In addition to the identification of confounding factors, there is the problem of measuring *changes* in health status. We have seen how many difficulties are posed in the measure of levels of health status; the measurement of changes in health status merely adds to these problems. As an illustration of these problems, we present the categories of disease severity (ranked, but not indexed) in Figure 1–1 on the vertical axis (for an index see Williams, 1974). Stages of disease range from no disease present to death (although it may well be that some states of health are worse even than death) (Hornbrook, 1983). On the horizontal axis we present the duration of the illness (see also Williams, 1974). In the chart we plot two courses of a given disease, a chronic disease with treatment and the same chronic disease with no treatment. In such a presentation, the output of medical care is the

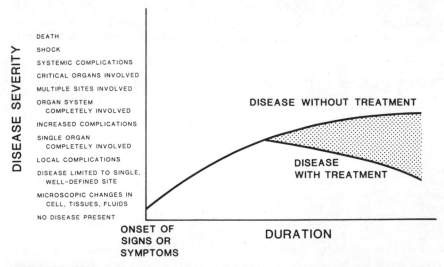

Figure 1–1 Representation of alternative courses of a disease in terms of stages of disease severity. In this example, treatment is associated with reduced severity. The difference between the "with treatment" and the "without treatment" curves represents the impact of medical care.

difference in disease states with and without the medical care. This is shown as the dotted area between the curves. In this version, output is depicted as differences in severity of illness.

It has been contended that, in general, there is a limit to how much good medical care can do: as more medical care is provided (to the same case, or as additional cases are treated), the *additional* output becomes less. This is illustrated in Figure 1–2, where health is shown on the vertical axis and the quantity of medical care on the horizontal axis. The medical care ''output'' curve showing the relation between health and medical care is drawn such that there would be some level of health without any medical care (H_0), and for additional levels of medical care there is some contribution to health; but this *additional* contribution declines as the output of medical care increases. Such an output curve assumes all other factors (environmental, genetic, personal) are held constant, and only medical care varies. The additional output is expressed as $\Delta H/\Delta M$, where ΔM is the additional medical care and ΔH is the additional health. Note that the way we have drawn the curve $\Delta H/\Delta M$ declines in value as more medical care (M) is provided.

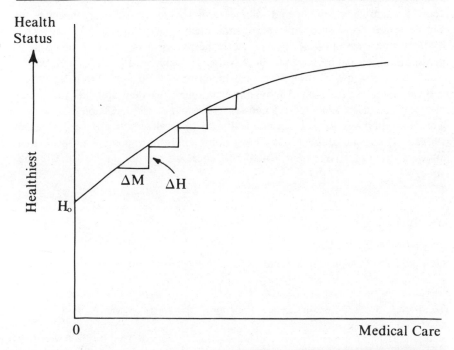

Figure 1–2 Hypothesized relation between health and medical care. In this representation, additional doses of medical care have diminishing impacts on health; eventually, a situation of low medical productivity, termed "flat of the curve medicine," is reached.

This eventual flattening of the output curve is referred to as being situated where "flat of the curve medicine" is produced (Enthoven, 1980). Drawing the curve in this way amounts to illustrating geometrically that, as one increases medical care provision, the additional effectiveness of medical care declines.

Researchers have attempted to establish the relation between medical care and health in different ways. Several early studies attempted to identify statistically a relation between mortality rates and various measures of medical input availability per capita using cross-state (Auster, Leveson, and Sarachek, 1969) and cross-national (Stewart, 1971) data. Both studies found a small or no relation. An explanation provided was that we may have reached the leveling-out point on the curve; furthermore, it was estimated that the self-care components of health care (e.g., smoking, diet, exercise) may indeed be much more important than the medical care components (Newhouse and Friedlander, 1979). However, subsequent statistical research that examined specific groups such as infants did find more significant results with regard to the impact of medical care (Hadley, 1982).

Because they are so broadly focused, the results of such studies are often difficult to interpret, and it may be that health output is more reasonably measured only by experimental means. The setting up of clinical trials by which one group receives a certain treatment and another group with similar characteristics (a control group) does not is an experimental method of establishing output. The differences in cure rates, if any, between the two groups could be taken as a measure of the output produced by the resources (Cochrane, 1972). In a number of instances, less aggregated studies have failed to turn up impacts on health of medical practices (e.g., no relationship was found between appendicitis death rates and appendectomies performed) (see Enthoven, 1980, Chapter 2). However, such findings cannot automatically be generalized to all medical care (Angell, 1985); although it may have some analytic appeal, a broad-brush approach may pass over many situations where we are not on the "flat of the curve."

REFERENCES

Measurement of Medical Care

Bailey, R. (1970). Philosophy, faith, fact and fiction in the production of medical services. *Inquiry, 7,* 37–53.

Berry, R.E. (1973). On grouping hospitals for economic analysis. *Inquiry, 10,* 5–12.

Freiman, M.P. (1985). The rate of adoption of new procedures among physicians. *Medical Care, 23,* 939–945.

Hornbrook, M. (1982). Hospital case mix: Its definition, measurement, and use. Part I: *Medical Care Review, 39,* 1–43 and Part II: *Medical Care Review, 39,* 73–123.

Hsiao, W.C., & Stason, W.B. (1979). Toward developing a relative value scale for medical and surgical services. *Health Care Financing Review, 1,* 23–39.

Lave, J.R., & Lave, L.B. (1971). The extent of role differentiation among hospitals. *Health Services Research, 5*, 15–38.

Phillip, P.J. (1977, April). HCI/HII—Two new AHA indexes measure costs, intensity. *Hospital Financial Management*, pp. 20–26.

Reder, M.W. (1969). Some problems in the measurement of productivity in the medical care industry. In V.R. Fuchs (ed.), *Production and productivity in the service industries* (pp. 95–131). New York: Columbia University Press for the National Bureau of Economic Research.

Russell, L.B. (1976). The diffusion of new hospital technologies in the United States. *International Journal of Health Services, 6*, 557–580.

Measurement of Health

Breslow, L. (1972). A quantitative approach to the world health organization definition of health: Physical, mental, and social well being. *International Journal of Epidemiology, 1*, 347–355.

Boyle, M.H., & Torrance, G.W. (1984). Developing multiattribute health indexes. *Medical Care, 22*, 1045–1057.

Culyer, A.J. (1972). Appraising government expenditure on health services: The problems of "need" and "output." *Public Finance, 27*, 205–211.

————— (1976). *Need and national health service*. London: Martin Robertson Co.

Goldsmith, S.B. (1973). A reevaluation of health status indicators. *Health Services Reports, 88*, 937–941.

Gonnella, J.S., Hornbrook, M.C., & Louis, D.Z. (1984). Staging of disease. *Journal of the American Medical Association, 251*, 637–644.

Hornbrook, M.C. (1983). Allocative medicine. *Annals, American Association of Political and Social Science, 468*, 12–29.

Israel, S., & Teeling-Smith, G. (1967). The submerged iceberg of sickness in society. *Social Policy and Administration, 1*, 43–57.

Kass, L.R. (1975). The pursuit of health. *Public Interest, 40*, 11–42.

Sullivan, D.F. (1966). Conceptual problems in developing an index of health. *Vital and health statistics*, Series 2, No. 17. (Publication No. [HRA] 74-1017). Washington, DC: U.S. Department of Health, Education and Welfare.

Williams, A. (1985). The nature, meaning, and measurement of health and illness. *Social Science & Medicine, 20*, 1023–1027.

Williamson, J.W. (1971). Evaluating quality of patient care. *Journal of the American Medical Association, 218*, 564–569.

The Health–Medical Care Relation

Angell, M. (1985). Cost containment and the physician. *Journal of the American Medical Association, 254*, 1203–1207.

Auster, R., Leveson, I., & Sarachek, D. (1969). The production of health. *Journal of Human Resources, 4*, 412–436.

Cochrane, A. (1972). *Effectiveness and efficiency*. New York: Oxford University Press, Inc.

Doessel, D.P., & Marshall, J.V. (1985). A rehabilitation of health outcome in quality assessment. *Social Science & Medicine, 21*, 1319–1328.

Doll, R. (1974). Surveillance and monitoring. *International Journal of Epidemiology, 3*, 305–314.

Enthoven, A.C. (1980). *Health plan*. Reading, MA: Addison-Wesley Publishing Co., Inc.

Hadley, J. (1982). *More medical care, better health?* Washington, DC: Urban Institute.

Newhouse, J.P., & Friedlander, L.J. (1979). The relationship between medical resources and measures of health. *Journal of Human Resources, 15*, 200–218.

Scheffler, R.M., Knaus, W.A., Wagner, D.P., et al. (1982). Severity of illness and the relationship between intensive care and survival. *American Journal of Public Health, 72*, 449–454.

Stewart, C.T. (1971). Allocation of resources to health. *Journal of Human Resources, 6*, 103–122.

Williams, A. (1974). Measuring the effectiveness of the health care system. *British Journal of the Preventive Medicine Society, 28*, 196–202.

Data Sources

American Hospital Association. *Hospital Statistics* (various years). Chicago: American Hospital Association.

U.S. Department of Health and Human Services. *Health United States*. Rockville, MD: National Center for Health Statistics (annual publication includes health and medical care trends).

_____ . *Morbidity and Mortality Weekly Report*. Atlanta, GA: Centers for Disease Control (weekly epidemiologic report).

_____ . *NCHS Monthly Vital Statistics Report* (monthly data on births and deaths).

_____ . *Vital and Health Statistics*. Rockville, MD: National Center for Health Statistics. (Periodical and occasional reports on a wide variety of topics, including population-based utilization data, mortality data, worker hours, and special studies. Known as the Rainbow Series. Early releases of data can be obtained in the "Advancedata" series.)

Chapter 2

Economic Dimensions of the Health Care Sector

2.1 INTRODUCTION

The purpose of this chapter is to provide basic concepts that will be used to describe the resource-allocation process in the health care sector. Section 2.1 sets out a framework identifying the economic dimensions of the sector. Using these dimensions as reference points, basic measurements of the capacities and activity levels of the sector can be made. These measurements provide the core of observations with which we are concerned in the remainder of this book.

In Section 2.2, concepts regarding the economic dimensions of health care activity are set out. In particular, two types of activity are distinguished: (1) *investment activity,* which involves the formation of new productive resources such as hospital equipment and specialist physicians, and (2) *service production activity,* which involves producing health care services. Section 2.3 uses the framework presented in Section 2.2 to describe three types of investment activity: basic medical education, postgraduate medical education, and hospital investment. In Section 2.4 we apply the framework to describe three basic medical production activities. We examine traditional physician and hospital activities, as well as the activities of the emerging alternative delivery systems (in particular Health Maintenance Organizations). Finally, in Section 2.5 we examine the role of middlemen in the health care delivery system (insurers and other types of contractors).

2.2 ECONOMIC DIMENSIONS OF HEALTH CARE

2.2.1 Production and Resources

To place health care activity in an economic setting, several concepts central to the analysis of resource use are presented. The first involves the distinction

15

between stock and flows. A *stock* is a quantity of resources present at a particular time; examples are the stock of radiologists in the United States at the end of a particular calendar year and the stock of x-ray machines in a state on a certain date. A *flow* is a quantity of activity occurring during a time period. Examples are the number of patients treated for cancer in 1974 and the number of radiologists trained in the United States during 1976; both are examples of *processes* (i.e., treating patients or training radiologists).

One type of stock central to economic activity is the stock of capital. Capital goods are goods produced in order to be used in further production. Generally, capital goods are considered to be those whose productive life is longer than one accounting period (e.g., 1 year). The capital goods available for production at any particular time are regarded as stocks. However, their importance in the role of producing output lies in the flow of services that stems from them. Two categories of capital goods are physical and human capital. Physical capital is the physical stock of productive means from which productive services flow. Examples are hospital beds and equipment and blood collection units. Human capital is the stock of skills, knowledge, and abilities embodied in individuals that enables the flow of services from these skilled individuals. Examples are trained surgeons and nurses. Both forms of capital are created through an investment process. Investment refers to the addition to capital stock produced during any one period. Examples of investment in physical capital are the production of x-ray machines during a period. This production flow adds to the stock of these machines. Medical education is an example of investment in human capital, the output of which results in skilled physicians.

Capital goods yield services that are used along with current inputs in the production process. *Production* is an act or process of creating output. Productive activity is a flow that entails combining input services to yield commodities (goods and services). These inputs can be services from various forms of capital, such as the services of an x-ray machine or a paramedic, or services of current inputs such as medical supplies; both types of inputs are called *factors* of production.

2.2.2 Classifying Output

Based on these concepts, the output of the health care sector can be divided into two groups: (1) investment output, which adds to the production of health care capital whose services will be used in future periods, and (2) the output of goods and services currently consumed. The link between these groups is that capital services enter the production of the current output of health care and depend on previous years' investment in skills and equipment. Current production techniques, referred to as technology, depend on the existing stock of human and physical capital, which in turn depends on earlier years' investment. An example is the intensive-care technology currently used to treat heart-attack patients.

Courses of treatment employing this technology depend on a heavy prior investment in intensive-care facilities and personnel training. Once this capital stock is
in place, coronary care patients will be treated using the inputs and technology
associated with this capital.

2.2.3 Cost of Activities

Having identified productive activities as those efforts involving resource inputs
whose aim is to create commodities, our next step is to find some common measure
of this activity's size. The concept of cost is a commonly used measure. Several
different meanings can be attached to the concept of cost. One definition, which
refers to *money cost,* is the money outlay that has been paid to the resources for
their services. For example, if an optometrist performs an eye-pressure test, the
money cost is simply what is paid for his or her services. Money cost is a
convenient way to measure the size of an activity, but it is not always a totally valid
measure. The same optometrist may provide free services while performing the
same test; then the money cost would be zero. Yet some activity has taken place,
and this activity has used scarce resources.

In the health care sector, many examples exist of free (i.e., zero money cost)
services provided. Clinical teachers in medical schools frequently donate their
efforts. Volunteer collectors for such organizations as the American Heart Association, United Way, and March of Dimes donate their efforts. The notion of
opportunity cost is used to obtain a measure of the size of activity that is invariant
as to whether or not the resources are paid in money for their services. Opportunity
cost is relevant when a resource has several alternative uses. If used in activity A,
the opportunity cost of an input is what that input would have earned in alternative
activity B, where B is the highest-valued alternative employment for that
resource. Let us say that an optometrist who performs a refraction for free in a
clinic could have obtained a fee of $20 had he or she performed it in the office. By
valuing this service at $20, we place it on a comparable base with all services
performed for a fee. Whenever a service is provided at a price below its alternative
value, the money cost will not take into account the portion of cost that is, in effect,
subsidized; opportunity cost is a better measure of the true size of the total resource
commitment to an activity.

2.2.4 Burden Sharing and Financing Output

The cost of a service or activity can also be examined from the point of view of
who bears its burden, that is, who incurs the cost. The *private cost* of a service is
the resource commitment that the individual who receives the service makes to
obtain it. Frequently, the money paid by the individual is taken as a measure of
private cost incurred by the individual to obtain the service. However, an indi-

vidual may expend time as well as money to obtain a service. For example, he or she may pay $20 and wait 60 minutes to see a doctor. In this case the private resource commitment is greater than the money paid.

Even if the money price were an accurate measure of the consuming individual's total cost, it may not be an accurate measure of the resource commitment made by *all* individuals, including those who do not consume the service. Let us take the example of Mr. A's medical care. A visit to a doctor may cost Mr. A $2. However, the total cost of the visit, as measured by the doctor's fee, may be $6. Let us say that the difference is made up by a government program. The government finances this program through taxes on Mrs. B or Mr. C. Thus Mrs. B and Mr. C bear the remainder of the cost for medical care. The cost to nonconsumers may be called the *external cost*. Since all costs must be borne by someone, the social cost is the sum of all costs borne by all individuals; that is, it is the sum of private and external costs. The social cost is a measure of the total resource commitment made by all members of society in the undertaking of any activity. In our example, the taxpayers bear $4 of the total burden of Mr. A's medical care, but Mr. A bears the rest.

Economic burdens, especially in the health care field, are often hidden, so those who bear the cost of an activity do not realize they are doing so. A commonly used government mechanism of shifting burdens is the tax subsidy. For example, an employee in the 50 percent tax bracket receives health insurance coverage from his or her employer that is valued (i.e., in terms of social cost) at $1,000. The individual would have had to earn $2,000 to purchase $1,000 of nonsubsidized goods; the cost to the individual of health insurance is half that of other goods purchased with after-tax dollars, such as food. In effect, employees who select more complete (nontaxable) health insurance instead of taxable money wages in their total compensation package pay less taxes, and hence their overall contribution to government expenditures is reduced. Such a policy of subsidies creates several discrepancies: it makes health insurance cheaper (relatively) than other goods for those who obtain their health insurance as employee benefits; furthermore, this insurance is less costly than for those to whom health insurance is unavailable as a tax-free benefit (i.e., who do not receive it as an employment benefit). In recent years there has been a movement toward making those who incur the costs of an activity bear the burden of the activity, that is, toward removing hidden subsidies as much as possible. Such a movement attempts to change the system's incentive structure so that consumers and providers bear a greater responsibility for their actions.

2.2.5 Institutional Setting of Economic Activity

The institutional setting in which economic activity occurs is concerned with the manner in which production, supply, commodity consumption, capital acquisition, and finance are organized. The descriptive task involves identifying the separate interacting units involved in the process of bringing the commodity to its ultimate users, outlining the major organizational characteristics of these units, and specifying their economic relation to one another. This last task includes tracing the flows of commodities and money among these units, as well as identifying any other relations (agreements) that may exist. This task is undertaken in Sections 2.3 and 2.4; however, one aspect, organizational characteristics, is briefly discussed here.

A transacting unit may be organized on a profit or not-for-profit basis. A profit-making unit can pay the surplus of revenues over expenses to its owners. Examples are profit-making hospitals and nursing homes. A not-for-profit organization may not pay its surplus directly to owners. This surplus must be retained by the organization or spent on activities relevant to the organization's operations. Such organizations can be operated by governments or nonprofit corporations set up primarily to operate the unit.

Organizations can be self-managed and under independent ownership or they can be a member of a chain. Chain membership is consistent with many types of operating arrangements, including contract management (management but not ownership by the chain) and chain ownership. Multiorganizational systems have become increasingly important in hospitals and health maintenance organizations in recent years.

Another facet of the institutional setting within which medical care is delivered is the role of competition. If more than one organization is serving a given market, these organizations can behave cooperatively or competitively. Competitive behavior is growing rapidly in health care markets in the United States.

2.2.6 Capacity

Capacity refers to the potential for producing output. Capacity is a function of the quantity of resources available (human and physical capital), the technology available, and the efficiency of combining resources. Capacity is often expressed in terms of potential output, which is the output rate at full capacity. The degree of utilization is the ratio of actual to potential output.

2.2.7 Size, Composition, and Distribution of Output

The final dimensional characteristics involve specifying the size, composition, and distribution of the output. Size involves determining how much output has been turned out; this output can be in the form of capital or health care services. The composition of the output consists of the proportion of the various ingredients or types of output. The total number of residents turned out in any single year is the total size; this output is composed of surgeons, medical specialists, and public health specialists. The distribution of output is primarily concerned with the quantities of a single type of output received by various groups. For example, the poor may receive fewer hospital services per capita than the rich, or males may receive more medical training per capita than females. Low-income regions may experience less hospital investment than wealthier areas. These are examples of the distributional characteristics of an activity.

2.2.8 Accounting for Output and Other Components of Cost

A major confusion in health care arises from the failure to clearly distinguish between total cost and the components of total cost. If we separate out total cost into two components, average cost per unit (called AC) and the number of units (called Q), then total cost is the product of AC and Q. It is mistaken to think that one is containing total costs when merely AC is being contained. If Q increases enough, the fact that AC has fallen may not be enough to contain total costs.

If the total cost of a program or activity has increased, it is often desirable to separate this change into components to determine the contribution of each component to the overall change. A useful technique that permits one to account for these relative contributions, provided the growth rate is small, is outlined next. Let us assume that the total cost of hospital care in 1977 is \$12,000 and in 1978 it rises to \$12,750. Knowing merely that total costs rose does not tell us whether unit costs or output increased, or by how much. To determine this, we must apply additional information to a formula. Let C represent total costs, Q represent units of output measured in bed days, and K represent unit cost, in terms of dollars per bed day. If subscript 1 stands for 1977 and subscript 2 for 1978, the total cost can be broken down as follows:

$$C_1 = K_1 Q_1 \quad \text{and} \quad C_2 = K_2 Q_2$$

Furthermore, let $K_1 = \$12$, $K_2 = \$12.50$, $Q_1 = 1,000$, and $Q_2 = 1,020$. If we let Δ signify "change in," then $K_2 = K_1 + \Delta K$, where ΔK is \$0.50 and $Q_2 = Q_1 + \Delta Q$, where ΔQ is 20 bed days. We can now express C_2 as

$$C_2 = (K_1 + \Delta K)(Q_1 + \Delta Q) = C_1 + \Delta C$$

Multiplying out the terms in parentheses, we obtain

$$C_1 + \Delta C = K_1 Q_1 + K_1 \Delta Q + \Delta K Q_1 + \Delta K \, \Delta Q$$

Since $C_1 = K_1 Q_1$, we can subtract this quotient from both sides and maintain the equality of both sides. Furthermore, by dividing both sides by C_1 (or $K_1 Q_1$), we obtain

$$\frac{\Delta C}{C_1} = \frac{K_1 \Delta Q}{K_1 Q_1} + \frac{\Delta K Q_1}{K_1 Q_1} + \frac{\Delta K \Delta Q}{K_1 Q_1}$$

Canceling terms, we have

$$\frac{\Delta C}{C_1} = \frac{\Delta Q}{Q_1} + \frac{\Delta K}{K_1} + \frac{\Delta K \Delta Q}{K_1 Q_1}$$

The expressions $\Delta C/C_1$, $\Delta Q/Q_1$, and $\Delta K/K_1$ are growth rates. That is, $\Delta C/C_1$ is 750/12,000 or 0.062, which means C changed by 6.25 percent over its base value. The last equation allows us to express this growth rate in terms of the two growth rates of the elements in the product and a residual term, $\Delta K/\Delta Q/K_1 Q_1$. Assuming ΔK and ΔQ are of a relatively small magnitude, this residual term can be approximated by a zero. We are then left with the approximation

$$\frac{\Delta C}{C_1} = \frac{\Delta K}{K_1} + \frac{\Delta Q}{Q_1}$$

This equation shows that the growth rate of total costs is approximately equal to the sum of the growth rates in unit costs and output. Applying this formula to the figures in our example, we calculate that unit costs rose by 4.1 percent (0.50/12,000) and output increased by 2 percent. Thus, the 6.25 percent growth in total costs was roughly attributable to a 4.1 percent increase in costs and a 2 percent increase in output.

This formula can be used to estimate the components' contributions to growth if, for example, only growth rates in total cost and unit cost are known. If $\Delta C/C_1$ is 5 percent and $\Delta K/K_1$ is 1 percent, then the difference, 4 percent, can be attributed to $\Delta Q/Q$. The formula can also be extended to account for contributions of separate elements to the overall growth of costs of expenditures when three or more elements form a product. Total cost can be expressed as the product of costs per bed day, the number of bed days used per capita, and the total population. The overall growth rate of total cost can be approximated by the sum of the growth rates in each element. Thus, if $\Delta C/C_1$ is 6 percent, $\Delta K/K_1$ is 2 percent, and population growth is 1 percent, we can approximate that per capita utilization rose by 2 percent. This formula is thus a useful way of organizing information about growth in overall costs and its determinants. It must be remembered, however, that this formula allows us to obtain estimates or approximations, not precise figures.

2.3 ECONOMIC DIMENSIONS OF HEALTH CARE CAPITAL FORMATION

In this section, the economic dimensions set out in the previous sections are used to describe three types of health care investment: undergraduate medical education, graduate medical education, and hospital investment in equipment and buildings. Some of these basic dimensions are summarized numerically in Table 2–1 to demonstrate the relative magnitudes of the various dimensions.

2.3.1 Undergraduate Medical Education

The goal of undergraduate medical education is to produce physicians; the output can thus be measured by the number of M.D. degrees granted. Undergraduate medical education takes place in medical schools and teaching hospitals. These institutions are complex, however, and the measurement of the economic dimensions is not straightforward. The resources that participate in the production of M.D.s can be divided into two groups: medical school and medical student resources. Medical school resources include medical school faculty, staff, equipment, and buildings; medical student resources include the efforts made and the equipment owned by the students.

Medical school resources are used for several purposes besides teaching; these include medical research and patient care. The functions are inextricably tied in with one another. The teacher presents his or her research findings to the students, and the clinician uses patients as teaching examples for the students. Because these activities occur together, any effort to separate research from education costs is bound to be arbitrary and of limited use for determining the costs of the separate components of medical school output (Fein and Weber, 1971). Thus the cost of medical school activity is really the cost of all functions that take place in the medical school.

In Table 2–1, resources used for undergraduate medical education are summarized in column 2. In column 3, the total money costs of operating medical schools in the United States in 1983/1984 are shown to be $8.7 billion (Jolly et al., 1985). This amount excludes the cost of services donated by clinical faculty, as well as the costs of efforts of medical students. The total amount of resources devoted to undergraduate medical education includes medical student efforts. If we were to value the costs of these resources at zero, we would be undervaluing their contribution to investment output in a manner similar to the undervaluing of donated services of optometrists (see Section 2.2.3). An approximate figure for valuing the costs of medical students' efforts (their opportunity cost) is the value of their services had they been employed in an alternative manner elsewhere in the economy. If these students had been employed, their wages would perhaps have averaged $20,000 annually. In 1984 there were about 67,000 full-time medical students; if we value the annual opportunity cost of each at $20,000, a rough figure for the cost of medical student time is $1.3 billion. The total annual cost of undergraduate medical education, including research and patient care functions, can be approximated at $10 billion (8.7 + 1.3 billion).

Table 2–1 Economic Dimensions of Selected Health Care Activities

(1) *Activity*	(2) *Resources used*	(3) *Cost of activity*	(4) *Output produced*	(5) *Financing sources*
Undergraduate medical education	Teachers (full and part time) Medical school facilities Medical students	Medical school expenses: $8.7 billion Opportunity cost: $1.3 billion	M.D.s and research	Medical school costs: Federal government, 24.7% Student fees, 6% Medical student costs: Self, 92%
Postgraduate medical education	Teachers Hospital facilities Interns and residents	Direct costs: $1.3 billion Indirect costs: $1.4 billion	Licensed doctors, specialists, research	Direct costs: 75% patient revenues
Hospital investment	Obtained from construction and medical equipment industries	$4 billion (1979) (equipment excluded)	Hospital equipment and buildings	Public, 4% Grants, 12% Private, 84% (80% debt)
Physician care	Physicians Nurses Paramedics Receptionists Supplies	$75.4 billion	Physician care	Government, 27.8% Private insurance, 44.4% Direct (patients) payments, 27.8%
Hospital care	Personnel: nurses, health service workers Purchased inputs: drugs, equipment, etc.	$157.9 billion	Hospital care	Government, 53.4% Private insurance, 36.9% Direct (patient) payments, 8.7%

The institutional characteristics of medical education include the organizational characteristics of producers and receivers of education and the financial arrangements. Medical schools are nonprofit organizations, with considerable variations in how they are organized. The major ownership classes of medical schools are those associated with state or private universities and independent schools. Correspondingly, the funding sources of medical schools are diverse. The role of the federal government, for example, has expanded and then declined in recent years; in 1984, revenues from all federal sources amounted to 24.7 percent of all medical school revenues.

Other major sources of revenue were state appropriations, at 21 percent, and professional fees earned by the clinical staff, at 33 percent. Student fees amounted to only 6 percent of medical school operating revenues. However, in addition to incurring these fee expenses, medical students incurred a large portion of the total costs (including opportunity costs) of their own education. With total money fees of $545 million and the large opportunity incurred ($1.3 billion), students received scholarships amounting to $120 million; in addition, loans (many of them subsidized) amounted to approximately $360 million. Thus the opportunity costs of medical students were not offset by outside funding; consequently, medical students bore most of the private cost of their own educations.

The trend in medical school finances is away from government subsidization and more toward the direct beneficiaries sharing the burden of costs. From 1975 to 1984, the federal role in financing medical schools declined from 36 percent to 24.7 percent of revenues. At the same time, student fees rose from 4.6 to 6 percent and receipts from faculty practice plans and other services rose from 18 to 33 percent. Student fees have increased slightly, and fewer student loans have been made at subsidized interest rates, which are indications of medical students paying a greater share of their education.

One of the prime distributional characteristics of medical school education is concerned with who receives the education. Undergraduate training has been largely confined to students from middle- and upper-income families (Harrison and Nash, 1974). The other characteristics of output, that is, size and composition, are discussed in relation to the total number of doctors produced in Section 2.3.2.

2.3.2 Graduate Medical Education

After receiving an M.D., a doctor must undertake an additional year of training, an internship, before receiving a license to practice medicine. In addition, many doctors continue their training in the form of a residency in either teaching hospitals or medical schools. Identifying the economic characteristics of postgraduate medical education is far more complex than identifying those of undergraduate medical education. Most postgraduate medical students (interns and residents) are involved in educational, patient care, and perhaps research functions simultaneously. Any accounting for the costs of separate functions would be arbitrary.

Two major costs are associated with graduate medical education: (1) the direct costs of residents', interns', and nurses' time and faculty salaries (Knapp and Butler, 1979), and (2) the indirect costs of *extra* resources used in teaching hospitals (through more extensive tests, record keeping, etc.) (Cameron, 1985). Direct costs, as measured by resident, intern, nurse, and faculty salaries, were roughly $1.3 billion in 1986. However, residents' and interns' costs were valued at their salary levels. It is likely that their salaries were less than they could have earned in nonlearning employment; that is, their salaries were less than their opportunity costs. Thus this figure understates the true direct costs of graduate medical education. Indirect costs, which can be established by comparing costs in similar teaching and nonteaching hospitals, were estimated at $1.4 billion (Kohlman, 1986). Financing for direct costs comes from direct payments from Medicare and Medicaid for their share of costs; state governments cover an additional amount, but the major portion comes from patient revenues, which are the prime source of indirect teaching costs.

One output of the entire medical education sector, both undergraduate and postgraduate, is trained doctors. The total number of trained doctors added to the existing stock comes from domestic undergraduate and postgraduate programs and from immigrant doctors entering the medical labor force. Table 2–2 presents figures relating to the growing number of active doctors. All figures are converted to a per capita basis to obtain estimates of the relative number of doctors in

Table 2–2 Selected Indicators of Capital in the Medical Care Industry

	Year				
Indicator	*1960*	*1970*	*1980*	*1983*	*1990 (projected)*
Physicians:					
Active physicians per 100,000 population	140	156.8	196.9	—	238
Primary care physicians as a percent of all active physicians	—	44.2	41.2	—	39.3
Hospitals:					
Community hospital beds per 1,000 population	3.6	4.3	4.5	4.4	

Source: Health United States 1985, U.S. Department of Health and Human Services. (Data are from Tables 64 and 72.)

practice. The first line in Table 2–2 shows that between 1960 and 1980 the total number of active physicians per 100,000 population grew from 140 to 196.9, an increase of 40 percent. Projected figures, based on existing rates of growth of medical school and postgraduate output and on trends in immigration, indicate that by 1990 this figure will be 238. If current trends continue, the composition of output will change considerably, and the percentage of all physicians in primary care will fall. In 1963 this percentage was 48; by 1970 it fell to 44.2; in 1980 it was 41.2; and by 1990 it is projected to be 39.3. This means that the number of physicians trained to perform highly complicated routines has grown and will continue to grow considerably both in number and as a percentage of the total, indicating a rapid increase in the capacity of the industry to provide specialized medical care.

2.3.3 Hospital Investment

Hospital investment involves the addition of equipment and buildings to existing capital stock. The actual production of capital goods takes place outside the hospital industry and is performed by medical equipment companies and construction companies. The cost of this activity for the hospital industry is the money outlays for the capital goods.

In 1979 new hospital construction amounted to over $4 billion. This activity was financed by a combination of public (12 percent) grants, private grants (4 percent), and other private means (primarily debt). (Equipment is excluded from this figure.) Over the years the sources of financing hospital capital have changed radically. Prior to 1946, philanthropy played a major role. With the passing of the Hill–Burton Act in 1946, direct government funds became the major source of funds. However, in recent years both private insurance and government programs (Medicare and Medicaid) have had generous reimbursement policies for hospitals' costs of debt, and so have encouraged hospitals to raise capital by borrowing. First, many insurers (including Blue Cross, Medicare, and Medicaid) have automatically reimbursed hospitals for the interest payments they incurred by issuing bonds, as well as for depreciation of assets. Such reimbursement methods have encouraged hospitals to borrow for investment projects. Second, nonprofit and government hospitals were permitted to issue tax-exempt bonds under Internal Revenue Service and state regulations. The purchasers of the bonds (in effect, borrowers) paid no tax on the interest income that accrued to them as bondholders. This gave the hospitals a competitive edge when floating bonds and permitted them to pay lower rates of interest than corporate borrowers (since interest on corporate bonds was taxable). These regulations permitted hospitals to borrow for lower interest rates.

Although the final proposals are not yet determined, Medicare has proposed a fixed rate of reimbursement for interest and depreciation, which would terminate the automatic pass through of capital costs from reimburser to payor. Furthermore, there is discussion of terminating or reducing the privileges of nonprofit and government hospitals in the bond market by having recipients of bond interest pay taxes on this income. These two regulations would put a lid on the hospital debt capital market, forcing hospitals to rely more on internally generated funds to finance investment projects.

Indeed, the generous reimbursement and tax policies with regard to hospital capital formation have resulted in substantial investment in the hospital industry. Indicators of how hospital capital has grown in recent years can be seen in the growth of short-term general hospital beds per capita between 1960 and 1983. According to these data, shown in Table 2–2, the number of short-term beds per capita grew from 3.6 per 1,000 resident population in 1960 to 4.5 in 1980. Most recently, bed numbers have been falling slightly. These statistics give a clear indication of the growth in short-term general capacity to admit patients on an inpatient basis.

The overall picture of capacity is much more complex, since quality is a key component of capacity to serve. In addition to investing in size of services, hospitals can also invest in widening the scope of the services they provide. A measure of the growth in capital equipment that has resulted from such investment in new technologies can be obtained from annual hospital survey data that report the extent to which specific hospital treatment facilities were available in selected hospitals. These data should be distinguished from the number of treatments performed annually with these facilities. Selected analyses of these data indicate rapid growth in hospital treatment facilities in recent years (Russell, 1976). For example, in 1980, under 1 percent of hospitals with bed sizes from 59 to 99 had CT scanners, and 6.6 percent of hospitals with bed size 100 to 199 had installed such units. By 1985 these numbers were 18.4 and 45.6 percent, respectively (American Hospital Association, *Hospital Statistics,* various years).

All the data presented in this section provide indications of the rapid growth in highly trained personnel and equipment available for use in the production of medical services. The next section describes the system of provision for such services.

2.4 ECONOMIC DIMENSIONS OF HEALTH SERVICE PRODUCTION

2.4.1 Health Care Expenditures and Costs

In 1984, total health care expenditures were $387.4 billion. This amounted to 10.6 percent of the Gross National Product, which is the dollar value of all final goods and services produced in the United States economy (Levit et al., 1984). The year 1984 was the first in many decades that saw health care costs begin to abate; in 1983, health care expenditures reached 10.7 percent of the GNP. Indeed, for several decades rising health care costs have been a matter of great concern.

Health care expenditures are a measure of the money outlays on health-care-related goods and services. They do not represent the total economic burden (economic costs) of illness. This burden consists of *direct* medical care costs associated with illness plus the indirect costs, which include lost earnings due to absence from work or premature termination of work. It should also be noted that some medical care is not related to illness, and so the total *money outlay* for medical care will be more than the money outlay for medical care due to illness. An estimate of the total economic costs of illness in 1980 was $415.9 billion. These costs were composed of $211 billion in direct (medical care) costs and $204 billion in indirect (work loss) costs due to mortality and morbidity. Mortality losses, it should be noted, include the present value of the future stream of lost earnings due to premature death (see Section 13.3.5). The illnesses with the largest costs were diseases of the circulatory system ($79 billion), accident, injury and poisoning ($57 billion), and cancer ($45 billion) (Rice, Hodgson, and Kopstein, 1985). These costs can be compared with the overall expenditures for medical care in 1980, which were $247 billion. Indirect costs of illnesses thus add a considerable burden to the economy.

As additional attention is drawn to medical care costs, the question that increasingly arises is, Where do these costs go? Two areas that have drawn considerable attention in recent years are (1) the unequal distribution of expenditures among recipients, and (2) the concentration of additional expenditures in "little ticket" items associated with new (and in some cases unproved) procedures. With regard to the first question, a number of studies have documented that a substantial portion of medical costs are spent on a small portion of patients (including terminal cases) (Zook and Moore, 1980; McCall, 1984; Anderson and Knickman, 1984; Scitovsky, 1984). As the population ages, a trend toward more high-cost patients is likely to continue (Rice and Feldman, 1983). Trends such as these seem to pose more difficult ethical problems than those of the second area, which relate to the "little ticket" items such as x-rays and lab tests that have been absorbing a considerable portion of hospital bills and whose overuse seems much easier to document (Angell, 1985).

2.4.2 Physician Care

Physician care is administered directly by, or under the direct orders of, the physician. With such a broad definition, this type of care could be understood to include most of what is medical care today. Traditionally, a delineation has usually been made to separate physician care from care provided by institutions. According to this distinction, physician care is regarded as care provided in the physician's office outside an institution and services provided directly by physi-

cians in institutions, although the latter have been distinguished from care provided by the institutions themselves. This delineation is based on the recognition
of the physician's professional independence. Two points should be noted, however. Recently, the distinction between physician and institution has become
blurred. Increasingly, physicians have become employees of institutions that
provide care (such as health maintenance organizations and hospitals). Additionally, although there has been a distinction between physician and institution,
much of institutional care (lab tests, x-rays, pharmaceutical consumption, length
of stay, etc.) has been under the direct orders of physicians. The economic impact
of physicians is much greater than their share of the economie pie.

Much physician care is still provided by independent practitioners who are, in
effect, self-employed. Under the circumstances of self-employment, physicians
can participate in a solo practice (a practice operated by a single physician) or a
group practice (a practice operated by two or more physicians). Self-employment
is a state of contract, not of locational circumstance: self-employed physicians can
treat patients in a number of settings (offices, hospitals, nursing homes), but they
maintain separate contracts with their patients and bill them separately.
Increasingly, physicians are practicing medicine under the auspices of an organization that employs them. (See Section 2.4.4.)

Overall expenditures on physician services in 1984 were $75 billion. This figure
includes the cost of private-practice physicians' services provided both in offices
and institutions. It also incorporates the salaries, supplies, and so on, that physicians pay to their staff and for noninstitutional services and materials that they use
in their practices. This figure was about 19 percent of all expenditures on health
services in 1984.

Data concerning the growth of physician expenditures are shown in Table 2–3.
Between 1965 and 1984, total expenditures on physician services grew by
11.5 percent annually (from $8.5 billion to $75.4 billion). Using the formula
developed in Section 2.2.8 we can gain additional insight in how much of this
increase was due to an increase in actual services provided and how much was due
to inflation. We will develop our analysis in terms of per capita expenditures,
which, as can be seen in column 3, grew by 10.4 percent annually during this
period.

Using a multiplicative formula, per capita expenditures can be expressed as
follows

$$\frac{\text{Expenditures}}{\text{per capita}} = \frac{\text{average price}}{\text{per service}} \times \frac{\text{services}}{\text{per visit}} \times \frac{\text{visits}}{\text{per capita}}$$

The growth in expenditures per capita can be approximated by the sum of the
growth rates in the three components (see Section 2.2.8). Note also that the
average price *per visit* is equal to the product of the average price per service and

Table 2-3 Selected Indicators Relating to Physician Expenditures, 1965–1984

(1) Year	(2) Total expenditures on physician services (billions of $)[2]	(3) Per capita expenditures on physician services ($) (index, 1960 = 100)[1]	(4) Consumer price index for physicians' services (index, 1965 = 100)[2]	(5) Number of physician visits per person[2]	(6) Consumer price index for all consumer goods[1] (1965 = 100)
1965	8.5	42 (100)	100	4.5	100
1970	14.3	67 (159)	138	4.6	123.5
1975	24.9	111 (264)	195	5.1	171.3
1980	46.8	199 (473)	304	—	262.2
1984	75.4	307 (730)	433	5.0	330.6
Average annual growth rate 1965–1984 (compounded)	11.5	10.4	7.6	0.4	6.1

Sources: [1] *Health Care Financing Review,* 7 (1), pp. 16–33, U.S. Department of Health and Human Services, 1985; [2] *Health United States 1985,* U.S. Department of Health and Human Services. (Data are for 1964, 1976, 1981, and 1983.)

the number of services per visit. Data are available on total expenditures per capita (see column 3, Table 2–3), the price of physicians' services (column 4), and the number of visits per capita (column 5) for all U.S. residents from 1965 through 1984. We can apply our growth formula to allocate the overall growth in per capita expenditures, which is 10.4 percent, to its components. It can be seen that the growth in the number of patient visits was only 0.4 percent, a very small portion of the total growth. Prices per service, as measured by the Consumer Price Index (CPI) for physicians' services, increased on average by 7.6 percent, which is about 73 percent of the total growth. The residual amounts to 2.4 percent (10.4 − 7.6 − 0.4), which we can attribute to the number of services per visit. We have thus accounted for the total growth in expenditure, and, according to these figures, very little of the increase is due to the quantity of services.

The validity of our price measure depends on how well the data measure the concepts with which they are associated. The CPI measures price changes for specific product or service components of consumers' expenditures. The overall CPI measures an average price level of a given basket of commodities, expressed in index form. In the present case, we present the index with a 1965 base, meaning 1965 = 100. The CPI for all consumer commodities is shown for various years in column 6 of Table 2–3. The CPI for doctors' fees measures in index form the average level of the customary fee doctors charge their patients for a given sample of selected services (Ginsburg, 1978). Over time, certain changes may take place in the nature of the services provided by physicians or in the method of charging patients, which cause the CPI-measured level of customary charges to be a biased estimate of the actual fees paid by the consumers (or their insurers). For example, doctors may provide a higher-quality service and may charge more for it. A doctor's fee for an examination in 1965, for example, might have been $65, whereas in 1977 the same doctor might charge $80. As measured by the CPI, examinations would show a 23 percent increase. However, if these examinations changed in quality, then the 23 percent figure would be an inaccurate measure of the price change of the same commodity over time. An additional problem, known as fee fractionization, involves the doctor changing his or her fee practices over time so that fewer services would be covered by the same fee. Thus, if the doctor formerly charged $65 for an examination that included a vaccination, but later charged separately for the vaccination itself, 23 percent would be a low estimate of the change in price. The presence of these problems indicates that the CPI index for physicians' services must be used carefully; this is true of many statistics in an area where difficulties exist in the measurement of product quality. The CPI and its components are compiled by the U.S. Department of Labor and are published in the *Monthly Labor Review* by the Department of Labor. The rapid upward movement of price indicators, one of the most striking characteristics of the entire medical care market in recent years, has abated lately, a phenomenon to be explained using the tools developed in Part II of this book.

To obtain a complete description of the dimensions of the physician care market, it is necessary to incorporate the financing structure of physician care into the overall picture. Because of the importance of third-party financing in the entire medical care sector, Section 2.4.5 is devoted to this subject.

2.4.3 Hospital Care

Hospital care is by far the largest portion of the health care sector. In 1984, expenditures for hospital care amounted to $157.9 billion, which was 41 percent of the health care dollar. The hospital industry has been undergoing tremendous changes in the past several years. Some of these changes have been institutional. Traditionally, hospitals have been independent, nonprofit agencies, individually owned and operated by local governments or nonprofit corporations. Among the changes are the growth of for-profit (investor owned) hospitals. In 1972, investor-owned hospitals represented 12.8 percent of all short-term hospitals and 6.4 percent of the beds; by 1984 the respective figures were 13.6 and 9.8 percent (American Hospital Association, *Hospital Statistics 1985*).

Perhaps more important than type of ownership is membership in a multi-hospital system. In a multihospital system, two or more hospitals are linked together by ownership, management, or leasing. According to a 1984 survey by *Modern Health Care* magazine (June 7, 1985), 1,411 acute-care hospitals were leased and 565 were owned by multiunit systems (which may be for profit or nonprofit). In total there were 5,800 acute-care hospitals in operation in that year. The rapid growth of this phenomenon, coupled with the large size of the biggest chains (over $3 billion in revenues for Kaiser Permanente and Hospital Corporation of America), has led some commentators to express concern that the health care industry may become controlled by a few dominant corporations (Relman, 1980).

Changes in medical practice are also changing the hospital. Prior to the 1970s, virtually all surgery was done on an inpatient basis. Recent advances in medicine, most notably the availability of shorter-acting anesthetic drugs, now allow many surgical operations to be performed safely on an outpatient basis, either in a hospital outpatient department, a doctor's office, or a free-standing surgical clinic. In 1979, 16 percent of all surgery done in the hospital setting was done on an outpatient basis; the comparable figure in 1983 was 31 percent. As a result, hospital admissions have been declining in the 1980s. This fact, coupled with the fact that the length of stay of admissions has been declining because of changes in medical practice, has resulted in a sharp reduction in the number of patients being treated in a hospital at any one time; as a result, the occupancy rate of community hospitals has declined from 75 percent in 1972 to 69 percent in 1984.

As can be seen in Table 2–4, expenditures for hospital care have risen rapidly from 1965 through 1984 (11.3 percent average annual growth rate), and this has caused a great deal of policy concern (although the increase abated somewhat in the middle 1980s). To gain a better picture of the inflation picture, we can break down total expenditures as follows:

$$\begin{array}{c}\text{Total} \\ \text{expenditures}\end{array} = \begin{array}{c}\text{cost per} \\ \text{input}\end{array} \times \begin{array}{c}\text{inputs} \\ \text{per day}\end{array} \times \begin{array}{c}\text{days per} \\ \text{admission}\end{array} \times \text{admissions}$$

The average annual growth rate for each of these components from 1965 through 1984 has been 7.6 percent for costs per input, based on the Hospital Input Price Index of the Health Care Financing Administration (Freeland, Anderson, and Schendler, 1979); 1.4 percent for admissions; and a minus 0.3 percent for length of stay. Data for inputs per day (which can be further broken down as the product of inputs per services and services per day and has been referred to as *service intensity*) are no longer available directly, but can be inferred as the residual.

Since the equation is multiplicative, the total growth rate can be approximated by the sum of the components. Of the total growth in expenditures, 7.6 percent, which is 67 percent of the total annual growth of 11.3 percent, can be attributed to input prices. The next largest category is the residual, which approximates service intensity (inputs per day); 28 percent of the growth in expenditures was due to this factor. The other two components, length of stay and number of admissions, together accounted for about 10 percent of the annual growth. The overall picture of hospital expenditure growth is that the major contributing components are input price inflation and service intensity per patient, while quantity factors play a small role.

2.4.4 Alternative Delivery Systems

A very recent feature of the health care industry is the emergence of alternative delivery systems, which are so named because they differ in structure from traditional physician and hospital organization. The most prominent of such systems is the health maintenance organization (HMO). The major distinguishing characteristics of the HMO are that it performs both insurance and medical care provision functions and that membership is purchased on a fixed annual capitation fee.

With regard to structure and ownership, HMOs vary considerably. The two major forms of structure are (1) the *group or staff* HMO, which contracts with a medical group practice to provide care for HMO members (usually on a capitation basis) or which hires its own physicians on a salary basis, and (2) the *independent practice association (IPA)*, which contracts with community doctors (usually on the traditional fee-for-service basis) to serve its patients.

Health maintenance organizations can be either local, independent operations or members of a multi-HMO chain; and they can be organized on a for-profit or

Table 2–4 Selected Indicators Relating to Hospital Expenditures, 1960–1984

(1) Year	(2) Total expenditures on hospital services, billions of dollars, (indexed, 1965 = 100)[1]	(3) Price per input (1965 = 100)[2]	(4) Days per admission (average length of stay)[3]	(5) Admissions (millions) to nonfederal short-term general hospital	(6) Residual (inputs per day)
1965	18.4 (100)	100	7.8	26.4	
1970	28 (152)	138.5	8.2	29.5	
1975	52.4 (284)	200	7.7	33.4	
1980	101.3 (550)	315.6	7.6	36.1	
1984	157.9 (858)	439.4	7.3	35.1	
Average annual growth rate, 1965–1984 (compounded)	11.3	7.6	-0.3	1.4	3.2

Sources: [1] and [2] *Health Care Financing Review*, 7 (1), p. 33, U.S. Department of Health and Human Services, 1985; [3]*Hospital Statistics*, American Hospital Association, 1985. (Data for [3] are for community hospitals).

nonprofit basis. In 1981 the typical plan had between 5,000 and 15,000 members, but generally the industry is quite concentrated in the sense that a few large chains have the bulk of HMO membership. Of the 243 plans surveyed in 1981, the 17 largest had over 60 percent of the national membership (InterStudy, 1981). A striking feature of HMO membership is its recent, rapid growth. In 1980, 4 percent of the U.S. population was enrolled in an HMO; by 1985, this number had increased to 19 million, which is roughly 8 percent of the U.S. population (Inter-Study, 1985). An annual census of HMOs is conducted by InterStudy, a Minnesota research center, which releases its data each January.

Two other types of alternative systems are emergicenters and surgicenters. Emergicenters are clinics that offer episodic, ambulatory care. They are characterized by their marketing efforts with regard to hours of operation and location and by their identification as a commercial enterprise rather than as a professional office. Emergicenters are not a significant advance in health care. While they may be a thorn in the side of hospital emergency rooms and some primary practice physicians, they practice traditional fee-for-service medicine. Thus their prime contribution to patient welfare seems to be in terms of convenience for relatively healthy patients.

Surgicenters are free-standing organizations where outpatient surgery is performed. The major difference between surgicenters and hospital-owned outpatient surgery clinics is in terms of ownership. Surgicenters may be independently or chain owned.

2.4.5 Third-Party Finance

The introduction of third parties into the health care picture enables us to obtain a more complete description of the health care market. Our description will initially be of the traditional hospital care sector of the market. Subsequently, we will show how the introduction of new forces is altering this traditional view.

The role of third parties in the traditional hospital care sector can be illustrated by tracing the payments for hospital expenses to three major sources. The first is direct fees paid by the consumer to the hospital. Direct (out of pocket) payments by patients amounted to 8.6 percent of all hospital revenues in 1984. The second source of payment is through private health insurance. With this source of payment, consumers or corporations pay premiums to private intermediaries who offer coverage of expenses in the event of hospitalization. This form of payment amounted to 37.9 percent of all hospital expenses in 1984. The third major type of payment is via government programs, which amounted to 53.4 percent of expenses in 1984 (Levit, et al., 1985). Such government programs are supported by taxpayers whose tax revenues are used to pay for hospital care. Considerable growth has occurred in recent years in the government financing of hospital care. The watershed year was 1966, when two federally sponsored programs, Medicare and Medicaid, were instituted (see Chapter 11). Traditionally, some hospital care has been unfunded and hospitals made up the deficits by higher revenues from insured patients. There is some concern that this cost shifting will meet resistance from third parties and will lead to a growing indigent care problem.

A simplified version of the flow of funds under the traditional arrangements in the hospital care market is shown in Figure 2–1. In this diagram, solid lines refer to money payments and intermittent lines refer to services provided. The three sources of payments for hospitalization are shown as direct fees, payments via private insurance, and payments via government programs. In the case of government programs, the private intermediaries (insurance companies) are shown as reimbursing agents for the government. Hospitals pay their service suppliers and employees with receipts from the three payment sources. The intermittent line from the physician to the hospital service line illustrates the physician's influence on the flow of hospital services. Payments to physicians are ignored since they are considered distinct entities from institutions (at least in the traditional view). The difference between revenues and benefits plus administrative costs is the *contribution to surplus* (or profit) of the intermediary. This could be negative, indicating a loss on current operations.

There are two major types of private, traditional health insurers in the United States (HMOs are considered nontraditional). These are commercial insurance

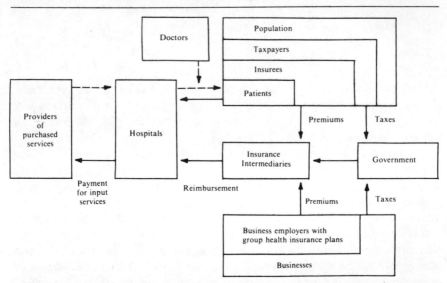

Figure 2–1 Flow of funds and services in the hospital care market. Figure shows flow of funds from consumers to employees to hospitals via third parties, and the flow of services from hospitals to patients. While doctors are included in the picture to demonstrate their influence on the service flow, payments to doctors are made separately and are not shown here. The solid line indicates money flow, and the broken line represents service flow.

companies and Blue Cross and Blue Shield. Commercial insurance companies are stock or mutual companies. *Stock companies* are those owned by stockholders; profits are paid to these stockholders in the form of dividends. *Mutual companies* are owned and controlled by policyholders, to whom any profits revert (in the form of lowered premiums). The second type of traditional insuring agency is Blue Cross and Blue Shield. Both are nonprofit organizations. Blue Cross initially began operations in the 1930s under the auspices of hospitals to ensure that hospitals would be paid for their services. Over the years, Blue Cross plans have become increasingly independent of hospitals. Blue Cross has been primarily associated with hospital insurance. Blue Shield is associated with the insurance of surgical, major medical, and regular medical expenses. *Surgical coverage* involves the coverage of doctors' operating fees. *Major medical* coverage is for treatment expenses in excess of a given amount. *Regular medical* coverage involves coverage of doctors' fees for nonsurgical hospital care and nonhospital care.

Data for the commercial insurers show that roughly 15 percent of policies are individual policies (in which the individual contracts separately with the insurer), and the remainder are group plans (in which the individual contracts through an employer or some other entity such as a professional association). Blue Cross has a slightly higher proportion of its policies as group policies.

Data for 1977 show that, for employer group plans, about 80 percent of the premium was paid by the employer (Taylor and Lawson, 1981). Persons with no employment-based insurance and who cannot get insurance through a group may pay an unusually heavy burden for health insurance. First, employer health insurance premiums are nontaxable for income tax purposes; individuals who buy individual policies can deduct premiums only if they itemize deductions and only an amount in excess of a basic amount. Second, group plans are less costly to administer (13.3 percent of premiums is the average for group contracts and 46 percent for individual contracts) (Carroll, 1978), and thus premiums will be much lower. Indeed, employment-based plans are characterized by their generous coverage, and tax reform discussion includes examining the possibility of putting a cap on the tax-free (employer paid) portion of premiums.

Although two major public programs (Medicare and Medicaid) provide health insurance for those who are "in need," such programs are limited. As a result, a substantial portion of the population, about 25 million in 1977 (see Section 11.2.3), is uninsured. Many of these, although they do not qualify for public funds, do incur medical costs that they cannot meet. With public funds becoming ever tighter, this has created a growing *indigent care* problem. In the past the health care system itself (through higher charges on patients and insurees) has subsidized much unpaid care, but payors of care may increasingly resist paying premiums to cover others' expenses. Alternative sources of funds for this case will have to be found.

Data on health insurance coverage and expenses are obtained from several sources. The Health Insurance Association of America issues an annual statistical book, *Source Book of Health Insurance Data*. Blue Cross–Blue Shield data are in the *Fact Book,* published annually by the national Blue Cross Association. Information is also published through occasional studies in *Health Care Financing Review* and the *Monthly Labor Review*.

2.4.6 Nonfinancial Intermediaries

A new arrival on the health care scene is the preferred provider organization (PPO) or agency (PPA). A PPO is a bargaining intermediary that mediates between providers and insurers. A PPO can be established by provider groups, community groups, businesses, insurers, or independent entrepreneurs.

A successful PPO must be able to obtain agreements from providers and insurers to offer something to each. Providers (doctors, hospitals) may offer "preferred fees" or charges (e.g., guaranteed) to selected patients; they may also be willing to submit to reviews of patient use by a committee set up by the PPO designed to control utilization.

Insurers can deliver large blocks of patients to providers. The mechanism by which they do this is to set up policies that reward insurees if they use the preferred providers. For example, insurers can set up policies such that, if insurees receive treatment from providers in the preferred group, there are lower patient charges; if they choose to go to providers in the nonpreferred group, they must pay a copayment of, say, 20 percent of charges. Such arrangements encourage insurees to go to the preferred providers.

Preferred provider organizations are very new on the scene. Perhaps the major innovation they make is that under these arrangements insurers permit patients to choose their providers (although with a penalty if it is not a preferred provider). Many HMOs do not reimburse patients if they see non-HMO doctors. The PPO increases the flexibility of the patient and thus increases the range of choice.

REFERENCES

Overall Dimensions

Angell, M. (1985). Cost containment and the physician. *Journal of the American Medical Association, 253,* 1203–1207.

Bauerschmidt, A.D. (1969). Sources and uses of health care funds in South Carolina. *Business and Economics Review of the University of South Carolina, 3,* 2–7.

Fuchs, V.R. (1984). "Though much is taken": Reflections on aging, health, and medical care. *Milbank Memorial Fund Quarterly, 62,* 143–166.

Levit, K.R., Lazenby, H., Waldo, D.R., et al. (1985). National health expenditures 1984. *Health Care Financing Review, 7,* 1–35.

Mullner, R., & Hadley, J. (1984). Interstate variations in the growth of chain-owned proprietary hospitals, 1973–1983. *Inquiry, 21,* 144–151.

Rice, D.P., & Feldman, J.J. (1983). Living longer in the United States: Demographic changes and health needs of the elderly. *Milbank Memorial Fund Quarterly, 61,* 362–396.

Sutcliffe, E.M. (1972). The social accounting of health. In M.M. Hauser (Ed), *The economics of medical care,* (pp. 238–257). London: George Allen and Unwin.

Costs, Prices, and Expenditures

Anderson, G., & Knickman, J.R. (1984). Patterns of expenditure among high utilizers of medical care services. *Medical Care, 22,* 143–149.

Freeland, M.S., Anderson, G., & Schendler, C. (1979). National hospital input price index. *Health Care Financing Review, 1*(1), 37–61.

Ginsburg, D.H. (1978). Medical care services in the consumer price index. *Monthly Labor Review, 101,* 35–40.

Klarman, H.E. (1972). Increases in the cost of physician and hospital services. *Inquiry, 7,* 22–36.

Long, S.H., Gibbs, J.O., Crozier, J.P., et al. (1984). Medical expenditures for terminal cancer patients during the last year of life. *Inquiry, 21,* 315–327.

McCall, N. (1984). Utilization and costs of medicare services by beneficiaries in their last year of life. *Medical Care, 22,* 329–342.

Rice, D.P., Hodgson, T.A., & Kopstein, A.N. (1985). The economic cost of illness: A replication and update. *Health Care Financing Review, 7*(1), 61–80.

Scitovsky, A.A. (1984). "The high cost of dying": What do the data show? *Milbank Memorial Fund Quarterly, 62,* 591–608.

———, & McCall, N. (1977). Changes in the cost of treatment of selected illnesses. (Publication No. [HRA] 77–3161.) Hyattsville, MD: National Center for Health Services Research.

Zook, C.J., & Moore, E.D. (1980). High-cost users of medical care. *New England Journal of Medicine, 302,* 996–1002.

Health Capital Formation

Cameron, J.M. (1985). The indirect costs of graduate medical education. *New England Journal of Medicine, 312,* 1233–1238.

Fein, R., & Weber, G.I. (1971). *Financing medical education.* New York: McGraw-Hill Book Co.

Freiman, M.P. (1985). The rate of adoption of new procedures among physicians. *Medical Care, 23,* 939–945.

Harrison, J.L., & Nash, K.D. (1974). Redistribution effects of publicly supported medical education. *Mississippi Valley Journal Economics and Business, 9,* 1–16.

Jolly, H.P., Taskel, L., & Elliott, P.R. (1985). US medical school finances. *Journal of the American Medical Association, 254,* 1573–1581.

Knapp, R.M., & Butler, P.W. (1979). Financing graduate medical education. *New England Journal of Medicine, 301,* 749–755.

Kohlman, H.A. (1986, January). Who's picking up the tab for graduate medical education? *Health Care Financial Management, 10.*

Mullner, R. (1981, July). Funding sources, costs of 1979 hospital construction reported. *Hospitals, 1,* 59–62.

Perry, D.R., & Challoner, D.R. (1979). The rationale for federal support of medical education. *New England Journal of Medicine, 300,* 66–71.

Russell, L.B. (1976). The diffusion of new hospital technologies in the United States. *International Journal of Health Services, 6,* 557–580.

Sykes, C.S. (1986). The role of equity financing in today's health care environment. *Topics in Health Care Financing, 12,* 1–3.

Wilson, G., Sheps, C.G., & Oliver, T.R. (1982). Effects of hospital revenue bonds on hospital planning and operations. *New England Journal of Medicine, 307,* 1426–1430.

New Institutions

Adams-Ryan, D., Peddecord, K.M., & Root, G.L. (1985). Operational and legal implications of preferred provider organizations. *Hospital and Health Services Administration, 30*(3), 44–57.

Burns, L. (1982). Ambulatory surgery growing at a rapid pace. *AORN Journal, 35,* 260–270.

———, & Ferber, M.S. (1981). Ambulatory surgery in the United States. *Journal of Ambulatory Care Management, 4,* 1–13.

de Lissovoy, G., Rice, T., & Gabel, J. (1986). Preferred provider organizations. *Inquiry, 23,* 7–15.

Ermann, D., & Gabel, J. (1985). The changing face of American health care: Multihospital systems, emergency centers, and surgery centers. *Medical Care, 23,* 401–420.

Relman, A. (1980). The new medical-industrial complex. *New England Journal of Medicine, 303,* 963–970.

Schroer, K.A., & Taylor, E. (1985). PPA's fewer startups but better operations. *Hospitals, 59,* 68–73.

Health Insurance

Arnett, R.H., & Trapnell, G.R. (1984). Private health insurance: New measures in a complex and changing industry. *Health Care Financing Review, 6*(2), 31–41.

Carroll, M.S. (1978). Private health insurance plans in 1976. *Social Security Bulletin, 41,* 3–16.

Kasper, J.A., Walden, D.C., & Wilensky, G.R. (1980). Who are the uninsured? *National health care expenditures study* (data preview 1). Hyattsville, MD: National Center for Health Services Research.

Rublee, D.A. (1986). Self-funded health benefit plans. *Journal of the American Medical Association, 255*(6), 787–789.

Taylor, A.K., & Lawson, W.R. (1981). Employer and employee expenditures for private health insurance. *National health care expenditures study* (data preview 7). Hyattsville, MD: National Center for Health Services Research.

Data Sources

American Nurses' Association. *Facts About Nursing.* Kansas City, MO: American Nurses' Association (biannually, national data on the nursing profession).

Health Insurance Association of America. *Source Book of Health Insurance Data.* Washington, DC: Health Insurance Association of America (annual data on health insurance).

InterStudy. *National HMO Census.* Excelsior, MN: Interstudy (annual data on HMOs).

Part II

Explanatory Economics

Chapter 3

Demand for Medical Care: A Simple Model

3.1 THE CONCEPT OF DEMAND

The purpose of explanatory economics is to predict economic behavior. When analyzing demand behavior, our attention focuses on the quantity demanded by consumers of a specific commodity or service. To perform the analysis, we use a demand model that serves two purposes: it provides a categorization of the separate factors that might cause demand or quantity demanded to increase or decrease, and it provides a specific hypothesis about how economic factors (e.g., price and income) influence demand or quantity demanded.

A model is the device we use to obtain our results; it is a representation of reality, not a complete description of it. The purpose of a model, however specified, is to present us with an "if . . . then . . ." type of explanation. In the case of the demand model, the reasoning tells us something like "if factor x increases, then demand or quantity demanded will increase (or decrease, depending on what factor x is)." A good model screens essential causal factors and welds them into a logical, coherent system.

Even though the model is conjectural, it should tell us something about movements in real phenomena (e.g., the quantity of medical care demanded). In assessing our model, it is therefore sufficient to examine whether its predictions concerning movements in selected phenomena are realized by comparing our predictions with actual movements in the phenomena as measured by data movements. Accuracy of prediction is the test of an explanatory model. Thus, no model is complete without having been tested against actual events.

This chapter introduces a simple model of the demand for a commodity in light of this accuracy-of-prediction criterion. Section 3.2 sets forth the model, using an individual's demand for medical care as an example. Section 3.3 takes us behind the scenes and shows a derivation of a simple theoretical explanation of these hypothetical statements to clarify some of the explanatory variables. Several key shortcomings of the simple model when applied to the medical care context are emphasized; these objections are central to the analyses of Chapter 4. Section 3.4 examines the factors influencing the market demand for the commodity. Section 3.5 develops the concept of elasticity, a tool used to measure the magnitude of the hypothesized movements, and Section 3.6 presents the demand analysis when insurance is present. Finally, Section 3.7 presents some actual estimates of the demand relationship.

3.2 INDIVIDUAL DEMAND: THE PRICE–QUANTITY RELATION

3.2.1 Demand and Quantity Demanded

We begin our exposition of the price–quantity relation with a specification of the terms of reference and definitions of the variables used. The unit of analysis is the individual consumer. In the present context, we examine the economic behavior of a typical or representative consumer. This behavior involves attaining or attempting to attain commodities. Since our focus is on health care, the commodity *physician care* is used as the major example. Physician care is defined as examinations and treatments administered by physicians to their patients. Physician care is only one of many commodities in the health care sector. Thus, when following the analysis, keep in mind that the relations specified in this chapter can be applied to other health-related commodities as well, including hospital services, pharmaceuticals, dental care, home care, preventive measures such as inoculations, and health foods.

Having identified the commodity in our analysis, we must next find an appropriate unit of measurement. Here we encounter a problem that is pervasive in medical care organization analysis: it involves the definition and measurement of quality differences among units of medical care. Examinations and treatments can vary in thoroughness, in the physician's technical competence, and in his or her bedside manner, among other factors. Quality differences constitute differences in these characteristics. When analyzing physician care as a commodity, all these variations should be kept in mind. In this chapter we will abstract from quality differences to avoid complicating our initial entrance into explanatory economics. Our commodity, physician care, is measured by the number of visits to a physician by the typical consumer. Each visit is taken as identical with all others. Finally, we specify the time span as being 1 year; placed in a time frame, our commodity measure becomes the number of physician visits per year.

With this background, the demand hypothesis used to predict the effect of a change in direct per unit price on the quantity demanded of a commodity can be presented. The hypothesis is that *the lower the direct price offered to the consumer (all other factors held constant), the greater the number of units of that commodity he or she will demand.* A number of conventions or interpretations are related to this hypothesis. This hypothesized relation is known as the demand relation. By "quantity demanded," we mean quantity demanded at any specific price, all other causal factors held constant. By "demand," we mean the *set* of quantities demanded at various prices, all other causal factors held constant. By "direct price,"we mean the price paid directly by the consumer for a particular unit of the commodity; this is sometimes referred to as *out-of-pocket price*. By "all other factors," we mean those variables other than price that influence consumer demand behavior. The economic approach to consumer behavior is to specify an initial relation between direct price and quantity demanded, and then to introduce other causal factors in terms of how they affect the basic demand relation.

One such demand relation, assuming all other factors remain unchanged, is illustrated diagrammatically as line d_1 in Figure 3–1. The specific relation shown by this line, or curve, is that, at a price of $7 per visit, the consumer would be willing to visit the doctor twice a year; if the price were $6 per visit, the consumer would be willing to make three visits; and so on. Assuming that the quantities demanded at all other prices trace out a straight-line relation, d_1 represents a particular demand curve at one specific level of demand. The lower case d is used to indicate that we are representing the behavior of a single individual.

The rationale behind the downward sloping demand curve lies in the possibility of substitution. The economic approach implies that very few, if any, commodities are absolute musts. Substitutes exist for most commodities; some are quite similar and others are only vaguely so. The longer the time span during which the consumer adapts his or her behavior to these substitutes, the more relevant these alternatives become. A sore throat, for example, can be treated by a physician or by resorting to other substitutes, such as drugs or home remedies. Furthermore, even if treated by a physician, alternative types of broad-spectrum antibiotics can be used. Many suspected illnesses, such as tonsillitis, can be treated with substitute types of care, including surgery and drugs. In recent years the possibility of outpatient treatment instead of hospitalization has been suggested for many types of ailments. In the long term, health foods and other preventive services are substitutes for medical care in maintaining desired health levels. In these, as well as in other instances, the hypothesized relation applies: the lower the price of any specific alternative, the more it will be demanded.

Other hypotheses might be put forward to explain consumer demand behavior. One such alternative specification, which has received much attention in the medical care literature, is that at higher prices individuals will still demand and pay for the same quantity of medical care; that is, their need does not change simply because direct price has changed. This alternative hypothesis would be represented by a vertical demand curve. Similar vertical demand curves have also been

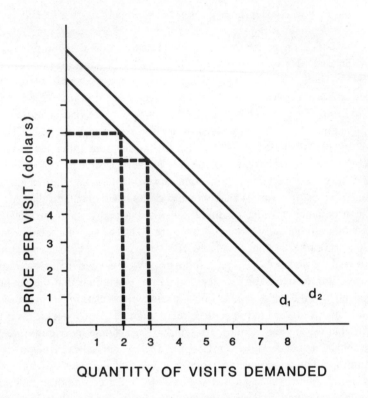

QUANTITY OF VISITS DEMANDED

Figure 3–1 Graphic representation of the demand relation, the famous downward sloping demand curve. Curves d_1 and d_2 show quantity demanded increasing as the direct price decreases. Each curve represents a separate level of demand. With reference to curve d_1, curve d_2 represents an increase in demand.

hypothesized for other items considered necessities, such as housing, basic foods, and even alcohol.

Having two alternative hypotheses, we are faced with the problem of determining which is the more useful in terms of explaining actual behavior. No amount of arguing will resolve the issue, however. The ground rules are that the more useful hypothesis will better explain actual data movements. The subject of empirical tests is discussed later in Section 3.7.

Before proceeding with qualifications to our hypothesis, we emphasize that we are focusing solely on consumer behavior. Our hypothesis relates only to how much the consumer is willing to buy at any price. We are not inquiring at this stage about whether or not the amount demanded will be supplied or available. (Such an inquiry is relevant to producer behavior, discussed in Chapter 6.) At present, we are examining part of the total picture of scarcity—the part relating to demand.

3.2.2 Changes in Demand

The effects of factors other than direct price on the economic behavior of consumers are introduced by way of their influence on the basic price–quantity relation. These other factors can be placed into three broad categories: (1) income, (2) prices of related commodities, and (3) tastes. Each category is considered next.

Income

The income of the consumer is generally assumed to be positively related to demand. That is, if income increases, quantity demanded at each price will be greater. The basic relation between income and demand can be illustrated with the use of demand curves. In Figure 3-4, curve d_1 can now be interpreted as a level of demand at an initial income level. Let us suppose that the income level increases. The hypothesized effect on demand is such that at $7 there will be three visits demanded instead of two, at $6 four visits will be demanded instead of three, and so on. The new demand level, corresponding to the higher income level, can be represented by curve d_2. In the diagram the relative position of the two curves summarizes the net influence of income on consumer behavior. A shift in demand from curve d_1 to curve d_2 is called an *increase* in demand.

and the curve d_2 represents the demand at a higher income level

The same reasoning can be applied in reverse to a fall in income. This decline causes the consumer to demand less of the commodity at each price. The demand curve in this case shifts inward, moving from a level such as d_2 to one such as d_1. This is called a *decrease* in demand.

Income is frequently defined as an individual's earnings in a specific time period. It is a variable used to measure the ability of the consumer to afford medical care. As such, earnings are an approximate measure. Another approximate measure is the level of wealth of the individual, which includes bonds, bank deposits, real estate, and other assets, less any liabilities such as loans. A third measure of ability to afford medical care is after-tax income. This measure is particularly important when considering changes in tax rates and their effects on purchasing power. Whatever the measure used, it should be a good approximation of the ability to afford medical care.

Prices of Related Commodities

The demand for a particular commodity is also influenced by the quantities consumed of related commodities. The quantities consumed of these related commodities are, in turn, influenced by their prices. Two classes of commodity relations are of concern to us. These are complements and substitutes. A *complementary* commodity is one whose use is generally accompanied by the use of the commodity in question. Examples might include penicillin and syringes, the services of a surgeon and a hospital's surgical services, and the services of a radiologist and the use of x-rays. The hypothesis relating the demands of complementary commodities is as follows: a fall in the price of a commodity increases the quantity demanded of that commodity; this also leads to an increase in the demand for commodities that are complements. That is, at each price, the quantity demanded of the complementary commodity increases. Similar reasoning, in reverse, holds for a decline in the price of one commodity in a complementary set. As an example of this relation, we can hypothesize that a fall in the direct price of surgical fees for tonsil removal will lead to an increase in the quantity demanded for such services; it will also increase the demand for hospital room services. Complements are of particular importance with regard to medical care demand. The close relation between physician care and hospital care has frequently led to the assertion that much hospital demand is really determined by the quantity of specific physicians' services consumed.

The second type of commodity relation is that of *substitution*. A substitute is a commodity whose use can replace that of the original commodity. The hypothesized relation is that a fall in the price of a commodity increases its quantity demanded; this leads to a reduced demand for substitute commodities. This relation can be illustrated using an example of two substitute services, postoperative recuperation time in the hospital or home care. A rise in the price the patient pays for an additional day of hospital care decreases the quantity demanded of hospital days. At the same time, it increases the demand for home care.

Substitution was also the reason given in Section 3.2.1 for the downward slope of the demand curve for any commodity. That is, the reason the quantity demanded for inpatient care is negatively related to patient price is because of substitution of inpatient care for home care when the price of inpatient care falls. However, this assumes that the price of home care remains constant. When home care's price rises, this will lead to additional substitution, which is accounted for in our model by an outward shift in the inpatient-care demand curve. The slope of the demand curve of any commodity, as well as how much it shifts when substitute prices change, depends on how similar the patient perceives the substitutes to be. Services like inpatient and outpatient surgery (e.g., for hernia repair and tonsillectomy) are very substitutable, as are nursing home care and home care in many instances.

Tastes

Taste is a catchall category covering all other factors that might influence demand. Tastes have sometimes been called *wants*, a term connoting the intensity of desire for particular commodities. The elements that influence the intensity of an individual's desire for medical care include health status, educational background, sex, age, race, and upbringing. Any of these can explain differences in the intensity of desire for medical care among individuals, that is, with other factors (incomes, other prices, and so on) held constant, these differences can offer explanations as to why one individual's demand curve will be d_1 (Figure 3–1), while that of another will be d_2. This would be the case if the health status of the d_2 individual were lower than that of the d_1 individual.

Tastes are usually considered to be a given from the standpoint of economic analysis. Although tastes differ among individuals, they are hypothesized for most commodities to be stable over fairly short periods of time. If this is the case, once the factors that underlie tastes are accounted for, differences in individual demands can be identified as being attributable to differences in incomes, other prices, and factors influencing tastes. However, controversy exists over the stability of individual tastes for medical care. In addition to the dependence of tastes on health, which is itself a transitory element, physicians potentially can exert considerable influence over tastes for medical care. Changing tastes have played a large role in health economics. Because of this, it is necessary to go behind the scenes to discover the role of tastes in medical care demand.

3.3 DERIVING THE DEMAND RELATION

In Section 3.2, the demand for medical care was analyzed as if it were an ordinary commodity like carrots or shoes. However, certain aspects of medical care make it unlike many ordinary commodities that an individual consumes. We must pay closer attention to these characteristics to determine if and when the standard analysis is an appropriate representation for the case of medical care. To do this, we present a theoretical model focusing on the conditions that are required for the demand relation to hold; special attention is paid to whether these conditions are likely to be met in the case of medical care.

The factors influencing a consumer's behavior with regard to the demand for a commodity can be placed under categories called income, prices, and tastes. Let us assume that a typical individual receives a given income of $100 per year and has a choice of only two commodities on which to spend this income. These two commodities are carrots and physician care; because our individual is swayed by the reputed health-stimulating powers of carrots, they will be regarded to some degree as being substitutes for medical care. The prices of medical care and carrots are assumed to be fixed at $10 per physician visit and $2 per carrot. At these prices and this level of income, the combinations of the commodities available to our individual are shown in columns 1 and 2 of Table 3–1. For example, the individual can purchase 9 visits and 5 carrots, or 8 visits and 10 carrots, while using up his or her budget.

Table 3–1 Schedule of Alternative Combinations of Medical Care and Carrots Available and of the Intrinsic Value of Medical Care

(1) Units of medical care	(2) Number of carrots	(3) Number of carrots that the individual is willing to give up in order to obtain one more unit of medical care
9	5	0
8	10	1
7	15	2
6	20	3
5	25	4
4	30	5
3	35	6
2	40	7
1	45	8
0	50	9

Although we can calculate the alternative combinations of commodities available to our individual, we do not have enough information to determine which of these combinations he or she will choose. To determine this, we must know the individual's tastes for the two commodities. Let us assume that the individual obtains "well-being" or "satisfaction" from only these two commodities and from only his or her own consumption (and no one else's). Since the consumption of these two commodities is all that provides well-being, our individual will presumably consume as much of them as possible. We thus conclude, from these assumptions, that the individual will use up the entire budget on carrots and medical care. That is, he or she will consume one of the available combinations shown in Table 3–1, columns 1 and 2. To say anything more than this, we must make additional specific assumptions about the intensity of desire for each commodity. We will limit this taste assumption to the individual's ranking of these available combinations, since they are relevant to the consumption decision, given these prices and income. Furthermore, we will characterize such tastes in relative terms, that is, in terms of how many carrots our individual would be willing to give up to obtain one more unit of medical care. We expect that this will depend on how many carrots and how much medical care he or she is consuming. The taste assumption in our model is that the more carrots the individual is consuming relative to medical care, the more carrots the individual will be willing to give up in order to obtain one more unit of medical care. In other words, an additional unit of medical care will be worth more to the individual. This assumption is illustrated in column 3 in Table 3–1, with reference to the combinations in columns 1 and 2.

Column 3 shows how many carrots the individual would be willing to give up to obtain one more visit. If the individual is using his or her entire budget on 50 carrots, he or she would be willing to give up as many as 9 carrots to obtain the first visit. If the individual is consuming 1 visit and 45 carrots, he or she will give up as many as 8 more carrots for one more visit, and so on. It should be stressed that column 3 represents the individual's intrinsic, relative valuations of the two commodities, which are a representation of his or her tastes. By saying that they are stable, we are saying that these relative valuations remain unchanged for their corresponding combinations.

Using a model that incorporates price, taste, and income assumptions, we can obtain considerable insight into some of the hypotheses stated in Section 3.2. First, we can determine which combination is optimal from the consumer's point of view. This depends on both the "willing" and the "able" parts of our model. The able portion states that, for every 5 carrots given up, the individual can obtain 1 unit of medical care since the price of medical care is five times that of carrots. Thus, if our typical individual begins with a potential combination of no medical care and 50 carrots, the first visit would be worth 9 carrots, but he or she would have to give up only 5 to obtain it. Assuming the individual is out to maximize well-being, he or she would certainly consume at least 1 visit. Using similar reasoning, the individual would consume the second visit because it would have a value of 8 carrots, and only 5 more would have to be given up to obtain it. In fact, the individual would similarly continue until he or she was consuming 5 visits and 25 carrots. The individual would not consume the sixth visit, however, because he or she would have to give up 5 more carrots to obtain it, and it is worth only 4 additional carrots.

Furthermore, we can examine the impact of a price change on the quantity of a commodity consumed. One of the virtues of such a *relative terms* model is that it focuses attention on an important dimension of prices: they determine how much one can obtain of a unit of one commodity in terms of another. Let us assume that income remains the same but prices change so that medical care now costs $9 per visit and carrots cost $3 each. The terms at which additional units of medical care can be obtained are more in favor of medical care now; 1 more visit can be obtained with only 3 more carrots. The available combinations will now differ somewhat from those of columns 1 and 2 in Table 3–1; and slightly different relative values will represent tastes, since these will have to correspond to the new combinations. Nevertheless, these relative values will retain magnitudes similar to those of column 3, and we can predict that more medical care and fewer carrots will be consumed at the new prices. This is because medical care is less costly, thus encouraging less substitution of carrots for it.

With this model, we can explain several important underlying conditions of our analysis. The first relates to the relative valuations themselves. Tastes, that is, the entire constellation of valuations at all relevant combinations of commodities, depend on a number of factors, but for most commodities they can be considered stable over short periods of time. The situation with medical care is somewhat different. With regard to an individual's tastes for medical care, perhaps the most important determining factor is his or her health status. An individual with acute appendicitis or pneumonia will have a different set of tastes from that of a "healthy, normal" individual. The tastes of the ill person will be characterized by giving more weight to medical care for all possible combinations; in Table 3–1, column 3, for example, the first unit of medical care might be valued at 12 carrots, the second at 11, and so on. The effect of this in terms of the demand curve would be to shift out the demand curve for medical care. In reference to taste differences across individuals, these differences may be systematically influenced by factors such as age, sex, race, and health status. Age, for example, will be negatively related to health status and can be expected to increase the valuations of medical care and thus the demand.

A second assumption relates to the conditions under which ill health is expected to occur. The analysis in this section focused on tastes for any given level of individual health; that is, it treated tastes as if the individual who forms these tastes could foresee his or her health status. In fact, illness is a risky event; its onset can seldom be predicted accurately for any individual. The present analysis does not recognize that the individual formulates his or her tastes and the demand for medical care by taking the risk of the situation into account. Yet this is an important consideration, for we find the presence of insurance against such risks to be widespread. This characteristic of medical care demand is treated in Chapter 4.

A third assumption of this analysis concerns the relationship between the product, medical care, and the phenomenon that it attempts to influence, health. In positing that our individual has a known set of valuations for medical care and carrots, the model implicitly assumes that he or she knows the benefits to be obtained from both. To do this, the individual must be aware of the benefits in health terms that will accrue from the various units of medical care. In reality, the individual seldom possesses such a high degree of acumen. Indeed, part of an individual's reason for visiting a doctor is to have the doctor explain what he or she "needs." The analysis in this chapter disregards the high level of consumer ignorance that may, in fact, exist.

3.4 MARKET DEMAND

The model developed previously was an explanation of an individual's demand for medical care. To generalize the model to explain market demand, we must make an additional assumption, one concerning the number of individuals who participate in the market. By *market* we mean the network of buyers and sellers of a commodity. The assumption we must make refers to how many buyers are vying for the product. The more individuals who seek the product, the greater will be the market demand and the quantity demanded in the market at any price.

This is illustrated geometrically in Figure 3–2. Here three individuals' demand curves are shown. d_b is Mr. D's demand schedule, d_k is Ms. K's demand curve, and d_j is Mrs. J's. At a price of $20 per visit, Mr. B will demand three visits, Ms. K will demand two, and Mrs. J will demand none. At $15 per visit, Mr. B., Ms. K, and Mrs. J will demand five, four, and one visit, respectively. At $10, these visits will be seven, six, and four. With this information on individual demand curves and the number of individuals, we can derive a market demand curve.

Given our three individuals' curves, the market quantity demanded at any price will be the sum of the individuals' quantities demanded at that price. At a price of $20, the quantity demanded in the market will be five visits. At a price of $15 per visit, ten visits will be demanded, and at $10 per visit seventeen visits will be demanded. The market demand curve is shown in Figure 3–2 as D_m.

We can now divide the factors influencing market demand into two categories: (1) those influencing individual demands only and (2) those influencing market demand. The former includes prices, incomes, and tastes. If any of these change, individual demands or quantities demanded will also change. If individual demand curves shift out, market curves, being based on individual curves, will shift out as well. In addition to individually caused factors, market demand will shift out when the number of participants in the market changes. An influx of people into an area will cause market demand to increase.

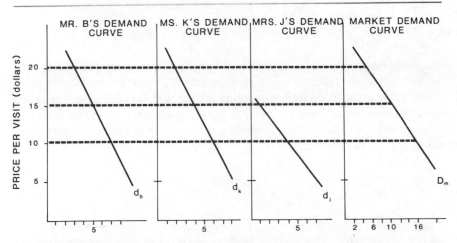

Figure 3–2 Derivation of the market demand curve from individual demand curves. The quantity demanded at each price by all consumers in the market together is equal to the sum of individual quantities demanded at each price. The market demand curve is the horizontal sum of all individual demand curves.

3.5 MEASURING QUANTITY RESPONSIVENESS TO PRICE CHANGES

In the preceding sections, we developed a model that enabled us to predict the direction of change a particular factor would have on quantity demanded or demand. Thus, we can predict that, when price falls, quantity demanded will rise.

We now inquire further and ask, By how much will the quantity demanded rise? For policy purposes, the answer to this question is important, because it enables us to obtain ballpark estimates of changes in quantity demanded, whereas we were totally in the dark before. Obviously, having some idea of the order of magnitude of these changes is better than having none at all. The concept used to measure quantity responsiveness to price changes is that of the *price elasticity* of demand. Price elasticity is designed to measure the responsiveness of a price change at a given point, or between two given points, on a single demand curve. That is, it attempts to measure responsiveness when only price, and no other influencing factor, changes to influence quantity demanded.

The elasticity of demand was designed to measure changes independent of the units of measurement. That is, the measure of elasticity is a measure of relative magnitudes and will not change if cents rather than dollars are used to measure price, or units rather than thousands are used to measure quantity. Elasticity is thus a pure measure of magnitudes of changes. The formula used for small changes in price is the percentage change in quantity demanded over the percentage change in price. In symbolic terms, this is written

$$\frac{\Delta Q/Q}{\Delta P/P} = E$$

where E is elasticity, Q is the original quantity, P is the original price, and ΔQ and ΔP are changes in Q and P. This formula is known as a *point elasticity* formula.

The point elasticity formula is appropriate for very small changes along the demand curve. If the change in price is at all appreciable, an average elasticity measure over the range of the demand curve covered by the change is more appropriate. This measure, known as the *arc elasticity* of demand, is written as

$$E = \frac{(Q_2 - Q_1)/(Q_2 + Q_1)}{(P_2 - P_1)/(P_2 + P_1)}$$

where Q_1 and P_1 refer to one set of price and quantity, and Q_2 and P_2 refer to a second set at another point on the same demand curve. [In fact, both the price and quantity changes are expressed in terms of average price and quantity levels, that is, $(P_1 + P_2)/2$ and $(Q_1 + Q_2)/2$; in the preceding equation, the 2's would cancel out and so we are left with this formula.]

An example will help to illustrate the use of this formula. Assume that the Richland County Health Department charges $3 per syphilis test and that in May it performed 1,200 tests. In June the County Council decided to raise the charges to $3.25 per test. Only 1,150 people requested tests in June. What is the elasticity of demand?

The elasticity measure of a price change is supposed to be a measure of responsiveness *along a demand curve*, that is, when all factors other than price remain constant. If this has been the case, we can use the elasticity formula as an approximation of the responsiveness of quantity demanded to price changes. If other things have changed, we must make some adjustment to take into account the extent to which these other factors influenced quantity demanded. Assume in our example that these other factors have been constant so that only price influenced quantity. In this case, we can use the elasticity formula directly:

$$E = \frac{(1,150 - 1,200)/(3.25 - 3)}{(1,150 + 1,200)/(3.25 + 3)} = -0.53$$

The elasticity of demand at that point is -0.53. (The minus sign is frequently dropped from discussions, so one will often see the price elasticity quoted as the absolute value, that is, 0.53. The reader should remember that in the case of price elasticity the negative sign, if dropped, is taken for granted.) We thus have a figure indicating the responsiveness of quantity to price.

Price elasticity is related to how total consumer expenditures respond to a price change. For any elasticity measure whose absolute value is less than 1, total direct expenditures will increase with a reduction in price; at these points on the demand curve, demand is said to be *inelastic*. In our example, total expenditures ($P \times Q$) were $3,600 before the price change and $3,737.50 after. Receipts from this source rose by $137.50 because of the nature of the responsiveness at that point on the demand curve. An elasticity measure of -0.53 is thought of as relatively unresponsive; that is, a small relative price rise or fall will generate a smaller relative quantity change. If price increases by 1 percent, quantity will decrease by only about 0.5 percent, and the total amount spent on syphilis tests will increase. With an elasticity of -0.53, a price *fall* will lower total expenditures (i.e., total consumer expenditures in terms of dollars) because the relative increase in quantity purchased will not be sufficient to overcome the relatively *greater* price decrease; this is so even though the number of units bought is increasing. Thus, if the Richland County Health Department wants more revenue and does not care about how many tests are made, it should raise its price to $3.25.

Demand curves can also have *unitary elastic* and *elastic* portions. Where the elasticity formula measures -1, demand responsiveness is said to be unitary elastic. For a small change in price, total expenditures will remain constant. When the demand responsiveness is elastic (i.e., greater than 1 in absolute value), it

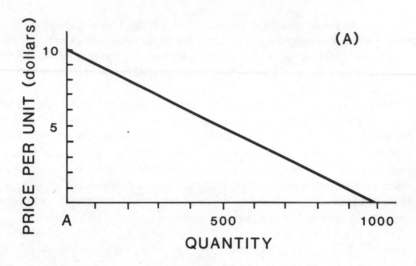

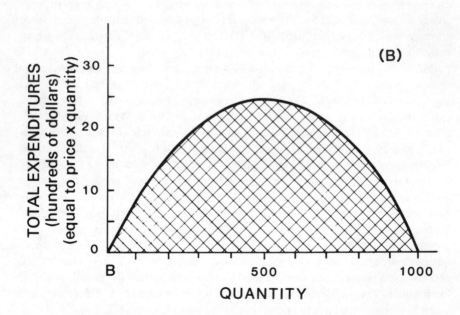

Figure 3–3 Relation among price, quantity demanded, and total revenue. (A) The basic relation between quantity demanded and price. (B) The relation between total expenditures (which equals price times quantity) and quantity. Part (B) is derived from part (A).

means that the relative change in quantity consumed exceeds the relative change in price. For a small increase in price, the decrease in quantity will be relatively greater, and total expenditures will fall. For a small decrease in price, total expenditures will rise.

These relations are shown in Figure 3–3. A straight-line demand curve for vaccinations is shown in Figure 3–3A. At a price of $10, no vaccinations are demanded, while as price falls in $1 increments, vaccination demand increases by 100. Thus, at a price of $9, 100 vaccinations will be demanded; at a price of $8, 200 will be demanded, and so on. Figure 3–3B shows the total expenditures generated at each level of sales. Thus, if 100 vaccinations are sold, $900 in expenditures is generated, and so on (see Table 3–2 for the actual values). Over a range, total expenditures increase but eventually the increase in expenditures levels off to a maximum, and beyond that point total expenditures begin to decline.

There is a connection between the elasticity along a specific segment of the demand curve and the total expenditure specific to relevant points on the curve. At relatively high prices and low quantities on a straight-line demand curve, only a relatively small change (in percent) in price is needed to induce a relatively large change in quantity demanded. The lower expenditure resulting from the fall in unit prices is therefore more than offset by the large increase in quantity demanded, and so total expenditure will decrease with a fall in price. Thus, in Table 3–2, for a reduction in price from $9 to $8, the arc elasticity of demand along that segment of the curve is -4.76; demand is said to be elastic, and for a reduction in price, total expenditures increase (in this case, from $900 to $1,600). As one moves down the demand curve, the relative price change becomes smaller in relation to the associated quantity change. Thus the absolute value of elasticity falls. But as long as this value in absolute terms is greater than 1 (i.e., we are on the elastic portion of the curve), total expenditures will increase, although not by as much as in higher-priced segments. Eventually, the elasticity takes on a value of -1; at this point, price and quantity changes just offset each other, and total expenditures will stay constant (the top of the total expenditures curve). As prices fall further, the consumer moves onto the inelastic portion of the demand curve. Price reductions offset quantity increases, and total expenditures fall. Thus, along any single straight-line demand curve, the elasticity of demand will decrease with successive reductions in price.

Further insight into the elasticity concept can be gained by examining elasticity for two *different* demand curves at a single price. Assume that two demand curves in two different markets for physician visits cross at a price of $3 as in Figure 3–4. The consumers in market 2 are more responsive to price reductions than are those in market 1. Let *AD* be the demand curve in market 1 and *BC* be the demand curve in market 2. Now let the price fall by 10 cents. Consumers in market 1 demand 10,300 visits, while those in market 2 demand 10,500. The arc elasticity in market 1 is

Table 3–2 Quantity Demanded, Price for Vaccinations, and Relation to Total Expenditures

Price	Quantity demanded	Total expenditures
$10	0	0
9	100	900
8	200	1,600
7	300	2,100
6	400	2,400
5	500	2,500
4	600	2,400
3	700	2,100
2	800	1,600
1	900	900

$$E = \frac{300/20,300}{-0.10/5.90} = -0.87$$

The arc elasticity in market 2 is

$$E = \frac{500/20,500}{-0.10/5.00} = -1.44$$

As can be seen, demand curve BC is for a more responsive group of consumers, and the elasticity for a given quantity will be greater in absolute value than that of a less responsive group.

3.6 INSURANCE, DIRECT PRICE, AND QUANTITY DEMANDED

A major factor in considering the demand for medical care is the role that insurance plays in influencing the direct price of medical care. There are a number of different types of insurance arrangements that consumers can obtain, and these will affect direct price and hence demand in different ways. We will examine the important alternatives.

In analyzing the effect of alternative insurance arrangements, we initially specify a demand curve in which the consumers have no insurance and hence pay the full price charged by the provider (say, a physician). This curve, where full price equals direct price, is labeled curve D_n in Figure 3–5. Now let us introduce the first type of insurance arrangement, a copayment.

A *copayment* is a payment of a proportion of the charged price paid by the patient; the insurance company pays the remainder of the charged price. For example, with 20 percent copayment and a charged price of $20 per visit, the

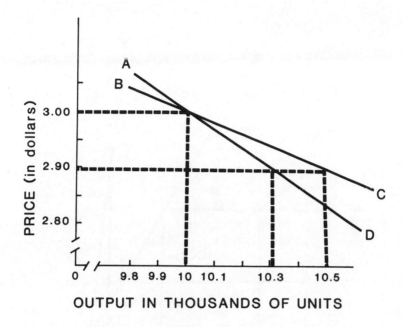

Figure 3–4 Responsiveness of quantity demanded to price for differently sloped demand curves. Curve *BC* shows a greater responsiveness of quantity demanded to price than does curve *AD*.

patient pays the provider 20 percent of the charged price, $4, and the insurance company pays the remainder. In analyzing the impact of a coinsurance contract on demand, we assume that, even though the consumer has purchased an insurance contract, demand behavior is still governed by the demand curve, D_n. What changes is that the direct price and charged price now differ from one another. At any given charged price, the consumer faces a lower direct price, and hence will move down the demand curve, D_n.

If the coinsurance rate is 50 percent, the demand curve facing the provider in Figure 3–4 is D_{50}. Here, at any charged price, the direct price is one-half the charged price, and the consumer demands a quantity determined by the direct price and the demand curve with no insurance, D_n. Thus, if the provider's charge were $8 per visit (in Figure 3–5), the consumer with a 50 percent coinsurance contract would pay a $4 out-of-pocket price, and the quantity demanded would be six visits. If the coinsurance rate were 20 percent, the market demand curve facing the providers would be D_{20}, showing a 20 cent direct price for each $1 charge. A charged price of $10 would mean a direct price of $2 and a quantity demanded of

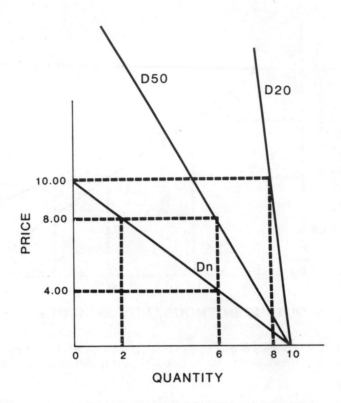

Figure 3–5 Representation of demand curves with no insurance (D_n), with 50 percent copayment (D_{50}), and with a 20 percent copayment (D_{20}). When there is a copayment, D_n also represents the relation between quantity demanded and direct patient price.

eight. As the coinsurance rate falls, the market demand curve facing the providers shifts out.

Next we examine the impact of an indemnity contract. An *indemnity* contract involves a fixed per unit amount that the insurer pays in the event of a service being used. For example, if an individual has pediatric coverage, an indemnity contract specifies that the insurer will pay x per visit (say $x = 4$) as long as x is less than the charged price. If the price is greater than x, the consumer is responsible for the balance. In Figure 3–6, D_n is again the demand curve with no insurance coverage. Now let the individual purchase an indemnity contract by which the insurer reimburses the provider up to $4 per visit. The demand curve facing the provider becomes D_{n+i} which is the D_n curve raised by $4 at all points. The position of D_{n+i} is such that, at each price charged, the direct price will be $4 less than this,

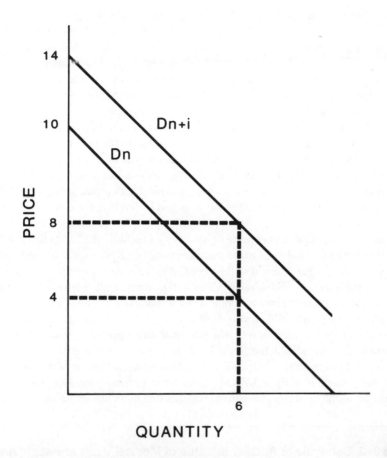

Figure 3–6 Representation of demand curves with no insurance (D_n) and with an indemnity of $4 ($D_{n+i}$). When there is an indemnity, D_n also represents the relation between quantity demanded and patient's direct price.

and the quantity demanded will reflect this lower *direct* price. In Figure 3–6 a charged price of $8 means a direct price of $4 and a quantity demanded of six. An increase in the amount by which the insurer indemnifies the consumer would shift D_{n+i} upward. The curve D_n would remain the same.

Finally, we examine the impact of a deductible. A *deductible* is a fixed amount that the insurer deducts from the total bill; the consumer must spend up to this amount before coverage begins. Until the consumer spends this amount, he or she pays the full price for each additional unit consumed (the price paid for the next additional unit is called the *marginal direct price*). The marginal direct price before the deductible is reached is the charged price. If there is no copayment in addition to the deductible, the marginal direct price, after the deductible is met, is zero.

To analyze the impact of a deductible on demand, we will slightly reinterpret the demand curve. Assume that the curve shows the value to the consumer of each additional visit (the marginal value). If the patient consumes one visit, the value of the additional visit is $9. The second visit has a smaller marginal value, in this case $8. In addition to consuming the first visit, the value to the patient of the second visit is $8. The two visits together would have a worth of $17 for the patient. These numbers and the worth for the third, fourth, and so on, visits, are shown in Table 3–3. The table assumes a declining marginal value placed on successive visits, which is consistent with what we assumed in deriving the demand hypothesis.

Let us now assume a market price of $8 and a deductible of $32. At this market price, the direct marginal price to the consumer will be $8 per visit until (and if) the deductible is met. Thereafter, it will be zero (if there is no copayment as well). In answering the question of how many visits will be demanded, we must look at the consumer's valuation of visits in Table 3–3 and compare these with the marginal direct price and the deductible level. At first, one might be tempted to say that only the first two visits are worth *at least* the marginal direct price and so only two will be demanded. One would then conclude that, having spent $16 in total, the consumer did not meet the deductible, and so demand will be at two visits.

But our patient is truly a logical ''economic person'' and will look more carefully at all the options. The patient realizes that he or she could buy the third

Table 3–3 Schedule of Additional Value of Medical Visits to Patient and of Total (Summed) Value of All Units of Care

Quantity	Value of additional unit of care to consumer	Total value of all care received up to given quantity
1	9	9
2	8	17
3	7	24
4	6	30
5	5	35
6	4	39
7	3	42
8	2	44
9	1	45
10	0	45

and fourth units and, in doing so, use up the deductible of $32. The patient would then be in a position where the rest of the visits demanded would be free! Indeed, if the patient consumed nine units, the value to him or her of *all of them* would be $45, well in excess of the outlay of $32 for the first four units. In general, we can say that, with a deductible, the amount demanded will be determined by having the consumer compare the additional value of all extra units with the additional out-of-pocket cost of all extra units. Even if the marginal value of the next (third in this case) visit is less than its marginal direct price, overall it will pay the individual to spend more in order to receive the benefits of the postdeductible units. If, however, the deductible were $100 and the charged price $8, the consumer would stop consuming at two units, because there would be no quantity of consumption above that where additional outlays exceeded the additional value to the consumer.

Frequently, deductibles and copayments are found together in the same policies. In our example, one can have a $32 deductible along with a 20 percent copayment (on units of care after the deductible has been reached). With a charged price of $8, the consumer would then pay a marginal direct price of $1.60 for each unit consumed after four. The consumer would overspend the deductible in this case, but would demand only eight visits because the ninth would cost $1.60 but would have a marginal value of only $1.

3.7 MEASURING DEMAND RESPONSIVENESS

Two different routes by which demand responsiveness can be measured are by natural experiments and controlled trials. A *natural experiment* (in the demand context) occurs when a change in insurance coverage is implemented by an insurer. We can use the results of such a policy action to determine demand responsiveness by conducting before/after comparisons of the data. Assuming all else has remained the same (e.g., that an increase in a deductible has not driven the sicker insurees to buy more complete insurance elsewhere), we can use this experiment to measure the influence of the change. Often the natural experiment will not give us sufficient information. The investigator has no control over insurer policy decisions and is therefore tied to the changes in price and coverage introduced by the insurer.

A more flexible, but also more expensive, approach is the *controlled experiment*. Using this approach, study groups are selected randomly (to avoid any self-selected characteristics, such as sicker individuals choosing more complete insurance coverage) and assigned to specific categories (such as 20 percent copayment, 40 percent copayment, etc.). Differences in utilization (which are assumed to be caused by differences in *demand*) can be measured between groups with different copayment levels, and thus a measure of demand responsiveness can be obtained.

An example of a natural experiment in the demand field occurred in 1977 when the United Mine Workers introduced a $250 deductible for inpatient services and a 40 percent copayment for physician and outpatient visits, up to a maximum family liability of $500. Prior to this, the insurees had no out-of-pocket expenses. Scheffler (1984) conducted a study of the impact of this cost sharing on hospital admissions, average length of stay in a hospital, the probability of insurees having at least one physician visit, and the number of times a patient visited a physician.

The results of this analysis showed that, in the five months prior to the hospital deductible (the comparison period), the hospital admission rate was 6.8 per 1,000 enrollees and the average length of stay per hospitalization was 5.42 days. The respective figures for the five months after the deductible were 4.8 per 1,000 for admissions and 6.45 days per hospitalization. The higher length of stay in the study period may have been because sicker cases were hospitalized, requiring longer stays. With regard to physician visits, the study's results indicated that the proportion of the population seeing a doctor at least once fell from 44 percent in the comparison period to 28 percent in the study period, while the average number of visits of those who did see a doctor at least once fell from 2.3 to 1.6.

The results of such an experiment, as with other such studies, have been convincing regarding the *immediate* utilization impact of cost-sharing policies. But do the reductions in utilization last? Are there longer-term ill effects farther down the line? One study (Scitovsky and McCall, 1977) verified that reductions in physician visits did materialize over several years, but several others have questioned whether longer-term impacts on ill health might arise (see Section 4.2).

By far the best known controlled experiment in this area is the six-site Health Insurance Experiment conducted by the Rand Corporation (Newhouse et al., 1981). In this study, 2,756 families were contracted with to participate in an experiment by which each family was assigned to one of five groups with a given copayment rate. The rates in the five groups included free care; 25, 50, and 95 percent coinsurance; and a deductible with 95 percent coinsurance (all services such as physician and hospitalization were covered under the single copayment). Those families with greater potential out-of-pocket expenses than their pre-experiment coverage were compensated accordingly. Upper limits were placed on each family's out-of-pocket expenses. The families participated for 3 to 5 years.

The results indicated dramatically the *differential* impacts of higher out-of-pocket expenses. For example, those with free care incurred average expenditures for all services of $401, while those with 25, 50, and 95 percent coinsurance incurred expenses of $346, $328, and $254, respectively. Furthermore, these differentials held up over several years. Since the entire purpose of such an experiment is to control for all other intervening factors (such as health status, income, etc.), the results have had a considerable impact in health policy circles, because such controlled results are seldom obtained.

Several questions have been raised in response to the applicability of the study's results. First, these experiments affected only a small portion of all the health care market in each of the six communities where it was studied. If copayments were raised on the entire market, or on a substantial portion of the market, would providers (doctors) react and generate additional demand, thus obviating the results? (see Section 4.11) (Stoddart and Labelle, 1985). Furthermore, the aged (and presumably the fragile) were omitted from the study. Would their response be any different?

Despite the unanswered questions, such studies have moved us closer toward developing a quantitative measure of the impact of direct price on demand. As seen previously, demand elasticity depends on the starting point on one's demand curve, which in turn is affected by one's level of insurance (see Section 3.5). A rough estimate of demand elasticity when consumers have 0 to 25 percent coinsurance is -0.2 (Newhouse, Phelps, and Marquis, 1980).

The use of such an estimate can be seen as follows. If the price for a physician visit is $100, the copayment rate is raised from 10 to 20 percent, and initially there are 120 visits; what would be the expected number of visits by raising the copayment rate? The answer (assuming an elasticity of -0.2) is obtained by solving for Q_2 (visits in period 2), where

$$E = \frac{(Q_2 - Q_1)/(Q_2 - Q_1)}{(P_2 + P_1)/(P_2 + P_1)}$$

or:

$$-2 = \frac{(Q_2 - 120)/(Q_2 + 120)}{(20 - 10)/(20 + 10)}$$

The result gives a value for Q_2 of 105 visits. In this case the total price did not change, although the copayment rate, and therefore the direct or out-of-pocket price, did. A similar analysis could be made by changing the charge or both the charged price *and* the copayment rate.

REFERENCES

Consumer Demand: Analysis and Surveys

Frech, H.E., & Ginsburg, P.B. (1975). Imposed health insurance in monopolistic markets. *Economic Inquiry, 13*, 55–69.

Ginsburg, P.B., & Manheim, L. (1973). Insurance, copayment, and health services utilization. *Journal of Economics and Business, 25*, 142–153.

Joseph, H. (1971). Empirical research on the demand for health care. *Inquiry, 8*, 61–71.

Mushkin, S.J. (1974). *Consumer incentives for health care.* New York: Neale Watson Publishers.

Phelps, C.E. (1977, October). NHI won't control costs, quality, or access. *Hospital Progress,* 79–84.

Empirical Studies

Barer, M.L., Evans, R.G., & Stoddart, G.L. (1979). *Controlling health care costs by direct charges to patients.* (Occasional paper 10) Toronto: Ontario Economic Council.

Beck, R.G. (1974). The effect of co-payments on the poor. *Journal of Human Resources, 9,* 129–142.

Davis, K., & Russell, L.B. (1972). The substitution of outpatient care for inpatient care. *Review of Economics and Statistics, 54,* 109–120.

Freiburg, L., & Scutchfield, F.D. (1976). Insurance and the demand for hospital care. *Inquiry, 13,* 54–60.

Gold, M. (1984). The demand for hospital outpatient services. *Health Services Research, 19*(3), 384–412.

Goldfarb, M.G., Hornbrook, M.C., & Higgins, C.S. (1983). Determinants of hospital use: A cross diagnostic study. *Medical Care, 21*(1), 48–66.

Hellinger, F.J. (1977). Substitutability among different types of care under medicare. *Health Services Research, 12,* 11–18.

Hershey, J.C., Luft, H.S., & Gianaris, J.M. (1975). Making sense out of utilization data. *Medical Care, 13,* 838–854.

Holtmann, A.G., & Olsen, E.O. (1978). The economics of the private demand for outpatient health care ([NIH] 78-1262). Bethesda, MD: John E. Fogarty International Center of the National Institutes of Health.

Keeler, E.B., & Rolph, J. (1983). How cost sharing reduced medical spending of participants in the health insurance experiment. *Journal of the American Medical Association, 249,* 2220–2222.

Nelson, A.A., Reeder, C.E., & Dickson, W.M. (1984). The effect of a Medicaid drug copayment program on the utilization and cost of prescription services. *Medical Care, 22,* 724–736.

Newhouse, J.P., Phelps, C.E., & Marquis, M.S. (1980). On having your cake and eating it too. *Journal of Econometrics, 13,* 365–390.

————, Manning, W.G., Morris, C.N., et al. (1981). Some interim results from a controlled trial of cost sharing in health insurance. *New England Journal of Medicine, 305,* 1501–1507.

Reeder, C.E., & Nelson, A.A. (1985). The differential impact of a copayment on drug use in a Medicaid population. *Inquiry, 22,* 396–403.

Scheffler, R.M. (1984). The United Mine Worker's Health Plan. *Medical Care, 22,* 247–254.

Scitovsky, A.A., & McCall, N. (1977, May). Coinsurance and the demand for physician services. *Social Security Bulletin, 40*(5):19–27.

Stoddart, G.L., & Labelle, R.J. (1985, October). *Privatization in the Canadian health care system.* Ottawa: Health and Welfare Canada.

Warner, J., and Hu, T-W (1977). Hospitalization insurance and the demand for inpatient care. In B.C. Martin (Ed.), *Socioeconomic issues of health* (pp. 27–43). Chicago: American Medical Association.

Chapter 4

Demand for Medical Care: Additional Topics

4.1 INTRODUCTION

In Chapter 3, the demand for medical care was introduced as if it were an ordinary everyday commodity. Some types of medical care *are* ordinary everyday commodities. Pediatric visits, the consumption of aspirin, and visits to a dentist are routine occurrences for many people. However, the conditions underlying many types of medical care demand are quite unlike the conditions surrounding the use of everyday commodities. In these instances the traditional model must be modified to incorporate these special circumstances. This chapter brings these additional factors into consideration by showing how they influence the demand relation as developed in Chapter 3.

Section 4.2 examines one alleged characteristic of medical care, that medical care is indispensable for life and health. Section 4.3 analyzes the implications for medical care demand when individuals other than the direct consumers are concerned with the consumption of medical care of these direct consumers. In this context we examine the relations among private, external, and social demand. Section 4.4 examines another characteristic, the uncertainty of the occurrence of illness. A model is developed that examines the circumstances under which the presence of this characteristic leads individuals to demand insurance. Section 4.5 extends the results of Section 4.4 to examine the market demand for health care insurance. Section 4.6 examines an issue that arises once the individual has purchased insurance; with the insurance policy in effect, the direct price for insured health care services falls and the quantity demanded increases. This phenomenon of an increase in the postinsurance quantity demanded is known in insurance circles as *moral hazard*. Section 4.7 compares the demand for traditional insurance with that when the consumer simultaneously contracts for insurance and medical care (i.e., in the case of prepaid care). Section 4.8 discusses the influence on the demand relation of the patient's beliefs concerning the efficacy or quality of medical care in producing health, assuming that this efficacy is known by the patient.

Section 4.9 is concerned with situations when the money paid for medical care is not an adequate reflection of the total resource commitment made by the patient in acquiring medical care. In particular, patients devote a great deal of traveling and waiting time to obtaining medical care. This section incorporates a more general picture of the cost of medical care that also includes time cost. Section 4.10 analyzes the demand for health rather than the demand for medical care. In this analysis, medical care and other resources are viewed as inputs in producing a more fundamental commodity, that is, health. Finally, Section 4.11 discusses the possibility of the doctor's influencing patient demand under conditions of consumer ignorance.

4.2 IMPLICATIONS OF HEALTH CARE FOR LIFE AND HEALTH

One of the most widely espoused characteristics of the commodity medical care is its implications for life and health. Stated bluntly, if one does not obtain medical care when ill, one may die or become permanently ill. In cases where this condition does hold, for example, after a heart attack or a serious traffic accident, the question of substitutes will have little importance. The demand curve in these instances will be vertical, and presumably the patient would pay out all of his or her wealth to receive the lifesaving medical care.

However, such instances amount to a very small portion of the total number of situations that cause individuals to seek medical care. For the vast majority of cases, individuals do have time to react; and in most of these instances, alternative courses of action are available, although in a few cases they may be somewhat unpalatable. In terms of the range of available substitutes, medical care should be viewed as a spectrum of services and products, rather than as a commodity with only emergency characteristics. The less the situation is an emergency and the greater the relevance of substitutes, the less steeply sloping will be the demand curve for medical care. Thus, for example, dental checkups can be given annually, monthly, or weekly. Few would consider the latter two to have emergency characteristics.

Even though most forms of medical care utilization may not have emergency dimensions, in many instances a reduction in medical care consumption may influence subsequent health status. In these instances it may be desirable to analyze medical care demand from the longer perspective of a multiperiod analysis. The imposition of a copayment on drugs or physician visits will generally lead to a reduction in quantity demanded in period 1. There is nothing in the theory of demand that says *which* units of medical care will be less demanded. Some may have been unnecessary to begin with, but some may have been highly desirable (from the point of view of their effects on health status). In those instances when medical care is desirable, a reduction in its consumption in period 1 may lead to subsequent reductions in health status (say in periods 2, 3, or 4; there seems to be no general rule as to when) and possible increases in medical care demand in those subsequent time periods.

This phenomenon was first examined with regard to the imposition of a $1 copayment for each of the first two doctor's visits and $0.50 for each of the first two prescriptions in the California Medicaid program. An original study (Roemer et al., 1975) stated that reductions in doctors' office visits and diagnostic tests after the copayment's introduction were accompanied by increases in hospitalization rates in subsequent periods. Although the data methods of the study were questioned, with no conclusive results (Chen, 1976; Dyckman, 1976; Hopkins, Gartside, and Roemer, 1976), the study raised the issue of the importance of examining demand-reducing measures in a more general context. A subsequent study based on the national Rand Health Insurance Experiment (Brook et al., 1983) examined the effects of reductions in use due to copayments on subsequent consumer health status and found that, in general, there were no adverse effects, but for certain groups there were. In particular, for poor individuals with hypertensive conditions, free care was associated with better blood pressure control and reductions in the risk of early death. Neither group of studies focused on populations who might be particularly susceptible to disease (the poor, elderly, or chronically ill), and so there is the likelihood that for selected groups reductions in demand can have considerable implications for subsequent health status and medical care demand (Relman, 1983; Fein, 1981; Stoddart and Labelle, 1985).

4.3 EXTERNAL AND SOCIAL DEMAND FOR MEDICAL CARE

In the analysis in Chapter 3, it was assumed that each individual's demand for medical care was the same as the demand for medical care by all members of society. The relevance of this assumption to certain social goods such as medical care, education, and some recreational services has been questioned. For these commodities, it has been asserted that individuals would be willing to pay something to enable others to consume them. This is not true for all commodities. Many individuals would be willing to pay something to help ensure that a heart attack victim could reach a hospital on time; they would not be so generous if the victim's car had broken down and he "needed" $400 for repairs. Furthermore, this is probably true for only certain types of medical care: medical care with health implications for the recipient (e.g., inoculations or care for the aged) elicit concern; cosmetic surgery is not likely to elicit a great deal of concern.

To formalize the analysis of this phenomenon, let us assume we are concerned only with individual A's consumption. The commodity whose demand we are analyzing will now be defined as individual A's consumption of medical care. This may also be called *own consumption*. Individual A's demand for his or her own consumption may be called private or internal demand.

Assume that the rest of society, other than A, can be characterized as individual B. According to our assertion, B may also have a demand for A's own consumption of medical care. Such a demand can be characterized in the same way as A's own demand: that is, the lower the price, the more of A's consumption of medical care will B demand. This demand is in addition to A's own demand and can be called an external demand, because it comes from a source external to the consumer of the commodity.

If we define society as the sum total of A and B, then society's demand for A's consumption of medical care will depend on the private demand of A and the external demand of B. This demand can be called *community* or *social demand*. The effect of the external demand is to increase the quantity demanded of A's consumption at any given price, assuming that this external demand is greater than zero at that price. (It may well be, as in the case of the external demand for auto repair, that this external demand is zero at a particular price or at any price.) The old phrase that "society wants everyone to have a decent level of medical care" can be rephrased in terms of this analysis. Society is the sum of all individuals, and the social demand for an individual's consumption of a given commodity is the sum of all the private and external demands. Saying that "society wants everyone to have a decent level of medical care" can be interpreted as saying that, at the given price, the social demand is such that a decent standard is demanded.

There are a sufficiently large number of manifestations of external demands for medical care to impress on us how real this phenomenon is. Philanthropic giving to organizations such as the American Heart Association, the United Way, the American Cancer Society, and the National Research Foundation is evidence that people do give to enable consumption by others of the services of these organizations, which include health education and research. The majority of hospitals in the United States began as nonprofit organizations with large charitable components. In recent years these charitable components have decreased because of the growth of government health programs such as Medicare and Medicaid. Such programs themselves may be an expression of external demands expressed through the "political marketplace." Before the introduction of Medicare and Medicaid, physicians contended that a great deal of their medical services were given under charitable circumstances, with doctors making the resource commitments to this end. The risk of communicable diseases will also create free care to be offered (or required) in the form of immunizations.

4.4 UNCERTAINTY AS TO THE OCCURRENCE OF ILLNESS: INDIVIDUAL DEMAND FOR INSURANCE

In Chapter 3 the analysis of demand was developed under the condition that the consumer would maintain a given state of health that would exist with certainty during the relevant time period. This underlying condition is not a good representation for many medical problems. There are types of illnesses and medical conditions for which consumers cannot be certain of the particular period during which the problem will occur (if it occurs). However, they do know that they might be sick during a particular period and that, if so, they will have to visit a doctor and possibly be hospitalized.

These types of situations can be characterized by viewing consumers as facing choices of whether or not to prepare for these contingencies. A simple analysis predicting consumer behavior under these circumstances involves specifying consumer tastes, wealth, the probability of illness, the cost of medical care, and a hypothesis as to how the individual will behave when faced with this uncertainty. Based on these assumptions or conditions, which make explicit some of the key variables associated with the uncertainty aspect of medical care demand, we can derive specific conclusions concerning consumer behavior.

To characterize consumer tastes with regard to the alternatives that an illness may bring, let us assume that when an illness occurs it leads to medical care expenses that we will regard as a loss in wealth to the individual. To specify what this loss means to the individual, we must introduce a term to characterize the individual's well-being under alternative levels of wealth. This term is *utility*. Utility is presented in index form. Let us present our taste assumption for wealth in the form of an index of utility in Table 4–1. This index shows what level of well-being is associated with each specific level of wealth. Thus a level of wealth of

Table 4–1 Relation between Wealth and Utility

Wealth ($)	Total Utility	Marginal Utility[a]
850	76.0	3.2
860	79.0	3.0
870	81.8	2.8
880	84.4	2.6
890	86.8	2.4
900	89.0	2.2
910	91.0	2.0
920	92.8	1.8
930	94.4	1.6
940	95.8	1.4
950	97.0	1.2
960	98.0	1.0
970	98.8	0.8
980	99.4	0.6
990	99.8	0.4
1,000	100.0	0.1

[a] Marginal utility is the change in utility from moving between income levels. For example, 3.0 measures the change from moving from $850 to $860.

$1,000 is associated with a level of well-being of 100, a level of wealth of $990 leads to a level of well-being of 99.8, and so on. The exact level of numbers in our utility index is totally arbitrary. That is, we could have picked 389.4 to be our utility level at $1,000. What is important is the assumption of the change in utility that is associated with a given change in wealth. Our assumption is that the taste function can be characterized by diminishing marginal utility. That is, as one moves to higher levels of wealth, an additional $10 of wealth beyond that will mean successively less additional well-being. Thus, beginning at a base of $850, an extra $10 will yield three extra units of utility, and so on. The actual numbers we use for utility levels do not matter; we can take any number to represent utility at $1,000 and any lower number to represent it at $850. To be consistent with our assumption, the increments in utility must be successively smaller for equal additional increments of wealth.

Diminishing marginal utility of wealth is referred to as *risk-averse* behavior. An individual is referred to as risk averse when, beginning from a given wealth level, a loss of a given amount is of greater subjective importance to the person than would be a gain of an equal amount. Holding on to what the person has becomes more important (is given more weight) than increasing wealth. Utility is the subjective index of the relative importance of wealth.

We are not saying that additional wealth means more to one rich person than it does to another poor one. This comparison, called an *interpersonal comparison,* involves our specifying different people's utilities on the same scale. Such a comparison involves specifying values as to how much different people are to count. This topic is discussed in Part III, which deals with Evaluative Economics.

Our second assumption is that our individual initially has a level of wealth of $1,000. We use a wealth rather than income variable because people derive satisfaction from all their assets, and health care expenses can potentially affect the level of peoples' assets, not just their annual income. Our third assumption is that, if the individual is sick, he or she will face medical expenses of $100. This financial loss can be broken down into two components: (1) a unit cost component and (2) a component representing the number of units consumed. We will assume that the unit cost is $10 per visit and that the individual requires ten visits.

A fourth assumption relates to the uncertainty element. Assume that we can assign probabilities to the various possible health states the individual may experience. Let us say there is a 1/10 chance the individual will be ill and will demand ten units, and a 9/10 chance the individual will be well and will not "lose" $100 to become better. These are the only two possibilities, so the sum of the probabilities equals 1. (See Section 4.5 for the meaning of probabilities.)

The fifth assumption is that the individual wants to maximize his or her utility level. Thus the individual will choose that course of action for which he or she can expect to receive the highest level of utility.

The model's conclusions are obtained by determining how, under these conditions, the individual will behave so as to maximize utility. The model predicts that if health insurance is available on the right terms, the individual will buy it to reduce the variability of his or her income. To see how this conclusion is derived, let us examine how much wealth and utility the individual would expect to have with and without insurance. Without insurance, our individual is 90 percent certain of having $1,000 in wealth and 10 percent certain of having only $900 because of the payout for medical care. The expected value of wealth will be 90 percent of $1,000 plus 10 percent of 900, or $990. This is the sum of the amounts the individual expects to receive under various conditions, adjusted for the probabilities that those conditions will arise. If $1,000 is the wealth level, the utility will be 100 units. If $900 is available, the utility will be 89 units. But our individual is only 90 percent sure of having 100 units of utility and 10 percent of obtaining 89 units. The expected value of the utility achieved will be 90 percent of 100 and 10 percent of 89, or 98.9. This is approximately the same utility that a 100 percent certain wealth of $970 would yield.

If our individual had wealth of $970, it would yield about the same utility as the present situation when no insurance is purchased. Let us say for $20 he or she could buy insurance coverage against the $100 loss. This would yield a certain wealth of $980. This is because the individual's wealth would be reduced by the amount of the premium, $20, and if he or she became ill, the insurer would bear the risk. A certain wealth of $980 would yield the individual a 100 percent probability of receiving 99.4 units of utility, which is a higher expected utility than that accompanying the uncertain situation. Being a utility maximizer, the individual would buy the insurance on these terms. Indeed, he or she would pay up to $30 in premiums to avoid such a risky situation.

Why is the risky situation so unpleasant that the individual would be willing to pay so much to avoid it? The reason is the diminishing marginal utility of wealth. Even though the individual faces only a 10 percent chance of losing $100, the losses in terms of utility become significant at lower levels of wealth. The "pain" of losing $10 when wealth is $910 is greater than the "pain" of the loss when wealth is $1,000. Thus, our individual is willing to pay a premium rather than face the risk of suffering such large losses.

Let us now assume that if he or she were sick, the individual would demand 10 units of care at any price, and that the price of medical care is now $15 instead of $10 per unit. The individual now faces an expected loss of $150 if he or she becomes sick. That is, wealth in this case would be $850. The individual would face an expected wealth of $985 (10 percent of $850 and 90 percent of $1,000) from all situations and an expected utility of 97.6 units (10 percent of 76 and 90 percent of 100). If the individual had a certain wealth of $960, he or she would obtain a certain utility of 98 units. The individual would pay something over $40 for insurance in this case. The conclusion is that, as the expected loss increases because of the rising price of medical care, the amount of money the individual is willing to pay to avert these expected losses increases as well, and the individual will be willing to buy additional insurance coverage, if terms are right.

The size of the financial loss in relation to the individual's wealth and the associated utilities is called the *financial vulnerability* factor. A second factor, relating to the probability of illness, is referred to as the *risk-perception* factor (Berki and Ashcraft, 1980). In the preceding example, if the probability of becoming sick increased from 10 to 20 percent, the expected utility in the no-insurance situation would fall to 97.8 (80 percent of 100 + 20 percent of 89). This is associated with a wealth level of close to $960, indicating that the individual would be willing to pay a premium of up to about $40 to avoid the risk of the $100 loss.

4.5 MARKET DEMAND FOR INSURANCE

For insurance to be available, it must be possible for our individual to pool risks with other people. That is, some organization must exist that will accept the risks and pay the benefits when they arise. To determine under which market conditions this will occur, let us assume an insurance company is being formed to cover the risks of 1,000 people with tastes, incomes, and health experience exactly like those of our representative individual in Section 4.4. We can now give a more definite meaning to the "probabilities" assigned there to the alternative health states. Assume that, with a large sample of 1,000 people, the insurance company can be almost certain that 100 will become ill and require medical care during the month. Because pooling a large number of risks yields a considerable degree of certainty, it becomes possible to assign a risk to each individual and evaluate his or her expected loss experience in terms of the group.

At a price of $10 for medical care, the insurance company knows that, with a group of 1,000 insurees, 100 will most likely become ill and will require 10 visits each. The expected medical expenses will be $10,000 for the group. The actuarially fair rate, the expected loss per individual insured, is $10. If each insuree pays a premium of $10, the expected losses of the group will just be covered. According to the analysis in Section 4.4, our individual, and every other insuree, would be willing to pay a premium of at least the actuarially fair rate to reduce the risk of large losses. Indeed, they would be willing to pay somewhat more, as seen in Section 4.4.

The insurance company cannot charge only the fair rate for the premium rate because resources are necessary to administer an insurance business and profits are wanted. The insurance company must charge more than the actuarially fair rate to cover its administrative costs and profits. As long as these add up to less than the amount that the individual insuree is willing to pay for insurance, the individual will be willing to pay the premium and buy health insurance. In this case, if the total premium is $30 or less when medical care costs $10 per unit, the individual will purchase the insurance to have risks of loss covered.

Several issues arise when individuals differ by risk perception or financial vulnerability factors. The first of these is cross subsidization. Let us assume that there are two groups, I and II, of 5,000 people with the same utility–wealth relation as in Table 4 1, each with a probability of 10 percent of being ill, and each facing prices per visit of $10. Only now group I members will use five units of medical care and group II, who are sicker, will use ten. The expected utility for group I is 99.7 (90 percent of 100 + 10 percent of 97) and that of group II is 98.9 (90 percent of 100 and 10 percent of 89). Group I members will pay up to $10 for insurance coverage, while group II will pay up to $30.

Let us say that the insurance policies are *community rated;* that is, everyone pays the same premium. A $10 premium rate would induce all members to join and would yield the insurer premiums of $100,000, well in excess of the expected payout of $75,000 for both groups. But group I is more than covering its full costs (including administrative costs), while group II is just covering its expected medical cost payout and is not covering its full costs. Group I is subsidizing group II.

Under such conditions there would be room for a competing insurance company to offer the entire group a "low-option" policy, covering just five visits, for a premium of $6 (allowing for a 20 percent loading factor). If all else were the same, all of group I would benefit by switching to the low-option policy. This would leave the initial company offering the high-option policy with only group II (high cost) members; to cover its costs, the company would have to increase the premium rate of its "high-option" policies.

The problem of *adverse selection* arises from a simple extension of this example. Adverse selection refers to higher-risk groups choosing policies with higher coverage. If one envisages a series of groups who vary by the probability of being ill and/or the amount of utilization when they are ill, a range of policies can be offered, varying from very low to very high coverage. The groups with higher expected usage (e.g., the unhealthy, the aged) will have higher expected losses and higher demands for insurance coverage. They will therefore select coverage that is more extensive (e.g., smaller deductibles, higher limits). Of course, in the absence of subsidies, higher coverage policies cost more, and this places a limit on the degree to which high-risk individuals can insure (Anderson and Knickman, 1984).

Parenthetically, we might add that when we observe one group using more medical services than a second group that has less, the difference in insurance coverage may explain only part of the difference in usage. The heavier using group may have been a high-risk group to begin with, and would have used more services even if coverage had been the same.

4.6 INSURANCE AND MORAL HAZARD

Once our individual has purchased health insurance, the direct price he or she pays for medical care falls. If the individual has purchased full insurance, this price is zero. Medical care still costs $10 per unit, but in paying the premium the individual ensures that the insurer will pay this cost. When the individual is ill, he or she faces a zero price for medical care. At a price of $10, the individual would visit the doctor 10 times. Assume that the demand relation is such that at a price of $5 the individual will consume 11 units and at a price of zero, 12 units.

This phenomenon of increased quantity demanded under insurance is known as moral hazard in the insurance industry. The connotation of the term is that individuals ''shirk'' their responsibilities and consume recklessly when they are insured. Interpreted from the point of view of economics, they are simply behaving in accordance with the principle of the downward sloping demand curve.

Increased consumption because of insurance must have effects on the insurance company, which has contracted to finance the insurees' medical care. Indeed, since the expected number of units of medical care of the insured population is greater with insurance, and since the insurance company must pay for this number of services, it must charge for them in the premium rate. With the moral hazard element taken into account, the insurance company will pay out $12,000 to service providers, since each of the 1,000 insured will consume 12 units of service if they are ill, and we can expect 100 will be ill. We assume, of course, that the number of people seeking medical attention will not increase after insurance, although this remains a possibility.

The premium rate per insured member will now be $12 plus the fee for administrative expenses and profit. If this fee is still less than what the consumers are willing to pay, the consumers will buy insurance. The effect on the medical care market in this case will be to increase the quantity of medical care demanded. However, there is also the possibility that individuals will not insure, but will retain the risk themselves. In this case they will face the full price of medical care should they become ill.

4.7 CHOICE OF HEALTH PLAN

Many employers provide their employees with a selection of health plans and allow the employees to make their own decisions about the types of coverage and service they will obtain. These choices have economic dimensions and may be analyzed with economic tools.

Each plan has associated with it a series of characteristics, such as range of choice of provider. As well, each plan has an *expected* financial expense associated with it: this expense includes any out-of-pocket premiums paid by the employee, and any other out-of-pocket expenses incurred for deductibles, copayments, and the like. The employee will make a decision as to which plan to choose by weighing the expected financial costs and evaluating the characteristics of each. He or she will choose the package that offers the greatest net benefit (the value of benefits minus costs).

Let us create a simple example by assuming that an employer offers its employees a choice of two plans, a full-coverage (no copayments) HMO and a traditional plan with a 20 percent copayment. We further assume that all characteristics for the two plans (convenience of each, choice of provider, etc.) are valued equally by the employees, so only financial considerations will weigh in their decisions as to which plan to choose. For the HMO, assume that the total annual premium for each employee's family is $300, that the company pays half of this, and that therefore the total out-of-pocket expense for the HMO is $150. As for the traditional plan, assume that the total premium is $200, that the employer pays half of this (so that the out-of-pocket premium is $100), and that for each unit of medical care consumed there is a charge of $50 (and therefore an out-of-pocket copayment of $10).

The features of this model are drawn in Figure 4–1. Out-of-pocket costs do not increase with demand for HMO members, but they do for traditional plan members. Let us assume that employees differ in the amount of health care they expect to demand. Those who are sicker or who have larger and younger families will expect to demand more episodes of care. Those who expect to demand exactly five episodes will have the same level of expenditures under either plan: they will be indifferent as to which plan to choose. Those who expect to have under five episodes demanded will choose the cheaper (to them) traditional plan; those who expect relatively heavy use (over five visits) can expect lower out-of-pocket costs with the HMO, and so on purely financial grounds they will select that option. Thus, there will be a bias in the selection process in favor of heavy users selecting the HMO option; the HMO enrollment, that is, will contain a larger proportion of heavy users.

The assumption that the characteristics of the two plans are identical is not realistic. Plans can vary in a number of ways, including their access (incorporating factors such as locational convenience and waiting time), the comprehensiveness of care offered by the same provider, the continuity of care (whether the patient can establish a relationship with a given physician), and the quality of care (Berki and Ashcraft, 1980). Each of these characteristics will be valued to some degree by the consumer. If a consumer places a greater overall value on the characteristics of the traditional plan rather than the HMO, some or all of the financial advantage that the HMO may have over the traditional plan will be eroded. For example, a consumer expecting seven visits, and all else being equal, would choose the HMO in our example. But if the traditional plan allowed the individual to retain his or her physician (to which he or she attaches a high value), this may outweigh any cost advantage that the HMO has. Our analysis predicts, then, that consumers who are likely to place high values on certain characteristics of any particular plan will be more likely to make a choice that is financially less advantageous.

In particular, when choosing an HMO, two choices are being made simultaneously: (1) the individual is choosing a certain level of insurance coverage, and

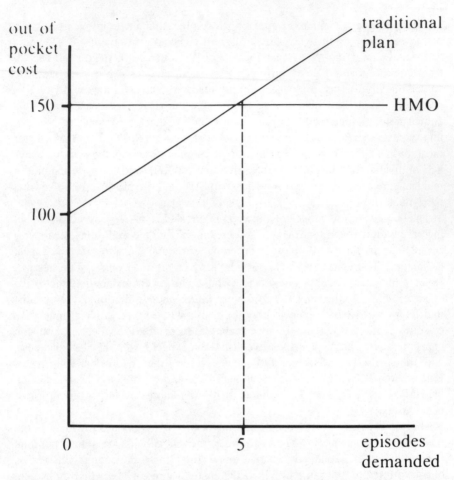

Figure 4–1 Out-of-pocket costs for two types of health plans. The traditional plan has an initial premium of $100 and subsequent copayments. Under the HMO (prepayment) plan, the consumer pays a fixed fee of $150 and no additional payment for use. In this example, for low usage levels the traditional plan costs the consumer less; for heavy users (above five visits in this example) the HMO costs less.

(2) the individual is choosing a specific set of providers (this choice is left open to the individual until the time of consumption under traditional insurance coverage). The HMO choice is therefore more complex and, accordingly, more complex to model.

4.8 INFLUENCE OF QUALITY ON THE DEMAND FOR MEDICAL CARE

In Chapter 3 the demand for medical care was analyzed under the condition that each unit of the commodity was like any other unit. Of course, this is not always the case. One of the more problematic tasks in analyzing resource allocation in medical care is coming to terms with quality differences.

Quality is not a single attribute but rather a series of attributes, any of which can make the product appear better or worse to the consumer. We will assume, in this section, that the consumer is fully aware of how each of these attributes that make up the quality level of a product will affect him or her. Furthermore, we will regard quality in a subjective sense, that is, in terms of how the consumer values these attributes of the commodity.

Two attributes of the commodity medical care will be used in identifying quality: (1) the comfort and luxury of the particular commodity or service, and (2) the level of medical excellence associated with the commodity. The former attribute can be associated with the doctor's bedside manner, the amenities in a hospital room, whether soft music is piped into the dentist's office, and so on. The medical excellence attribute can be associated with the level of accuracy of a diagnosis, the effectiveness of a treatment in restoring health, the effectiveness of a prescribed course of action in preventing illness, and so on. Assuming that these can be accurately assessed, a consumer can make a personal evaluation concerning the overall quality level associated with alternative units of medical care that incorporate different levels of these attributes. Thus the consumer can rank alternative units of medical care according to their level of quality.

If this is the case, we can hypothesize how the consumer would behave when faced with alternative qualities of medical care. Our hypothesis is that a higher quality level of medical care will increase the importance of medical care in relation to other commodities at all levels of medical care consumption. This will result in the shifting outward of the demand curve for medical care. We conclude that the higher the quality of medical care is, the greater the demand for the commodity.

Our qualification must be mentioned to this hypothesis. If the quality of care is low, the demand may be less. But if low-quality care results in subsequent illness (e.g., if rheumatic fever develops from a failure to check for strep throat, or if a patient with chickenpox contracts Reye's syndrome because he or she was pre-scribed aspirin), it may subsequently result in a greater demand for care.

4.9 TIME AND MONEY COSTS

Until now we have measured the resource commitment necessary to obtain a unit of commodity by the direct per unit money price of that commodity. Thus, if a unit of medical care costs $5, then $5 was treated as an accurate measurement of what one had to give up (the opportunity cost) to obtain a unit of medical care. Yet the resource devoted to consuming a commodity is more than the money price of the commodity; when obtaining medical care, one has to travel to and from the doctor's office and wait to see the doctor and to be examined. These efforts are personal resources and are part of an individual's total resource commitment to obtaining medical care.

The value of the effort involved in traveling and waiting is referred to as the *time cost* of obtaining medical care. The associated resource commitment can be measured by the amount that could have been earned if one had not visited the doctor, presuming that one does forego income in undertaking this activity. If one does not forego income, valuable time is still given up. In this case the opportunity cost of time would be measured by the value the individual would have placed on the activity that has been given up. This latter magnitude is much more difficult to measure, so for our purposes we will assume that all time spent in obtaining health care can be measured by the individual's wage rate.

An expression for the total cost or total resource commitment made by the person for each unit of health care can be expressed as $(w \times t) + p$, where t is the amount of time involved in obtaining a unit health care, w is the wage that would have been earned had one worked during this time, and p is the money price of the commodity.

The importance of this expression lies in its displacement of money price in a demand analysis. By regarding the commodity as medical care activity and the price of this activity as the total cost of medical care, we can develop a more general hypothesis about the consumption of medical care as a more useful explanatory device. Our new hypothesis becomes: as *total* per unit cost expressed as $(w \times t) + p$ falls, more medical care is demanded. To use an example, the time required for a visit to the doctor is 1 hour and the wage foregone is $4 per hour. The money price of a visit is $8. The total per unit cost, then, is $12. If the money price is set at zero by a government program, the total cost will fall to $4 per visit. Medical care may still be too costly for some people, even at a zero price. If the government wishes to encourage consumption beyond this point, it might have to undertake a policy that would lower waiting or travel time. One example would be to relocate a clinic in a central area.

Framing the analysis of demand in terms of total cost has offered new insights into distributional considerations regarding medical care. Even though money costs may be the same for all consumers, total costs may vary because of variations in w and t. For example, w may vary among consumers because some persons may have their wages docked if they take time off from work, while others may not. And t may change because of variations in distances from the provider of medical care. Our generalized demand hypothesis states that, with other things the same, the quantity demanded will vary inversely with the total per unit cost. When medical care is offered for "free," that is, at a zero money price, variations in quantity demanded will be determined by variations in time costs; those with the lowest time cost will demand the greatest quantities. Perhaps those with the lowest time costs and hence greatest quantities demanded are not the same as those with the most acute medical conditions. In this case, medical care would be rationed to those who are willing to wait and not to the most ill. This problem arises when a program lowers the direct money price to zero while failing to increase supply sufficiently to meet the increased quantity demanded. An excess demand results and queues may form. This raises the time cost, which becomes the mechanism by which medical care is rationed. The analysis of such a mechanism is actually one of a market mechanism incorporated by both supply and demand elements (discussed in Chapter 6).

4.10 THE DEMAND FOR HEALTH

Chapter 1 showed that the output of the health care sector can be regarded either as health care or as health. Recently, an alternative formulation of consumer behavior in this area has been presented in terms of the demand for health (Grossman, 1972). Health care can be regarded as an end in itself, something people want for its own characteristics, or as a means to an end. An example of an end that could be furthered by better health would be the consumption of other commodities; better health would enable one to earn more income to purchase these additional commodities.

In this analysis we assume health to be an end in itself that can be created or produced by the activities individuals undertake. These activities can include receiving medical care, engaging in self-care (exercise and proper diet), and so on. Such activities are substitutes for one another, each of which can further the desired end. The cost of each alternative activity can be expressed in terms of an individual's resource commitment required to produce one healthy day by that activity. Since each activity will normally require time and purchased inputs on the part of the consumer, the cost of one healthy day can be expressed as follows:

$$c = (a \times w) + (b \times p)$$

In this equation, c is the unit cost (cost per one healthy day produced) of the activity; a is the amount of time required to produce one healthy day by engaging in the activity; b is the amount of purchased inputs required in conjunction with a to produce one healthy day; w is the opportunity cost of the individual's time, and thus a measurement of the size of the resource commitment of one unit of time; and p is the price of one unit of purchased input.

C, the cost of one healthy day, will depend on these four factors. For each health-producing activity, there will be a different c. If one activity, say self-care, is very productive such that a and b are small, then the cost of producing an extra healthy day with this activity will be low. On the other hand, if self-care is not very effective in producing health, then a may be very high and c in turn will be high. Recall that, although the unit price of purchased inputs, p, may be high, the number of units required to produce a healthy day, b, may be low. In these instances, *purchased input-intensive* activities such as medical care may not necessarily be costly.

One prediction of this model is that, if the c of one type of health care rises relative to the c for another type, individuals will substitute in favor of the lower-cost alternative. For example, if waiting time in a doctor's office (a) becomes lengthy, the cost of medical care, if all other elements in the model remain constant, will rise. Self-care becomes less expensive under these circumstances, and individuals will obtain or produce more of it.

It is unlikely that a and b will remain constant over all levels of an activity. What is likely is that as more of an activity, say physician care or self-care, is undertaken a and b will decline. It will take successively larger doses of personal effort and purchased inputs to yield a unit of health. As one engages in more of any activity, the cost of an extra unit of health increases. For this reason, several health-creating activities will be demanded by an individual. An individual will demand some medical care and some self-care. However, if some outside factor changes, such as an increase in the amount of waiting time necessary to obtain medical care, this will still cause a shift to more self-care and less medical care demanded.

Viewing the demand for health-related resources in this way allows us to incorporate the full resource commitment of alternative ways to produce health. In such a framework, medical care becomes one of several alternatives, and a broader picture of the health-related resource picture can be obtained. However, while the health framework is broader in its approach, it is also more complex than merely focusing on one of the inputs, for example, medical care. And, for many purposes, such a broad and more complex picture is not required.

4.11 CONSUMER IGNORANCE REGARDING THE EFFECT OF MEDICAL CARE ON HEALTH

Section 4.8 serves as an introduction to the difficult topic of the consumer's ignorance about the effect of medical care on health. In many cases the consumer does not know this effect. In this context, the physician has been regarded as having two roles with respect to his or her patients: (1) the physician acts in an advisory capacity as an agent, informing the patient of his or her level of health and what alternative courses of treatment might change this level, and (2) the physician undertakes much of this treatment.

As we saw in Chapter 3, the patient's perceived level of health and the probable effect of medical care in altering this health level can have some influence on the patient's demand for medical care. Since the physician potentially has influence over how the patient views his or her health, as well as the patient's beliefs regarding the efficacy of medical care in altering this level, the physician conceivably can "induce" changes in the consumer's demand for medical care by providing demand-inducing information. For example, informing a patient that he or she has a dangerous but curable neoplasm can have a considerable influence on the demand for medical care.

Let H stand for the level of a patient's health (measured, for example, by the number of healthy days) and let M represent units of medical care. To analyze the physician's role as an agent, we make the following assumptions:

1. We assume that health creates utility (called U) in such a way that as one moves to higher health levels the additional satisfaction or utility from one additional unit of health, termed the marginal utility of health (or $\Delta U/\Delta H$), is declining. (Of course, the total utility is increasing with additional health. See Section 4.3 for a similar analysis in terms of wealth, rather than health.)
2. Other things being equal (life-style, environment, etc.), the additional health produced with an additional unit of medical care, termed the *marginal productivity of health* (or $\Delta H/\Delta M$), is declining with increases in medical care. More medical care, of course, produces more health, but at a diminishing marginal rate.
3. There is an initial level of health for the patient (although he or she may not know what it is).
4. Each unit of medical care is purchased at a cost to the patient, C_m.
5. There is also another commodity, X (say food), for which the patient also has a declining marginal utility ($\Delta U/\Delta X$) and a per unit cost of C_x.

Now the additional unit of medical care has an additional *utility* that is expressed as the product of the additional health produced by the unit of medical care ($\Delta H/\Delta M$) and the marginal utility of *health* ($\Delta U/\Delta H$), that is ($\Delta U/\Delta H$) $\times$ ($\Delta H/\Delta M$). Thus, if one extra doctor's visit produced 3 additional healthy days, and the additional utility for each healthy day is 5 units of utility, then an additional visit will have a marginal utility of 15.

The consumer's equilibrium for both commodities will be at that point where the marginal utility per penny spent on each commodity is the same. That is, the consumer cannot get more utility from switching from buying one more unit of M (thus lowering its marginal utility) and one less unit of X (raising its marginal utility). Of course, at the same time the consumer, if he or she gets utility from M and X, and nothing else, will also use up his or her budget. The expression for this equilibrium condition is

$$\frac{(\Delta U/\Delta H) \times (\Delta H/\Delta M)}{C_m} = \frac{\Delta U/\Delta X}{C_x}$$

If we rearrange the terms, we would have conditions similar to those in the relative terms model of Section 3.3; that is, the consumer would consume up to the point where the relative importance to him or her of the two commodities (the marginal utility of M divided by the marginal utility of X) equals the relative costs of the two commodities (C_m/C_x).

However, the patient may not know H and most certainly will not know the productivity of medical care in improving his or her health $(\Delta H/\Delta M)$. If we assume that the physician knows H and $\Delta H/\Delta M$ and that he or she has an awareness of the patient's tastes and other circumstances (prices and income), then *if* the physician behaves as a "perfect agent," he or she will prescribe and/or provide a quantity of M such that the consumer's equilibrium conditions are met.

But there are a number of possible deviations from this ideal. Even if the doctor knew H and $\Delta H/\Delta M$ and he or she could infer the other conditions regarding the patient's values and economic circumstances, the doctor's self-interest may deviate from that of the patient. The doctor could then provide the patient with estimates of H ("It could be a strep throat; we'd better take a culture") and $\Delta H/\Delta M$ ("I'd better have a look at that next week") that are distortions of the true values. Under these circumstances, the physician can "generate" or induce a demand for his or her services. If the physician exaggerated H, for instance, this would increase $\Delta U/\Delta M$ to the patient and increase the demand for M.

But there are limits to such a process. For one thing, with repeated events (such as common colds) the patient eventually gains some information to evaluate H and $\Delta H/\Delta M$. In addition, information sharing among patients, or between patients and other physicians, limits the degree to which a physician can present the patient with misrepresented information. The physician may also have some moral misgivings about such misrepresentations. As a result, there are limits to how much demand generation can take place, although these limits will vary with consumer characteristics (e.g., level of education) and type of condition. Finally, the assumption that the physician has perfect information about H and $\Delta H/\Delta M$ may not always be realistic. Diagnosis and treatment are often undertaken under conditions of uncertainty. Physicians then experiment to obtain the best treatment. While the physician can still generate demand, one cannot say with the same degree of certainty how much of the "experimentation" was purposive demand generation and how much was honest experimentation.

REFERENCES

Utilization and Subsequent Health Implications

Brook, R.H., Ware, J.E., Rogers, W.H., et al. (1983). Does free care improve adults' health? *New England Journal of Medicine, 309*, 1426–1434.

Chen, M.K. (1976). Penny-wise and pound foolish: Another look at the data. *Medical Care, 14,* 958–963.

—— (1976). More about penny-wise and pound foolish: A statistical point of view. *Medical Care, 14,* 964–968.

Dyckman, Z.Y. (1976). Comment on "copayments for ambulatory care: Penny-wise and pound foolish." *Medical Care, 14,* 274–276.

——, & McMenamin, P. (1976). Copayments for ambulatory care, "son of thrupence." *Medical Care, 14,* 968–969.

Fein, R. (1981). Effects of cost sharing in health insurance. *New England Journal of Medicine, 305,* 1526–1528.

Hopkins, C.E., Gartside, F., & Roemer, M.I. (1976). Rebuttal to "Comment on 'copayments for ambulatory care: Penny-wise and pound foolish.' " *Medical Care, 14,* 277.

Keeler, E.B., Brook, R.H., Goldberg, G.A., et al. (1985). How free care reduced hypertension in the health insurance experiment. *Journal of the American Medical Association, 254,* 1926–1931.

Relman, A. (1983). The Rand Health Insurance Study: Is cost sharing dangerous to your health. *New England Journal of Medicine, 309,* 1453.

Roemer, M.I., & Hopkins, C.E. (1976). Response to M.K. Chen. *Medical Care, 14,* 963–964.

——, Hopkins, C.E., Lockwood, C., et al. (1975). Copayments for ambulatory care: Penny-wise and pound foolish. *Medical Care, 13,* 457–466.

Stoddart, G., & Labelle, R.J. (1958, October). *Privatization in the Canadian health care system.* Ottawa: Health and Welfare Canada.

Demand for Health

Grossman, M. (1972). On the concept of health capital and the demand for health. *Journal of Political Economy, 80,* 223–255.

—— (1972). *The demand for health.* New York: National Bureau of Economic Research.

—— (1982). The demand for health after a decade. *Journal of Health Economics, 1,* 1–4.

Hay, J.W., Bailit, H., & Chiriboga, D.A. (1982). The demand for dental health. *Social Science and Medicine, 16,* 1285–1289.

Lairson, D., Lorimor, R., & Slater, C. (1984). Estimates of the demand for health: Males in the pre-retirement years. *Social Science and Medicine, 19,* 741–747.

Warner, K.E., & Murt, H.A. (1984). Economic incentives for health. *Annual Review of Public Health, 5,* 107–133.

Williams, A. (1985). The nature, meaning and measurement of health and illness: An economic viewpoint. *Social Science and Medicine, 20,* 1023–1027.

Choice of Insurance Plan

Anderson, G., & Knickman, J. (1984). Adverse selection under a voucher system: Grouping medicare recipients by level of expenditure. *Inquiry, 21,* 135–143.

Berki, S.E., Ashcraft, M., Penchansky, R., & Fortus, R.S. (1977). Enrollment choice in a multi-HMO setting. *Medical Care, 15,* 95–114.

——, & Ashcraft, M. (1980). HMO enrollment: Who joins what and why: A review of the literature. *Milbank Memorial Fund Quarterly, 58,* 588–632.

Bice, T.W. (1975). Risk vulnerability and enrollment in a prepaid group practice. *Medical Care, 13,* 698–703.

Supplier-Induced Demand

Feldstein, M.S. (1974). Econometric studies in health economics. In M. Intriligator and D. Kendrick (Eds.), *Frontiers in quantitative economics* (pp. 377–434). Amsterdam: North Holland Publishing Company.

Pauly, M.V. (1980). *Doctors and their workshops.* Chicago: University of Chicago Press.

Time Costs

Acton, J.P. (1973). *Demand for health among the urban poor* (No. R-1151-OEO/NYC). New York: New York City Rand Institute.

Culyer, A.J., & Cullis, J.G. (1976). Some economics of hospital waiting lists in the NHS. *Journal of Social Policy, 5,* 239–264.

Chapter 5

Behavior of Health Care Costs

5.1 INTRODUCTION

The present chapter focuses on the economic behavior of health care providers. The first aspect of provider behavior examined is concerned with how the resource commitment made by individual suppliers varies with the amount of production undertaken by the providing unit. The focus, then, is on the individual providing unit. The measure that we use to weigh the magnitude of the resource commitment of each providing unit is the cost to the unit of resource services. Here we examine how these costs vary as the size of operations of the providing unit varies.

Before embarking on the analysis of costs, a brief exposition of the relation between resource services and outputs, the production relation, is presented in Section 5.2. This presentation is made in purely "physical" terms and is designed to provide a brief summary of the role of production in determining cost. Section 5.3 discusses the basic cost–output relation and examines three alternative ways of looking at this relation. Using the cost–output relation as our basic reference point, Section 5.4 examines the various factors that change this relation, as changing technology, the quality of care given, the incentives offered to providers, and the size of the production unit. Section 5.5 presents a summary of some empirical estimates of the cost–output relation.

5.2 PRODUCTION: THE INPUT–OUTPUT RELATION

5.2.1 Basic Relation

The economic analysis of production involves the specification of alternative combinations of inputs that yield varying levels of outputs. The production process itself, its organization, and technology lie in the realm of administrative practice and medicine. This production process has considerable impact on economic variables (discussed in Sections 5.2 and 5.3) and can be influenced by economic factors as well, as seen in Section 6.6.

The production process chosen is determined by the technology used. Roughly defined, technology is a way of doing things. The production process in medical care is determined by what things are done to the patient as well as the way they are done. In this sense, there are many "technologies" even for the same illness. To bring out the essential characteristics of the production or input–output relation, we focus initially on one technology and later introduce complicating factors and determine how they affect this relation.

The simplest production process can be illustrated by a solo private-practice physician. In our example the physician treats patients with only one type of disease, all of the same degree of severity. The disease is a conclusively diagnosed common cold. Treatment involves an examination, diagnostic tests, and a prescription of two aspirins and a glass of water. A number of simplifying assumptions should be noted. First, the product is homogeneous because the *case mix* is made up of cases of a single disease, all of equal severity. Second, all treatments are of the same quality. All patients receive the same examination, the same tests, and the same banter from the physician. Under these conditions we will examine the production process.

The process involves the use of various resources in performing tasks. These resources can be divided into two groups, fixed and variable factors. *Fixed factors* are those whose use is restricted to their current occupation *for the time period under consideration*. Given their specialized nature, or high costs of transferring to other uses, or other contractual arrangements, fixed factors cannot be used elsewhere in the economy during the current period of production. Furthermore, the producer cannot increase the quantity during this period, which we will assume to be 1 month. In our example, fixed factors include physician office space, test equipment, and physician time.

Office space and equipment are rented annually, let us say, and so their use for a 1-year period is fixed. As for physician time, we assume that the doctor has by choice decided that during the month he or she will remain in his or her present position and will work 40 hours per week. Physician time is therefore a fixed factor. Whether or not a factor is fixed depends on the time period under consideration. If our time period was 5 years, office space, equipment, and even physician time might vary. The variable factor of production is nurses' time. This input can be purchased in varying quantities by the physician. It will be assumed that a nurse performs all tasks that the doctor does not.

The production process consists of three types of tasks performed by the available resources. The first are the administrative tasks of setting appointments, keeping records, moving patients through the office, and billing the patient. The second type involves technical tasks of performing blood tests with the rented equipment. These tasks are performed by the nurse. The third task, performed by the physician, is the examination itself. For simplicity, we will assume no patients can be processed without some nursing time. Generally, of course, the doctor is able to process some patients with no help, but we will assume this is not the case. We also assume that, within the current ranges of resource use considered, the doctor can treat all patients who are processed; his or her time limitations do not create a "capacity" problem.

We now inquire into the number of patients who can be processed using varying levels of the variable input in conjuction with the given fixed inputs. The specification of this production relation will be made under the conditions that, whatever the level of variable inputs used in conjunction with the fixed inputs, the maximum number of patients possible is being processed. This condition will only hold if the factors have incentives to produce as much as possible. This condition is discussed further at the end of this section. Under these conditions a *production function* that expresses how output will vary when inputs are changed in quantity can be specified. In specifying this function, let us call nurses' inputs, L, which are measured by hours worked. All other factors, which in our case are fixed, will be called F. Output, called Q, is measured by patient visits, implying that each "produced" visit involves the various tasks specified. The production function can be written in functional forms as $Q = Q(L, F)$, which means that Q depends on L and F.

The production function is a summary of what goes into the process and what comes out. With F fixed, only L can vary. By saying L varies, we are in fact specifying different combinations of L and F. With few nursing hours, the nurse must perform all the nonexamination tasks and as a result cannot afford to specialize. Few patients will thus be processed. In Table 5–1 we present this by showing only one patient processed with the first 8 nursing hours input. When additional patients are processed, the nurse can begin to perform some tasks for both patients together. This concentration of tasks allows added output to be produced with fewer additional resources. Indeed, in our example, only 7 additional nursing hours are required to process a second patient. The expression for the additional production yielded by the use of one extra unit of the variable input is the *marginal product*. This can be expressed symbolically as $\Delta Q / \Delta L$. As can be seen in Table 5–1, at the lowest level of output, one visit, an extra nursing hour adds one-eighth of a visit to the level of output. At a level of two visits, the additional output of an extra nursing hour is one-seventh visit. This fraction is an expression of the marginal product. The *increasing* marginal product (one-seventh is greater than one-eighth) means that as size of output increases additional nursing hours are more productive. This tendency toward an increasing marginal product, created initially by the gains that the concentration of tasks allows, is reinforced by gains created from the specialization of tasks as output continues to grow. As more patients are processed and more nursing hours are used, some tasks can be divided

Table 5–1 Relations between Cost and Output

(1) Total Nursing Hours (L)	(2) Total Visits (Q)	(3) Marginal Product (ΔQ/ΔL)	(4) Total Fixed Cost (TFC)	(5) Total Variable Cost (TVC)	(6) Total Cost (TC = TFC + TVC)	(7) Average Fixed Cost (AFC = TFC/Q)	(8) Average Variable Cost (AVC = TVC/Q)	(9) Average Total Cost (ATC = TC/Q)	(10) Marginal Cost (ΔTC/ΔQ)
8	1	1/8	$100	$ 16	$116	$100	$16	$116	$16
15	2	1/7	100	30	130	50	15	65	14
20	3	1/5	100	40	140	33.3	13.3	46.67	10
24	4	1/4	100	48	148	25	12	37	8
30	5	1/6	100	60	160	20	12	32	12
38	6	1/8	100	76	176	16.6	12.6	29.3	16
50	7	1/12	100	100	200	14.28	14.28	28.57	24
64	8	1/14	100	128	228	12.5	16	28.5	28
100	9	1/30	100	200	300	11.1	22.22	33.3	72
140	10	1/40	100	280	380	10	28	38	80

among nurses, resulting in gains from specialization. As seen in Table 5–1, the third patient is processed with only 5 extra nursing hours, the fourth patient with 4 extra hours.

But such gains cannot be reaped forever. Eventually, overroutinization can lead to boredom. In addition, the fixed amount of equipment in the office becomes heavily taxed and nurses have to wait to perform lab tests. This changes the relation between additional output and additional input; to produce successively more units of output at these higher levels of output requires larger doses of additional nursing hours. Placing the argument in terms of marginal productivity, at higher levels of output the marginal productivity of nurses' efforts begins to decline. Thus, in our example, at a level of output of four visits the marginal product is one-fourth; at a level of output of five visits the marginal product falls to one-sixth of a visit; and for six visits the marginal product is lower still, being one-eighth of a visit per nursing hour added. Production has reached the stage of *diminishing marginal productivity*. It should be noted that *total* output is constantly rising; the assumed relation in our production function stipulates that additional increases of output are harder and harder to come by as the size of output rises.

The figures used in our example were concocted to demonstrate the principle we are hypothesizing, that of eventually diminishing marginal productivity. Other examples could fit just as well as long as they are consistent with this principle.

5.2.2 Shifts in the Relation

We have now defined a production function and specified in general terms the most important property we would expect such a function to possess: the marginal product will eventually decline when the size of output increases. This relation was specified under restrictive underlying conditions. We can now examine the effect that might take place if some of these conditions did not hold. These changes will be examined using the basic input-output or production relation specified in Table 5–1 as a point of reference. A change in any of these underlying conditions will be regarded as causing one of two possible changes: it will either increase or decrease the amount of output that can be obtained from given amounts of inputs. Either change will be regarded as a *shift* in the production relation. An upward shift means that at each level of input more output can be produced; a downward shift means that less output is produced. Looking at an upward shift in marginal terms, at any level of *input use* more additional output can be produced with an additional unit of the variable input; or, expressed in *output terms*, at any *level of output* fewer additional inputs are required to produce one extra unit of output. In marginal language, we say that the marginal product is greater at any level of output. Thus, at a level of output of eight visits, the original production relation was such that an extra nursing hour employed led to an increase in output of one-fourteenth of a visit. With an upward shift in the production function, an extra nursing hour might now produce one-tenth of a visit. Of couse, the assumption that marginal productivity is diminishing still holds, but the entire relation is such that now more can be obtained at any level of output.

We will now examine the effect some of these underlying conditions have on the production relation if they change. The possible changes include a change in the case mix, in the severity of illness of patients, in the quality of care, in technology, in the amount of capital, F, that the employer uses, and in the underlying incentive structure.

First, a change in the case mix might occur when the physician is confronted with a number of rheumatic fever cases in addition to common colds. Such a case mix would require more resources per case than the original example and would shift the production relation downward. The same type of downward shift would occur if the physician were faced with more severe cases of the same illness. These cases would require more resources and would thus shift the production relation downward.

Second, the effect of a change in the quality of care will depend on the precise meaning attached to quality. If quality means a more thorough examination, leading to a more definitive diagnosis or a more likely recovery, then the effect of higher-quality care is to shift the production relation downward, and more resources are required for each examination. Similarly, if higher quality means more personal care, the same effect on the production relation will result.

Third, quality is frequently associated with technique or technology, which has come to be associated with highly trained specialists and sophisticated equipment. If such an association is drawn, then higher-quality care, translated into our framework, means a greater flow of services from more capital, both human and physical. More inputs are required to produce a single unit of output (measured as a visit), and therefore the measured relation between inputs and visits will shift downward. However, note that the more resource-intensive visits are not the same, qualitatively, as the less resource-intensive ones. We cannot say that medical resources are less productive in any of these instances. We are saying that a given amount of resources will produce a lower quantity of care, but this medical care is of a higher *quality*.

Fourth, this last interpretation of quality, as consisting of more resource-intensive examinations or treatments, should be distinguished from the type of resource intensity that occurs when more capital or other fixed resources are used in conjunction with variable resources to produce the same quality product. An example of this would occur when a larger piece of equipment, a computerized blood counter, replaces a smaller one, a Kolter counter. More output *of the same quality* per variable input can be processed with the larger piece of equipment. The production relation shifts upward in this case.

A final factor influencing the production relation is concerned with the incentive for the "manager" of the providing agency to ensure that tasks are performed with a minimum use of inputs. Our production relation was derived under the condition that the maximum output is obtained from any given level of resource use. Incentives enter the picture when we consider the benefits that management (the doctor, in our example) obtains from the resources themselves. If the profits of the enterprise, the management's reward, are related to how low production costs are, then the management will have an incentive to use as few resources per unit of output as possible. However, incentives can be structured in such a way that the use of inputs is encouraged. If, for example, the management receives a fixed rate of profit that is positively related to its costs, then it will have an incentive to use more resources to perform each task. This would raise its total costs and thus its profits. Even though the analysis of production lies very much in the realm of production management and medicine, the production relation cannot be analyzed in total isolation from the economic incentives under which the organization operates. Section 6.6 discusses further the analysis of incentive schemes.

5.2.3 Substitution among Inputs

The analysis of the previous section was conducted under the assumption that one variable input existed. In fact, there may be several variable inputs, and they may be substitutable for each other, at least to some degree. Let us suppose that there are two variable inputs, physician time, P, and nurse practitioner time, N, in addition to the fixed inputs, F. The production function is now expressed as $Q = Q(P, N, F)$. Substitutability among inputs is often analyzed by assuming the level of output, Q, is held constant and examining how much nurse practitioner time must be added to the process to offset a unit of physician time. This is referred to as the *marginal rate of substitution* of nurse practitioners for physicians.

Such a degree of substitution may well be possible in a number of instances, but it may be limited. Thus, if a given number of patients are being treated in an ambulatory setting, and initially there are ten physicians and one nurse practitioner, the tasks of the physicians may be such that a nurse practitioner may be substituted for a physician with no adverse effects on the quantity or quality of output. However, additional substitution may prove to be more difficult, and two nurses will be required to replace a physician. Eventually, no additional substitution may be feasible to maintain the quality and quantity of output. Nevertheless, within a given range, substitution is possible.

A number of areas have been identified in health care where substitution is possible. One study examined the role of paraprofessional surgical assistants in surgical operations who substituted for physicians or surgeons as assistants to the operating surgeon. The study found that trained assistants could replace physicians in this assisting role with no adverse effects on the operating surgeon's time (Lewit et al., 1980), particularly in less complex operations.

Another example of the substitutability of inputs is in the use of drugs and attendants for the care of mental patients. To some extent, increased utilization of drugs reduces the amount of effort required of psychiatric hospital attendants. For other examples, physician assistants and nurse practitioners can perform many of the tasks that doctors traditionally perform (Reinhardt, 1972), and dental technicians can perform simple tasks such as cleaning teeth and even some repair work.

Frequently, such substitution may be feasible and even economical, but barriers exist to limit it. For example, licensing laws may limit the degree to which nurse practitioners can substitute in tasks for doctors. In such cases, one must separate what is feasible from what is legally or institutionally permitted.

5.3 SHORT-RUN COST–OUTPUT RELATIONS

5.3.1 Production and Cost

The previous section focused on the relation between output and alternative combinations of inputs. In specifying the production relation, the inputs were presented as separate entities that work together. The next step in our analysis is to present a measure of the resource commitment undertaken by the provider in producing the output. One such measure, which places all inputs on a single scale measured in money terms, is *cost*. To a provider, cost means the value of inputs used in the production process. As discussed in Section 2.2.4, however, this value is not always well approximated by money outlays.

Therefore, a broader view of cost, one that measures what the provider gives up by using all the resources committed to production, not just the paid-for ones, is used in this section. This concept is the *opportunity cost*, defined as the value to the provider that was given up by *not* committing its resources to the next highest-valued use. Another way of putting it is that the costs of resources are measured by the market value that those resources can be sold for. This concept is particularly important when measuring the value of resources that are unpaid (e.g., resources that the producer owns) and hence that appear to be free. If the owner of these unpaid resources is giving up some return on them, then there is a cost associated with them, and this cost must be estimated by calculating the probable market value of the resources.

Since we are concerned with the functioning of an organization, the costs of resource use will be considered from the organization's point of view. An organization can undertake a resource commitment that does not appear in its *paid out* costs. Nevertheless, if the organization commits its resources to a particular use, they are part of the organization's costs and should be counted as such. On the other hand, some entity outside the organization may make a resource commitment that allows the organization to function. For example, a blood donor gives his or her time and blood to a blood donor clinic, a benefactor may endow a hospital with an operating room, or a doctor may volunteer teaching time to a medical school. In these instances, resources are used to undertake activities, but they are not part of the resource commitment undertaken by the blood clinic or the hospital. Rather, they are part of the *total* resource commitment required to undertake the activity. In this chapter we are concerned with the operations of health organizations and so focus on the narrow, partial resource commitment made by these organizations in their activities. This leaves the question of the total resource commitment made to perform any activity, including the commitment of the organization as well as that of donors, volunteers, benefactors, and government. For a discussion of the broader social viewpoint, see Section 13.3. In this section our focus is on the narrow, organizational point of view.

In the analysis that follows, the definitions presented are placed in a time frame of 1 month. Given this time frame, we can divide production costs into two groups: fixed costs and variable costs. *Fixed costs,* also called overhead costs, do not change with output over the relevant time frame. *Variable costs* occur when the value of the total resource commitment increases as output increases. In our example of the physician's practice, the fixed costs are those that do not vary during the month; they are the costs of the fixed factors, including space and equipment rental costs and the cost of physician time. We assume the rental values to be $50 during the period. We also assume that the physician could have earned $50 working in a clinic rather than in a private practice; this amount measures the opportunity cost of time he or she faced when making the decision to continue his or her practice. Given that the decision to practice privately has been made, it becomes a "sunk" cost, relevant more to past decisions than to present ones. Nevertheless, it is still a cost and is classified as a fixed cost. The total fixed costs are thus $100. (The cost curve of a company incorporates the return that the owners could normally get on their assets, including time, the portion of buildings they own, etc. This normal return is sometimes called *normal profits.* Any returns above this opportunity cost are called *economic profits.*)

Variable costs are costs of variable inputs. In our example, the only variable input is nursing hours. Assume that the price of nursing services is $2 per hour. Thus, 8 hours of services cost $16. We can now specify the relation between the value of resource commitment by the provider, that is, cost, and the level of output. This relation depends on the quantities of resources used (determined by the production relationship) and the money paid for, or the opportunity costs inputed to, these resource services. This relation can be viewed in three different ways. First, we can examine costs from the point of view of the *total* resource commitment required to maintain production at any specific scale of output. In this case, we determine how *total costs* vary with output. Second, we can look at the average value of resource commitment, that is, the value of the resource commitment required to produce a single unit of output. The value of this average resource commitment is called *average cost*. The third way of viewing costs is to examine the value of additional resources that must be committed to the production process to produce an additional unit of output. This concept is called the *marginal cost* and is defined as the additional cost required to produce one additional unit of output. We will now discuss how each of these alternative measures varies as the level of output changes.

5.3.2 Total Costs

Total cost (*TC*) is the sum of all costs incurred in producing a given level of output. Total variable cost (*TVC*) is the total cost of variable inputs for any level of output; total fixed cost (*TFC*) is the total cost of all fixed factors. Total cost is the sum of the two (i.e., *TVC* + *TFC*). We now look at these magnitudes with regard to our example, shown in Table 5–1. Total fixed costs are $100 whatever the level of output. Therefore, *TFC*, plotted on a graph in Figure 5–1, is depicted by a straight horizontal line at a level of $100.

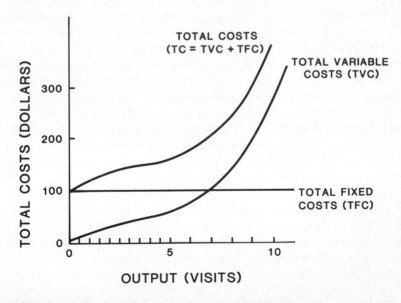

Figure 5–1 The relation between total fixed costs, total variable costs, total costs, and the level of output. At each production level, total costs can be divided between fixed and variable costs. Fixed costs do not vary with output. Based on data from Table 5–1.

The behavior of total variable costs depends on two factors: (1) the relation between output and variable inputs, specified in Section 5.2, and (2) the unit cost of these variable resources. These total variable costs are shown in the context of our example in column 5 of Table 5–1. In Figure 5–1, a *TVC* curve is drawn with properties similar to those of our example.

The total cost curve (*TC*) is the vertical sum of the two curves, *TVC* and *TFC*, at each output level. This is shown in Table 5–1 in column 6. The level of *TC* is determined by fixed costs; its shape is determined by the production function and the variation of output with variable inputs. Given the fixed per unit price of the variable input ($2 an hour), the production function relation, translated into a cost–output relation, means that the addition to total costs of the extra resource commitment levels off as output increases. Thus, *TVC* is $16 at a scale of one visit, $30 at a scale of two visits, $40 at a scale of three visits, and $48 at a level of four visits. Placed in diagrammatic terms, this leveling off of costs is shown in the output range of 0 to 4 with reference to curve *TVC* in Figure 5–1. If additional resources had been increasingly more productive beyond this scale of input, the *TVC* curve would have continued leveling off. At the extreme, if higher levels of production could be undertaken with the same resources, then *TVC* would be horizontal. But, beyond four units of output, diminishing marginal productivity begins to set in, and in terms of costs this means that successively greater resource commitments are needed to produce at successively higher levels of output. In Table 5–1, the *TVC* rises to 60, 76, 100, 128, 200, and so on. In terms of the total resource commitment, total costs are rapidly rising. As seen on the curve, beyond a scale of 4, *TVC* is curving upward; at the extreme, it would become almost vertical. Thus an enormous commitment in resources is required to move to a higher output level. The shape of the *TC* curve is similar to that of the *TVC* curve except that *TC* is higher by a level of $100.

5.3.3 Marginal Cost

Implicit in the total variable cost–output relation is the marginal cost–output relation. The marginal cost at any level of output is the additional cost required to move a unit higher on the output scale. It is thus defined as $\Delta TC/\Delta Q$. Since *TFC* is constant over all levels of output, the marginal *fixed* cost would be zero at any scale, since the *additional* fixed resource commitment is zero at all levels of output. Thus, the marginal cost is the addition to total *variable* cost for producing one extra unit of output. In Table 5–1 the marginal cost (*MC*) is shown in column 10. As can be seen, the extra cost of moving to one unit of output from zero is $16, to two units from one is $14, and so on. Until four units of output, *MC* is falling. However, because of the diminishing marginal productivity of variable inputs, coupled with the fact that the additional quantities of variable inputs used are all paid the same wage, producing additional units of output eventually requires a successively greater resource commitment. This is reflected in rising marginal cost after the fourth visit; the fifth visit costs $12 extra, the sixth, $16 extra, and so on. The marginal cost curve is shown in Figure 5–2. Note that beyond an output of 4, marginal costs cease falling and begin to rise.

The concept of marginal cost is central to the analysis of most economic decisions. For the most part, the types of decisions that concern economists are related to the consequences of whether to use additional (or fewer) resources for a particular use. For example, we might be concerned with the implications of placing additional surgeon-training facilities in either Boston or Boise; we might analyze the consequences of adding one or more paramedics to existing medical practices; or we might be interested in the consequences of decreasing the number

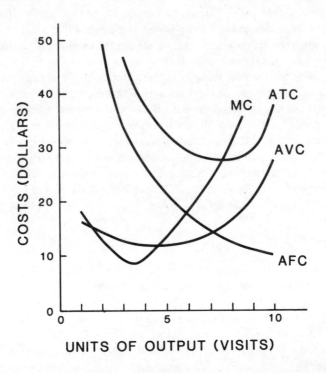

UNITS OF OUTPUT (VISITS)

Figure 5–2 Relation between cost and output. Average costs are shown in total (*ATC*) and in the two components of the total: fixed (*AFC*) and variable (*AVC*). Marginal cost (*MC*) is the addition to total cost of the next unit produced. There is a unique relation between *MC* and both *AVC* and *ATC*: when *MC* is below *ATC* (or *AVC*), the average cost is falling; when *MC* is greater than *ATC* (or *AVC*), the average cost is increasing; and when *MC* equals *ATC* (or *AVC*), the average cost is constant, that is, it has reached its minimum point.

of obstetrical beds in a particular region or hospital. In these instances, as in most other instances concerning the placement of resources, the allocational decision involves expanding a particular facility or service or increasing the quantity available of a trained input. In these cases, the concept used to measure the added resource commitment is the marginal cost.

5.3.4 Average Cost

The third way of looking at costs is to average the costs required to obtain a given level of output. The average total cost (*ATC*) is the total cost per unit of output and is defined for any level of output; it is expressed as *TC/Q*. It measures the value of the average resource commitment required to sustain a given scale of output. However, because it is useful in making comparisons, this measurement has been frequently used in empirical studies.

The behavior of the *ATC* depends on the behavior of the average fixed cost (*TFC/Q*) and the average variable cost (*TVC/Q*). Average fixed cost is lower at successively higher levels of output because the $100 in fixed costs is spread out over more output. Thus, at one visit average fixed cost is $100, at two visits it is $50, and so on. Average variable cost is initially lower at successively higher levels of output. At one unit of output it is $16, at two it is $15, at three it is $13.30, and so on. Falling average variable costs are made possible by the increasing productivity of additional variable inputs at low output levels.

Another way of viewing this relation is to show that *MC* is initially below *AC*, which brings down the average as output increases. The *MC* for the first visit is $16, and the average variable cost is $16. For the second visit, *MC* is $14. This brings down the average variable costs of the two visits to $15 (i.e., $30/2). The falling average variable and average fixed costs together ensure that average total costs (which is the sum of the two) will also fall as output expands. Eventually, after four visits in our example, *MC* increases as output expands. Expanding output from four to five visits costs an extra $12; expanding to six costs another $16; and *MC* at seven is $24. However, as long as marginal cost is lower than average total cost, a further expansion of output will continue to reduce *ATC*.

For example, in Table 5–1 we can see that at five units of output, total cost is $160 and *ATC* is thus $32. An expansion of output by one unit to a level of output of six would cost an additional $16. The new *ATC* at six units of output will *decrease* to $29.33 because the *MC* of the sixth unit of output is lower than the *ATC*, and so expanding output brings down the average. With a rising *MC*, this situation will not continue indefinitely. At some level of output the *MC* will just equal the average, and at a still higher level it will exceed it. The average must then begin to rise. In our example, the level where *MC* equals *ATC* is eight visits. As seen in Table 5–1, an expansion from seven to eight visits will cost an extra $28. With an *ATC* of $28.57 at the level of seven visits, expansion to eight visits leaves

ATC at about the same level. An expansion to nine visits has an *MC* of $72. This is above the *ATC* at eight visits. The *ATC* increases to $33.33 at nine visits.

The average cost curves are shown in Figure 5–2 in juxtaposition to the *MC* curve. These curves are based on the data presented in Table 5–1, but have been smoothed out. The average fixed cost (*AFC*) curve declines over all levels of output. The average variable cost (*AVC*) curve declines over small levels of output until four visits. At five visits, the *MC* just equals *AVC*, and so *AVC* bottoms out. For output levels higher than five, *MC* is above *AVC*, and so *AVC* increases with expansion of output. The curve *AVC* is thus shaped like a U, indicating that at lower levels of output *AVC* falls as output expands; it then bottoms (where *MC* = *AVC*) and begins to rise. The *ATC* curve (remember, *ATC* = *AVC* + *AFC*) is also U-shaped like the *AVC* curve. It is located above and slightly to the right of *AVC* and also bottoms out where the rising *MC* cuts it.

The *ATC* curve, as already noted, has a fixed and a variable component. The relative sizes of these two components will determine at which level of output the *ATC* curve will begin to slope upward. The fixed-cost component (*AFC*) always falls as output increases, because the same costs are spread over a greater output. The variable-cost component follows the rules of productivity and begins to rise because, eventually, higher marginal costs will raise the average. The larger the fixed-cost component, the greater the stage during which average total costs are falling. Hospitals have been identified as having large fixed-cost components. If this is indeed true, then over a large range of its potential output levels, hospitals should experience diminishing *ATCs*.

The fixed-cost component can be related to the use of capital equipment. A heavy investment in capital equipment will create large fixed costs. However, such equipment may permit additional tests to be undertaken with a small additional commitment of resources up to large scales of output. Thus, although fixed costs are high, marginal costs are low. For these types of productive processes, the *ATC* may fall over large scales of output. This type of phenomenon is called an *indivisibility;* the expensive equipment, available in a large dose, cannot be divided into smaller units. It is operated at small levels of output at a high *ATC*, and at large levels at a low *ATC*.

This section has identified the shapes of three related cost–output measures: total cost, average cost, and marginal cost. Their shapes are dependent largely on the production relation. As shown in Section 5.2, the production relation is subject to *shifts* caused by a variety of influences. These same influences can cause the cost curves to shift, that is, to change their positions. Section 5.4 outlines how the position of the cost curve reacts to changes in these various conditions.

5.4 POSITION OF THE COST CURVE

The position of the cost curve is determined by the same factors that influence the production relation. These factors include the case mix and the severity of cases treated, the quality of care provided, the technology used, the amount of fixed factors employed in the production process, and the incentives under which the provider is operating. Each factor will be considered separately.

Given fixed factors and fixed costs, a change in the case mix toward more complicated cases and an increase in the average severity level of diseases treated will increase the variable resources required per unit of output and will thus increase marginal and average costs at all output scales. The positions of both the *ATC* and the *MC* curves will now be higher; this is similar to saying that both the *MC* and the *ATC* relations will shift upward. These shifts are demonstrated in Figure 5–3. Here, ATC_1 and MC_1 are the average total cost and marginal cost relations before the change to a more complex case mix. The results of this change are shown by a shifting of *ATC* to ATC_2 and of *MC* to MC_2.

An increase in quality, if taken to mean more thorough examinations or treatments, will similarly shift the cost curves upward. The adoption of a technology that uses more resources per case will have a similar effect. Many recent technological innovations have been associated with a large capital investment for

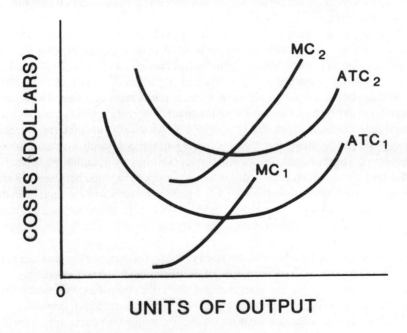

Figure 5–3 Diagrammatic representation of shifts in average and marginal cost curves. Curves ATC_1 and MC_1 form the initial relation between costs and output. With reference to this relation, ATC_2 and MC_2 represent an inward shift in costs, showing higher costs at every level of output.

equipment, as well as a larger flow of variable expenditures for the services of the more highly trained personnel who operate this equipment. Examples of such technological innovations are open-heart surgery, a technique that intrigued economists in the 1960s, and computed tomography (CT) scanning, a revolutionary and somewhat costly advance on x-rays. Both techniques require heavy investment in equipment and are costly in comparison with previously used techniques. The effect of introducing either of these techniques would be to shift both the fixed and variable components of the *ATC* upward, thus increasing the *ATC* for all levels of patients treated. However, it should be remembered that the quality of visits in terms of a more accurate diagnosis or a more certain improvement in health may accompany the introduction of the new technology. One physician visit or treatment or one length of stay of hospitalization is not the same as another in this case.

All technological innovations in medical care are not of this resource-using type, however. Innovations in pharmaceuticals have reduced the length of hospitalization required for some illnesses; two notable examples are tuberculosis treatment and mental illness treatment. Furthermore, some new laboratory equipment has allowed many tasks to be automated; this has led to falling average costs over large levels of output because of the low variable costs associated with the use of this equipment.

The effect of incentives that encourage resource use is to raise the level of average costs associated with any single level of output. Assuming that a single least-cost position is associated with each output level, and thus we can identify a least-cost average cost curve, these "perverse" incentives will encourage the provider to choose a position above this curve. It has been questioned whether a cost curve that measures the cost output relation when given resources are not used to maximize as much output, that is, a more-than-least-cost curve, is a meaningful concept. This is because more than one such average cost point may exist at any output level. There can only be one least-cost point, however, and in the least-cost case, a cost curve, which supposedly represents a *unique* relation between cost and output, can be uniquely determined. Once a provider chooses to use more than the least amount of resources to achieve a given output level, given the quality, he or she can use these excessive resources to varying degrees. There is no longer a *unique* cost curve.

Another factor that might cause cost curves to shift is the price the provider pays for the hired resources. In our example, if the physician had to pay $3 per nursing hour instead of $2, both the marginal and the average cost curves would shift upward. Conversely, if the price fell to $1, the curves would shift downward. A final factor that will influence the position of the average cost curve appears when two or more types of variable inputs exist. When these inputs can be substituted for each other, at least to some degree, then a substitution of a less costly for a more costly input can lower the cost curve. This need not always be the case, of course.

If a paramedic is substituted for a physician and, although less expensive per hour, takes much longer to do the same task, the total or average cost may not shift downward as a result of the substitution. Also, keep in mind that the quality of the product may booome lowor ao a rooult of tho oubotitution, and ovon though output costs less to produce, the output is not the same as before.

5.5 ECONOMIES OF SCOPE

We have proceeded with the discussion of costs as if the health care institution had a single output. While this helps to clarify certain relations between costs and level and scale of output, the assumption of a single product line needs to be altered with regard to certain types of institutions, notably hospitals. Hospitals are multiproduct firms that, in many cases, provide a large number of separate product lines, such as clinical laboratory services, emergency room services, physical therapy, and intensive care (Berry, 1973; Goldfarb, Hornbrook, and Rafferty, 1980).

The product-line dimension of output should be distinguished from the case-mix dimension. *Case mix* refers to the complexity of the types of diseases being treated. A hospital with a greater number of types of illnesses has a different case mix than one that specializes in a few types of illnesses. If, as is sometimes done, severity is included as a dimension of case mix, then case-mix indexes can be developed (Hornbrook and Monheit, 1985). The hospital has a number of services or product lines ready to serve patients with different types of severities of illnesses. The more different services that are available, the greater will be the scope of services of the hospital. In fact, two hospitals can have very similar case-mix measures, but very different service scopes. When the concept of scope is recognized as an added dimension of hospital output, a new concept is required to analyze how costs and scope are related.

The concept of *economies of scope* refers to possible savings from producing different products jointly in the same production unit, rather than producing them individually in separate production units. In notational terms, let X_1 stand for one output, say, family planning services, and X_2 stand for a second output, pediatric services; $C(X_1)$ stands for the total cost of producing X_1, $C(X_2)$ the total cost of producing X_2 in a separate setting, and $C(X_1, X_2)$ the cost of jointly producing X_1 and X_2 in the same production unit. Economies of scope arise when the cost of jointly producing specific quantities of the two services $C(X_1, X_2)$ is less than the sum of the costs of producing each service separately, $C(X_1) + C(X_2)$. In our example, economies of scope would exist if a clinic could jointly produce given quantities of family planning services and pediatric services more cheaply than they could be produced separately.

Economies of scope might arise when tasks in providing two separate services are complementary and so, if the services are produced jointly, production costs are reduced. For example, if providing both family planning and pediatric services requires a common core of services, say, blood tests and x-rays, then providing the two types of services in separate producing units would cause duplication. Savings could be achieved by combining the two separate services into a single service that serves both groups of patients. Of course, it is also possible to have diseconomies of scope. This would occur when two types of output are best produced in separate producing units. For example, if psychiatric patients are treated with one treatment regimen and home health services with a different one, combining the two units in a single producing unit may be more costly than single producing units specializing in each service.

In one of the few studies of economies of scope in health care, Cowing and Holtman (1983) estimated both scale and scope economies for 138 short-term hospitals in New York State. They divided the hospital output into five diagnostic categories (actually representing different case mixes rather than service scopes): medical–surgical, maternity, pediatric, other inpatient care, and emergency room care. For four of the services, excluding pediatric care, marginal cost fell over low ranges of output and then became constant. These results indicate substantial economies of scale in these services and suggest that merging of the services produced on a small scale into larger units could yield considerable savings. However, with regard to the existence of economies of scope, the findings were generally negative, indicating an absence of such economies. These findings, if they hold up in repeated trials, could indicate that, on cost grounds alone, hospitals should specialize rather than become multiproduct agencies. One must be careful in overgeneralizing in this case because, even though economies of scope may not be widespread, specific services may have production conditions that, when combined, yield scope economies.

5.6 LONG-RUN COST CURVES

The cost curves in Section 5.4 were derived under the assumption that some of the inputs were fixed. Suppose we take a longer perspective and allow enough time for the providing unit to change its fixed factors—to expand or contract its physical plant and equipment or its physicians. If one maintains a planning period of sufficient length, this is certainly possible. The analysis of such problems is called *long-run analysis*.

Indeed, the fixed factors in the short-run perspective are no longer fixed; they, too, can vary. From this longer planning perspective, all our resources are variable. Suppose a hospital board is planning to build a new facility from scratch. The board has a choice of facilities of three sizes: 60, 120, or 250 beds. Associated with each facility are given capital outlays of $2 million, $3 million, or $3.5 million. Associated with each size of facility is the given annual capital costs of depreciation and interest on the financial capital. During the planning period and until the decision is made as to which size to choose, these capital costs can be varied (in three different levels) and thus are variable. Associated with each scale of facility is an average cost curve (either ATC_1, ATC_2, or ATC_3 in Figure 5–4), including capital costs (remember that, in the long run, there are no fixed costs). Now assume that each scale of plant is least costly for given ranges of output. For fewer than 1,000 annual admissions, ATC_1 is the least costly; for over 3,000 admissions, ATC_3 is the least costly. Depending on which level of output is chosen, one scale of plant will be the least costly. The dashed curve in Figure 5–4 represents the least cost that can be produced at any given output level, given that we had the choice of scale of plant. This is called the long-run average cost curve (*LRAC*); it is made up of the minimum cost points at each output level.

The *LRAC* is usually hypothesized, if it were represented in a smooth fashion, to be U-shaped. Such a shape would be generated by falling long-run average costs (economies of scale) at low scales of plant size, followed by constant and finally increasing costs (diseconomies of scale). Before discussing such costs, one must specify whether one is talking about a single operating unit (e.g., an individual hospital, nursing home, or ambulatory care clinic) or an entire operating entity (e.g., a corporate chain).

A single operating entity may be subject to eventual diseconomies because the gains from specialization in certain tasks eventually run out. Or a single hospital

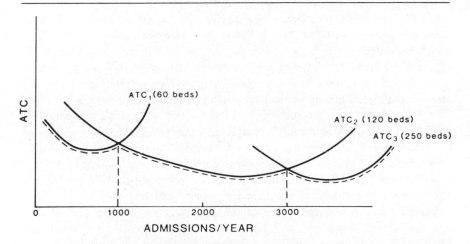

Figure 5–4 Relation between short- and long-run average cost curves. Short-run curves (ATC_1, ATC_2, and ATC_3) are shown for three plant size levels (expressed in terms of bed size). The long-run average cost curve (*LRAC*) is derived from these curves (shown as the dashed line). *LRAC* is the minimum cost point at each level of output. At 1,000 and 3,000 admissions, the *LRAC* becomes associated with different cost curves (different sizes of plant) because it becomes more economical to produce successively greater outputs with larger-sized plants.

unit may be able to expand only by the addition of diverse units (e.g., a CT scanning unit or a physiotherapy department), and such units may be costly to manage in a single unit. For these reasons, the long-run cost curve of the single operating unit may exhibit diseconomies of scale.

The multiplant firm, such as a multihospital corporation, may exhibit scale economies as it expands by acquiring additional distinct operating units. Certain functions, such as purchasing, may be run more efficiently on a scale that exceeds that of the individual operating unit. Furthermore, running a multiunit organization allows one to develop standardized procedures in patient records, accounting, and the like, and to make comparison between units. For these reasons, as a *chain* expands, it may exhibit economies of scale, at least up to a point.

5.7 EMPIRICAL ESTIMATION OF COST CURVES

Average or per unit cost is a convenient and accessible summary of a producer's performance. To obtain the average cost at any level of output, divide TC by Q. Given this convenient measure of performance, it is natural that analysts would use it to make comparisons of providers who produce roughly the same product but at different levels. Our simple, unqualified, short-run hypothesis would lead us to expect a U-shaped relation between average cost and output. However, inter-producer comparisions are fraught with complications.

Quality, case mix, and technology differences among producing units may make comparisons difficult. For these, as well as other reasons cited in Section 5.3, producers may be operating on different cost curves. This is shown in Figure 5–5 where ATC_1 is the average short-run cost curve of a producer under a given set of conditions. With reference to producer 1, producer 2 may be producing a higher-quality product or serving patients with a more severe case mix, but with the same amounts of *fixed* inputs, and so its cost curve would be ATC_2. ATC_2 would be above ATC_1 at all levels of output. To identify the shape of the short-run cost curve, one must control for factors that shift the curve. Assume, for example, that producer 1's cost–output point is at x, and 2's is at v. Without knowing how the producers' qualities and other factors differed, one would not know if points x and v are on the same curve or on different curves.

In the estimation of long-run cost curves, one encounters even greater difficulties. Let us say that producer 3 has a more capital–intensive operation than producers 1 or 2 in that producer 3 has invested more heavily in capital equipment to gain economies from automation. Also assume that the quality and case mix of producer 3 are similar to those of producer 1. The true long-run cost curve for the industry (assuming that these are the only two scales of operations available) is ATC_1 up to point t in Figure 5–5 and ATC_3 for scales of output above and beyond point t. But when we start out to estimate this curve, we do not know this. In the

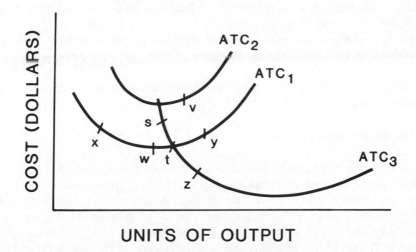

UNITS OF OUTPUT

Figure 5–5 Identifying points on the *ATC* curve. When data are gathered from producers on their average total costs at various output levels, care must be taken in interpreting these points. Data points collected from different producers may be on similar *ATC* curves (such as *x*, *w*, *t*, and *y*) or on different *ATC* curves (such as *v* and *y*). The clue to which is more likely lies in identifying extraneous circumstances (other than output) that might have caused producers to operate on different curves. These circumstances, if identified, would lead us to conclude whether pairs such as *w* and *z* or *w* and *y* are on different or similar curves. The circumstances that shift the cost curve (or lead to different cost curves) include differences in input prices, quality of output, and capital equipment.

---

data that are usually available for making such comparisons, we have only one observation from each producer. This observation tells us, for example, that producer 1 is producing at 1,000 units of output with an *ATC* of $50; producer 2 is producing at 1,200 units with an *ATC* of $80; and so on. (We may, of course, also have some information on some of the operating characteristics of each producer.) With this information, we have only one point on each producer's cost curve, but this is not enough information to tell us where on the cost curve each producer is operating.

If, for example, producer 1 is producing at point *x* and producer 3 at point *z*, then both are on the long-run cost curve, and an estimation of a long-run cost curve with points such as these will give us a reasonably accurate picture of what the long-run cost curve looks like. But there is no reason why we should be so lucky. Producer 1 could well be producing at a high capacity level, such as point *y*, and producer 3 could be at a low capacity level, such as point *s*. While both are on their *short-run* curves, neither is on its long-run curve. We would have no way of knowing this;

and if we assumed that we were estimating a long-run curve, we would end up with biased results.

In fact, where on its cost curve each producer is producing deals with the question of supply. This deals with the producer's goals or objectives as well as the conditions underlying costs and revenues, which is the topic of Chapter 6. We now present brief summaries of empirical evidence on producer cost curves for several health-related activities.

5.7.1 Physicians' Practices

Group practice in medicine has occasionally been held out as an institution that should yield considerable economies of scale and thus, if encouraged, should help in raising output at moderate increases in total costs. Since a fairly large number of group practices are in operation, it appears that the proposition of falling average costs might be easy to test. However, because of considerable variation among types of practices, difficulties in output measurements, and difficulties in gathering appropriate data, only tentative answers to this issue have been obtained. The first statistical analysis was made from data collected on solo and group practices in the field of internal medicine (Bailey, 1968), cast in physical rather than cost terms. Because the study compared practices in the same field, it circumvented problems such as different production techniques. The data collected showed that the average volume of services provided per physician, adjusted for the type of visit such as routine visit, annual examination, or complete examination, was greater for solo practices than for physicians working in groups. Although the sample size was small, it cast some doubt on the "obvious" economies of scale argument.

There are several reasons why this finding may not be so surprising. First, the technology generally used in internal medicine is such that the gains from task specialization and the use of capital-intensive techniques may be achieved at a low level of output. For the tasks involved in operating a practice of internal medicine, the *ATC* curve may reach a lower point at a scale of output supportable by one practitioner. Second, an incentive factor may be at work when several practitioners combine in a group practice that shifts the *ATC* curve upward when the group is formed. This factor arises when the members of the practice share revenues and costs; when this sharing occurs, the revenues that any single member of the group generates and the costs that he or she incurs are shared and borne by *all* the members. The individual member of the group does not personally incur the entire burden of the costs generated. Because of reduced burden, the individual physician can make a heavier use of nurses' time and of equipment while feeling less impact than in a solo practice. It is hypothesized that under these cost-sharing arrangements each physician in the group would generate more costs than in a solo practice; the cost curve for a group practice will then be higher than for a solo one.

Furthermore, the larger the group, the higher will be the cost curve *due to this factor alone* (there may be additional offsetting influences other than this incentive factor; see Scheffler, 1975).

Another study analyzed interpractice variations in staff salary costs with scale of output, measured as office visits, for a sample of single-specialty practices, although not all of the same specialty (Newhouse, 1973). The presence of cost sharing was found to shift the cost curve upward for group practices. Furthermore, after adjusting for this incentive factor, the cost curve was found to exhibit economies of scale, indicating that scale economies do exist either among practices with no cost sharing or with some cost sharing, each taken separately. Because of the small sample and the inattention paid to case mix and technology differences among practices caused by specialty differences, the results are more suggestive than conclusive.

5.7.2 Hospital Marginal Costs

The importance of the topic of hospital marginal cost is related to the objective of reimbursing hospitals for the extra resources they incur when their volumes change. If a hospital is being reimbursed at its level of existing costs in 1986 and its admissions increase by 5 percent, its additional costs may be greater than, equal to, or less than 5 percent. If the hospital were reimbursed by an additional 5 percent (ignoring inflation) to cover the volume differential and actual costs went up by 3 percent, the hospital would incur a windfall gain. On the other hand, the hospital would lose out if its costs increased by 10 percent.

The concept that is often used to measure marginal cost variation is the ratio of marginal to average costs (called M/A). Recall (Section 5.3) that if M is greater than A (or $M/A > 1$) then average cost will increase. For example, beginning from an initial output level of 1,000 admissions and an average cost of $200 per case, if output expands by 5 percent (50 admissions) and M is $220, then M/A is 1.1. Expansion has raised average cost; and if the hospital were reimbursed for the additional cases at $200 per case, it would incur a loss. If the hospital were reimbursed on the basis of its prior year's costs plus the marginal cost of its additional cases, it would be fully reimbursed.

This problem has arisen in a number of instances. During the early 1970s when price controls were set on hospital revenues, allowable revenues were set at the previous year's revenue levels, plus an inflation factor, plus a volume adjustment based on estimates of M/A (Lipscomb, Raskin, and Eichenholz, 1978). In the Finger Lakes region of New York State, a regional reimbursement experiment was set up by which hospitals were reimbursed based on a base year cost, plus an inflation factor, plus a volume adjustment that assumed that the value of M/A was 0.4 for inpatient care and 0.6 for outpatient care (Farnand, Jacobs, and Dickson, 1986). And, currently, under Medicare regulations, hospitals are given extra reimbursement for cases in a particular diagnostic group whose length of stay or costs are outside diagnostic limits (*outliers*). The additional reimbursement is based on a value of M/A for the extra days of 0.6.

One way of estimating hospital marginal cost is to take short-term (e.g., monthly) values of operating costs and volume for a given hospital over a period (2 to 3 years) and find the average variation in costs with a given variation in output. Another way is to relate variations in costs and outputs across hospitals. The former method will probably give a more accurate estimate than the latter of short-run marginal cost, but there are difficulties even with it. Among these are that the cost levels of inputs must be adjusted for (assuming they have changed) and that capital equipment and operating techniques must remain the same throughout the study period or the hospital will have moved from one short-run cost curve to another.

In addition, the marginal cost will depend on the measure of output (e.g., whether it is length of stay or by admission). It will vary with the amount of the volume adjustment (e.g., 2 or 5 percent) and how permanent the volume change is taken to be by the hospital administrator. For a volume increase that is small or short-lived, the administrator may decide to tax existing resources for a time, rather than immediately expanding and hence raising marginal cost. The estimate of M under these circumstances would appear to be lower than if the administrator responded more automatically.

For the preceding reasons, there is no accepted measure of the true short-run value of M/A (Lave and Lave, 1984). Estimates range from roughly 0.2 to 0.6, but remember that these will vary depending on a number of factors (Friedman and Pauly, 1983).

5.7.3 Hospital Scale Economies

A large number of studies have examined the possible existence of hospital scale economies, with very mixed results (Berki, 1972). Early studies identified scale economies for hospitals, but subsequent works have not exhibited any noticeable economies (Lave and Lave, 1984). There is an explanation for the differences in findings.

As discussed earlier, the typical hospital is an organization with a complex case mix and a large number of different services. Each service has its own cost–output relation, which may exhibit economies of scale. The *scope* of services is greater, the larger the hospital (Berry, 1973). But hospitals may have more varied case types as they grow larger, and so some specific services (e.g., cobalt therapy) that are devoted to specific case types may, in themselves, be operated at low capacity and high cost. A multiproduct hospital can be quite large, yet can have a number of specific services that are operating with considerable excess capacity (Finkler, 1979). As a result, as the overall hospital unit expands, it may take on a more complex scope of services; but because many of the services may not be utilized at a low-cost, high-capacity level, overall the larger hospitals may not exhibit lower-cost operations than smaller hospitals.

A recent study (Hornbrook and Monheit, 1985), which incorporated both case-mix and service-scope variables to investigate economies of scale, found no scale economies at the hospital level. But a number of studies of individual services, such as open-heart surgery facilities, CT scanners, therapeutic radiology facilities, and hospital laundries, have found evidence of scale economies (Gregory, 1976–1977; McGregor and Pelletier, 1978; Finkler, 1979; Schwartz and Joskow, 1980). Thus, while individual services may exhibit considerable scale economies, when operated together but at low-capacity levels, they may offer the appearance that large units are no more economical to operate than are small ones.

REFERENCES

Production of Medical Care

Cromwell, J. (1974). Hospital productivity trends in short-term general non-teaching hospitals. *Inquiry, 11*, 181–187.

Goldfarb, M., Hornbrook, M., & Rafferty, J. (1980). Behavior of the multiproduct firm. *Medical Care, 18*, 185–201.

Lewit, E.M., Bentkover, J., Bentkover, S.H., et al. (1980). A comparison of surgical assisting in a prepaid group practice. *Medical Care, 18*, 916–929.

Reinhardt, U. (1972). A production function for physicians' services. *Review of Economics and Statistics, 54*, 55–66.

———— (1973). Manpower substitution and productivity in medical practice. *Health Services Research, 7*, 200–277.

———— (1973). Proposed changes in the organization of health care delivery. *Milbank Memorial Fund Quarterly, 51*, 169–222.

Ruchlin, H.S., & Leveson, I. (1974). Measuring hospital productivity. *Health Services Research, 9*, 308–323.

Scheffler, R.M. (1975). Further consideration on the economics of group practice. *Journal of Human Resources, 10*, 258–263.

————, & Kushman, J.F. (1977). A production function for dental services. *Social and Economic Journal, 44*, 25–35.

Costs: Hospitals

Barer, M. (1982). Case mix adjustment in hospital cost analysis. *Journal of Health Economics, 1*, 53–80.

Bays, C. (1980). Specification error in the estimation of hospital cost functions. *Review of Economics and Statistics, 62*, 302–305.

Berki, S. (1972). *Hospital economics*. Lexington, MA: D.C. Heath Co.

Berry, R.E. (1973). On grouping hospitals for economic analysis. *Inquiry, 10*, 5–12.

Cowing, T.G., & Holtmann, A.G. (1983). Multiproduct short-run hospital cost functions. *Southern Economic Journal, 49,* 637–653.

Evans, R.G. (1971). "Behavioural" cost functions for hospitals. *Canadian Journal of Economics, 4,* 198–215.

Farnand, L.J., Jacobs, P., & Dickson, W.M. (1986). An evaluation of a program to regulate rural hospital costs. *Inquiry, 23,* 200–208.

Feldstein, P. (1961). *An empirical investigation of the marginal cost of hospital services.* University of Chicago Graduate Program in Hospital Administration.

Finkler, S.A. (1979). Cost effectiveness of regionalization: The heart surgery example. *Inquiry, 16,* 264–270.

——— (1979). On the shape of the hospital industry long run average cost function. *Health Services Research, 14,* 281–289.

Fraser, R.D. (1971). *Canadian hospital costs and efficiency.* Ottawa, Ontario: Economic Council of Canada.

Friedman, B., & Pauly, M.V. (1983). A new approach to hospital cost functions and some issues in revenue regulation. *Health Care Financing Review, 4,* 105–114.

Gregory, D.D. (1976–1977). Some evidence on the economic aspects of hospital cooperative ventures. *Journal of Economics and Business, 29,* 59–64.

Horn, S.D., Sharkey, P.D., Chambers, A.F., & Horn, R.A. (1985). Severity of illness within DRG's: Impact on prospective payment. *American Journal of Public Health, 75,* 1195–1199.

Hornbrook, M.C., & Monheit, A.C. (1985). The contribution of case mix severity to the hospital cost–output relation. *Inquiry, 22,* 259–271.

Kralewski, J.E., Dowd, B., Pitt, L., et al. (1984). Effects of contract management on hospital performance. *Health Services Research, 19,* 479–498.

Lave, J., & Lave, L.B. (1984). Hospital cost functions. *Annual Review of Public Health, 5,* 193–213.

Lee, M.L., & Wallace, R.L. (1972). Problems in estimating multiproduct hospital cost functions. *Western Economic Journal, 11,* 350–363.

Lipscomb, J., Raskin, I.E., & Eichenholz, J. (1978). The use of marginal cost estimates in hospital cost-containment policy. In M. Zubkoff, I.E. Raskin, & R.S. Hanft (Eds.), *Hospital cost containment* (pp. 514–537). New York: Watson Publishing International.

McGregor, M., & Pelletier, G. (1978). Planning of specialized health facilities: Size vs cost and effectiveness in heart surgery. *New England Journal of Medicine, 299,* 179–181.

Schwartz, W., & Joskow, P. (1980). Duplicated hospital facilities. *New England Journal of Medicine, 303,* 1449–1457.

Sloan, F.A., Perrin, J.M., & Valvona, J. (1985). The teaching hospital's growing surgical caseload. *Journal of the American Medical Association, 254,* 376–382.

Costs: Medical Practice

Bailey, R.M. (1968). A comparison of internists in solo and fee-for-service group practice. *Bulletin of the New York Academy of Medicine* (2nd. Ser.) *44,* 1293–1303.

——— (1970). Economies of scale in medical practice. In H. Klarman (Ed.), *Empirical studies in health economics* (pp. 255–273). Baltimore, MD: Johns Hopkins University Press.

Frech, H.E., & Ginsburg, P.B. (1974). Optimal scale in medical practice. *Journal of Business, 47,* 23–36.

Newhouse, J.P. (1973). The economics of group practice. *Journal of Human Resources, 8,* 37–56.

Rossiter, L.F. (1984). Prospects for medical group practice under competition. *Medical Care, 22*, (1), 84–92.

Costs: Other Areas

Anderson, D.L. (1976). Public sector output measurement problems: The case of the hospital clinical laboratory. *Inquiry, 13*, 71–79.

Bishop, C.E. (1980). Nursing home cost studies and reimbursement issues. *Health Care Financing Review, 1* (4), 47–65.

——— (1983). Nursing home cost studies. *Health Services Research, 18*, 382–386.

Blair, R.D., Ginsburg, P.B., & Vogel, R.J. (1975). Blue Cross–Blue Shield administrative costs. *Economic Inquiry, 13*, 237–251.

———, Jackson, J.R., & Vogel, R.J. (1975). Economies of scale in the administration of health insurance. *Review of Economics and Statistics, 57*, 185–189.

Hay, J.W., & Mandes, G. (1984). Home health care cost-function analysis. *Health Care Financing Review, 5* (3), 111–116.

Schlenker, R.E., & Shaughnessy, P.W. (1984). Case mix, quality, and cost relationships in Colorado nursing homes. *Home Care Financing Review, 6* (2), 61–71.

Ullman, S.G. (1984). Cost analysis and facility reimbursement in the long-term health care industry. *Health Services Research, 19*, 83–102.

Chapter 6

Behavior of Supply

6.1 INTRODUCTION

This chapter is concerned with the determinants of the quantity and quality of output of various health-related products. Our approach is framed in terms of the behavior of the organizations supplying these products; it provides hypotheses about what causes suppliers to produce particular quantities and qualities of output. These hypotheses are formulated in terms of models of supplier behavior. They incorporate and relate the key causes of supplier behavior, seeking to isolate the direction in which individual factors cause supply to move, while also allowing us to concurrently keep in mind other factors that may also be influencing supply movements.

In presenting these hypotheses about supply behavior, a distinction is made between the supply of a single producer and that of all producers in the market, that is, the difference between individual and market supply. The importance of this distinction becomes clearer in Chapter 7 when market behavior is discussed.

In this chapter no single model of supplier behavior is presented as the appropriate one to use in explaining movements in supply. The subject is complex, and our models offer suggestive rather than definitive answers. In particular, health care providers differ with regard to type of organization. Some organizations, such as proprietary-owned hospitals and nursing homes and physicians' practices, are profit-seeking institutions. Others, such as Blue Cross, voluntary hospitals, the Red Cross and independent blood banks, and philanthropic organizations such as the March of Dimes and the American Heart Association are nonprofit agencies. This means that their "owners" (referred to as governors or trustees) can neither appropriate for themselves any profits that the organization might make nor sell the rights to the assets of the organization for personal gain. Separate hypotheses are discussed for both types of organizations.

In this chapter a basic model of an individual profit-seeking supplier is first developed, followed by a model of the market supply behavior for a group of such firms. Because profit-seeking and nonprofit organizations are not the same types of organizations, the following three sections focus on the effects that the nonprofit organizational form has on the behavior of the nonprofit organization. Much disagreement exists over the analysis of nonprofit agency behavior. As a result, several alternative hypotheses about nonprofit agency behavior need to be presented. In Section 6.4 the nonprofit agency is examined as if it were an output maximizing agency. Section 6.5 extends this analysis to incorporate the role of the agency in producing quality as well as quantity output. Also in Section 6.5, the voluntary hospital, a peculiar form of nonprofit organization, is introduced in terms of its organizational structure. Section 6.6 develops a model in which the nonprofit agency is regarded as an instrument that is used to the benefit of its managers. In Section 6.7 another key economic variable, the method of financing the organization's activities, that can influence the output of the organization is introduced. Reimbursement plans for doctors, hospitals, and health maintenance organizations are analyzed with regard to the manner in which they influence the economic behavior of the various suppliers.

6.2 A MODEL OF SUPPLY BEHAVIOR OF AN INDIVIDUAL PROFIT-MAKING AGENCY

The assumptions of our supply model fall into three categories: revenue and cost assumptions and assumptions about the objectives of the organization. Our analysis will be conducted using an example of a laboratory owned by a pathologist that produces blood tests of a given quality.

With regard to revenue assumptions, revenue can come from two sources: (1) reimbursement for patient services (termed patient or *earned* revenue) and (2) other sources (grants, endowment funds, and other non-patient-related sources). We will initially assume that all revenues are from the former source; that is, nonpatient revenues are zero. This assumption will be altered later in the analysis.

With regard to patient revenues, we make the assumption that the organization is a ''price-taker,'' that is, a supplier that has no influence over the price of its output. This may be because the price is set by an independent, administrative agency over which the supplier has no influence or because the organization is operating in a competitive situation in which the best price it can get for its product is the price prevailing in the market. Higher prices in a highly competitive market will drive patients elsewhere, and lower prices will not enable the supplier to achieve its goal. The setting of price by market forces is discussed in Chapter 7. For the individual supplier in this section, it is taken as given.

Specifically, we will assume that the lab receives $12 for each test performed. Its marginal revenue (*MR*), defined as the addition to total revenue (*TR*) for one additional unit of output produced and sold ($\Delta TR/\Delta Q$), is 12. Total and marginal revenues are shown in Table 6–1, columns 11 and 12, for output levels from 0 to 10.

We assume that there are both fixed and variable costs. Our assumption regarding fixed costs is that the lab spends $7 monthly on equipment rental and mortgage payments; in addition, we assume that the pathologist/owner could earn a total of $5 if he or she worked elsewhere. This sum is at the same time a fixed cost and opportunity cost. That is, it incorporates a "normal" return to the owner's assets and efforts. The pathologist, once his or her time is committed to work in the lab for the period, gives up $5 per period. Total fixed costs are thus $12, and being fixed these do not vary as output changes. This is shown as column 2 in Table 6–1; the associated average costs (average fixed costs) are shown in column 5.

Variable factors are assumed to be employed in a least-cost manner such that the total minimum variable costs for operating the lab at each level of output are as shown in Table 6–1, column 3. The assumed variable cost–output relation is one of initially falling and subsequently rising average variable costs (column 6) and eventually rising marginal costs (column 8). Total cost figures, which are the sum of fixed and variable costs, are shown in columns 4 and 7 for total and average values.

These dollar figures are approximated in Figures 6–1A for total values and 6–1B for marginal revenue (*MR*), marginal cost (*MC*), and average total cost (*ATC*). Note that the *TR* curve rises at a rate of $12 per blood test, and that *MR* is constant at $12; these are merely two different ways of saying the same thing; that is, the revenue per unit of output sold is fixed at $12. This is a concrete expression of our assumption that suppliers are "price takers." Cost curves are shaped as hypothesized in Chapter 5. Note that we have drawn the curves as smooth functions, whereas in our numerical example the values jump in discrete steps. This is simply for geometric convenience.

Having specified our assumptions about revenue and cost, and remembering that we are analyzing the behavior of a profit-making organizational unit (hereafter referred to as ABC Labs), we are now in a position to answer the question that underlies our analysis: What quantity of output will be supplied? Many levels of output can be chosen by ABC Labs. It is our task to present a hypothesis that will enable us to predict which quantity will be chosen and how this quantity will vary when some of the underlying variables in our model, prices and costs, themselves vary.

Since ABC Labs is a profit-making organization, it seems reasonable to assume that its objective is to maximize profits. While this may not be absolutely realistic (ABC Labs may veer from this path somewhat), it nevertheless presents us with a

Table 6–1 Illustrative Data on Relation of Revenue, Costs, and Profits to Output

(1) Quality of Tests	(2) Total Fixed Costs (TFC)	(3) Total Variable Costs (TVC)	(4) Total Costs (TC)	(5) Average Fixed Costs (TFC/Q)	(6) Average Variable Costs (TVC/Q)	(7) Average Total Costs (TC/Q)	(8) Marginal Costs TC/Q	(9) Total Earned Revenue (P × Q)	(10) Total Grants	(11) Total Revenue	(12) Marginal Revenue (ΔTR/ΔQ)	(13) Profits (TR − TC)
0	12	0	12									
1	12	6.75	18.75	12	6.75	18.75	6.75	12	0	12	12	− 6.75
2	12	10.50	22.50	6	5.25	11.25	3.75	24	0	24	12	1.50
3	12	13.25	25.25	4	4.42	8.42	2.75	36	0	36	12	10.75
4	12	17.00	29.00	3	4.25	7.25	3.75	48	0	48	12	19.00
5	12	23.75	35.75	2.4	4.75	7.15	6.75	60	0	60	12	24.25
6	12	35.50	47.50	2	5.92	7.92	11.75	72	0	72	12	24.50
7	12	54.25	66.25	1.7	7.75	9.46	18.75	84	0	84	12	17.75
8	12	82.00	94.00	1.5	10.25	11.75	27.75	96	0	96	12	2.00
9	12	120.75	132.75	1.33	13.42	14.75	38.75	108	0	108	12	20.75
10	12	172.50	184.50	1.20	17.25	18.45	51.75	120	0	120	12	60.50

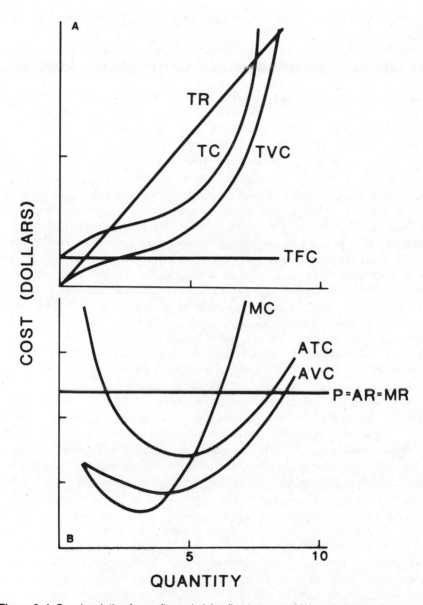

Figure 6–1 Supply relation for profit maximizing firm in terms of (A) total costs and revenues and (B) average and marginal costs and revenues. In (A), the supplier produces where total profits, equal to the difference between total revenue (*TR*) and total cost (*TC*), are at a maximum. In (B), the same conclusion can be derived in marginal terms. Here the profit-maximizing point is where *MR* = *MC*. In the diagram, since price per unit is constant, price and *MR* are the same thing.

working hypothesis, a first approximation, that will allow us to achieve specific, testable conclusions.

Referring to Table 6–1, we can now derive from our model a specific quantity of output that achieves the profit-maximizing objective for ABC Labs: profits are at a maximum of six units of output. Here they amount to $24.50. The reasoning used to obtain this conclusion can best be presented in marginal terms. Say that ABC Labs was initially supplying four units of output. Profits here, given by revenue and cost conditions, equal $19. If ABC Labs produces and sells one more test, additional revenue will be $12 (i.e., $MR = \$12$); the additional costs of production (MC) will be $6.75. The additional profit obtained by expanding output from four to five tests will be $5.25, bringing total profits to a new level of $24.25. ABC Labs, being profit maximizers, would expand production to at least five units. In fact, they will move beyond this amount because profits can be further increased by doing so. The best ABC Labs can do at the given price with their existing cost conditions is to produce six units of output for which their profit level will be $24.50. Expanding beyond six units still results in positive profits for awhile, but these profits would not be as great as at the level of six units of output. The conclusion of our model is that a profit-maximizing firm will expand production as long as MR exceeds MC by so doing. If we were dealing with smooth, continuous changes, our conclusion expressed in these terms would be that the profit-maximizing firm will expand output up to the point at which $MR = MC$, as long as MC is rising with output. At this point the firm is maximizing its profits, and so the quantity where $MC = MR$ is the supply position of the firm we are seeking.

This conclusion is shown diagrammatically in Figures 6–1a and 6–1b. In Figure 6–1a, profits at each level of output are shown in total terms as the vertical distance between total revenue and total cost at that level of output. Since profits are defined as $TR - TC$, then, where this vertical distance is at a maximum, profits are also at a maximum. This is at six units of output (allowing for small variations because we are dealing with continuous curves). In Figure 6–1b the same conclusion is drawn using marginal analysis. Here the point where $MR = MC$ is the profit-maximizing quantity, that is, the quantity that will be supplied. A movement in quantity supplied in either direction would detract from total profits and so would not be consistent with the profit-maximizing objective.

The first conclusion of our model, then, is that, given revenue (i.e., price) and cost conditions and given the profit-maximizing objective, a profit-maximizing firm will produce at the quantity where $MC = MR$. Using this information, we can now derive a supply curve or schedule that shows what the quantity supplied will be at *different* prices. This analysis is shown geometrically in Figure 6–2. If the price rises from $12 to $19, the lab will add to its profits by expanding output to a seventh unit, because, even though the cost of this unit is higher, the higher extra revenue will make it profitable to expand output. The same reasoning applies to additional price increases: higher prices will bring forth greater quantities supplied

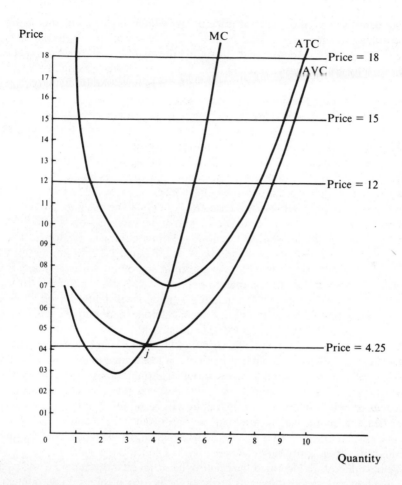

Figure 6–2 Profit-maximizing supply points at alternative prices. At each price above $4.25 the producer will maximize profits by supplying at the quantity where price = *MC*. If the price is at $4.25, the producer will just be meeting its variable costs. At any price below this, the firm's least unprofitable supply point will result in larger losses than if the firm shut down operations; the firm will not supply at any price below $4.25. Thus for prices above $4.25, the firm's supply curve and its *MC* curve are the same thing.

until $MC = MR$. The same reasoning in reverse holds for price declines, with one major exception: eventually the price could become so low that the owners of the firm would be better off, from the point of view of their profits (or losses), to shut down operations and produce nothing. For all prices below this level (represented by point j in Figure 6–2), the quantity supplied by the firm would be zero.

The identification of the critical price below which the firm will shut down is made with reference to the variable costs of the firm. Recall that fixed costs are the same thing as "already committed" costs, while variable costs are those that can be avoided by not hiring the variable factors; total costs are the sum of the two at each output level. If the price falls sufficiently, it is possible that even at its best level of output (from the profitability standpoint) the firm will be incurring a loss. The criterion the firm would use in deciding whether or not to continue operating under such unfavorable circumstances is not the mere fact that the firm is incurring a loss; rather, it is whether the firm is minimizing its losses—is the firm doing better by continuing to operate rather than by shutting down its operations? The critical importance of variable costs comes into play here; as long as the firm is at least meeting its total variable costs, it will be breaking even and perhaps running a surplus *on its variable costs*. In this case $TR - TVC$ will be positive. Even though total profits $(TR - TVC - TFC)$ may be negative, signifying a loss, the loss is less than it would be if the firm shut down entirely. For in the case of the firm's shutting down, both TR and TVC are zero and losses would equal TFC. In sum, as long as the firm is meeting its variable costs and adding something to cover some or all fixed costs, the firm should continue to operate; in this case, its supply curve is traced out by the MC curve. The quantity supplied will be where price equals marginal cost. Should the price fall so low that at no level of output could the firm meet all its variable costs, then it should shut down.

We can now present a complete analysis of the firm's supply behavior in terms of the curves of Figure 6–2: when the price is at least equal to the lowest point on the AVC curve, so that at some level of output all variable costs will be covered, the firm will produce some output. If the price is lower than this critical minimum price, called point j in our figure, no output will be supplied. If the price is above the critical minimum level, the firm will supply output at the quantity where $MR = MC$ (i.e., where price $= MC$). The MC curve of the firm, then, is its supply curve, relating price to quantity supplied.

We have therefore identified the relation between quantity supplied and price, showing how this quantity depends on the price the firm receives. In the context of this analysis, we can make some sense of the assumption that the costs of a profit-making firm are at a minimum. It was shown in Chapter 5 that the producer has a choice of producing a given quantity of output at the lowest possible cost or above the lowest possible cost. By choosing the lowest possible cost method of production, the firm can achieve its greatest profits, since profits are defined as the difference between total revenues and total costs. If costs were above the minimum, they would cut into profits and would be contrary to the assumed goals of the firm.

6.2.1 Nonpatient Revenues

Let us now introduce a new element into our analysis, nonpatient revenues. We will introduce a particular form of unearned revenue, a grant or subsidy, that is unrelated to output. Such a grant might be received from a donor or foundation. Our analytical task is to determine how it might affect the provider's supply.

The economic meaning of a grant unrelated to output is that if output expands or contracts the grant will remain unchanged. Such a grant can be treated analytically in one of two ways, either (1) as a fixed (for all outputs) addition to revenue, or (2) as a fixed reduction from total costs (a negative fixed cost). While the rationale for the former treatment seems clear-cut, that for the latter requires some explanation. A fixed subsidy in a sense reduces by a fixed amount the total costs that the provider must meet at each output level. For operational purposes, it will have the same impact on profits. We can therefore treat it as a reduction in total costs.

Let us say that the lab received a fixed subsidy of $5. This would increase non-patient revenues in Table 6–1 by $5 at each and every level of output. Profits would also increase by $5 at each level of output. In Figure 6–1, this would appear as an upward parallel shift in the *TR* function.

What is important from a supply standpoint is that neither patient revenues (including *MR*) nor variable costs are affected. Thus, while profits are higher by $5 *at every output level*, the maximum profitability level of output is the same—at six units of output. The fixed subsidy does not affect the *most profitable* level of output; it only affects the level of profits at that and every other level of output.

The same conclusion would not hold if the subsidy were related to output. For then, as output expanded, the marginal revenue would be the additional revenue from patient sources plus the additional (output related) grant revenues. When estimating the most profitable output level, the firm would have to consider both sources of additional revenue and relate them to marginal cost.

The conclusion, then, is that a grant that is not output related, which is given to a profit-maximizing firm, will not influence the supply decisions of the firm; the firm's supply position will still be where its marginal patient revenue equals marginal cost.

6.2.2 Shifts in the Supply Curve

Our final portion of this section shows what happens to the supply curve of the firm when factors that influence the position of the *MC* curve change. In general, it is shown in Figure 6–3 that any factor that causes the *MC* curve to shift upward from MC_1 to MC_2 will amount to an inward or upward shift in the supply schedule of the firm. The quantity supplied at any price will be reduced from Q_1 to Q_2. Such shifts can occur because of higher input prices or a higher quality of product being produced, to cite two of the factors discussed in Section 5.4 that might cause the firm's cost curve to shift. In the case of a higher-quality product being produced, for example, the net result will be that a lower quantity supplied will be produced by the firm at any given price. The same reasoning in reverse holds for outward shifts in the *MC* curve. For example, an increase in the capacity of the firm to

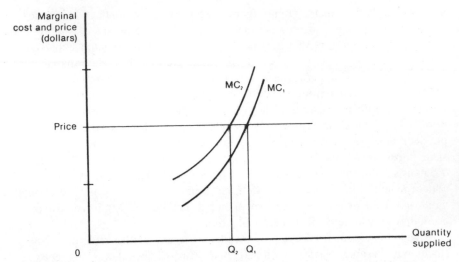

Figure 6–3 Shifts in the supply curve for a profit-maximizing supplier. An upward shift in the *MC* curve of a profit-maximizing firm will mean a lower quantity supplied at any price. In this figure, a shift from MC_1 to MC_2 means a decrease in supply. At the prices shown, quantity supplied decreases from Q_1 to Q_2.

produce output, caused by additional capital expansion, will cause the *MC* and thus the supply curve to shift outward, indicating a willingness on the part of the firm to supply more output at any given price. Such expansion is likely when the firm is operating on the downward sloping part of its long-run average cost curve. An expansion in output would allow it to move to a lower point on its LRAC curve (i.e., to a lower cost short-run curve).

6.3 MARKET SUPPLY

We now demonstrate how the analysis of individual supply movements can be extended to form a hypothesis of movements in product supply in a specific market. Our extension involves two assumptions in addition to the previous ones concerning individual supply behavior: (1) there is a set number of suppliers in the market, and (2) there are no agreements on the part of suppliers to restrict supply. The latter assumption is discussed in more detail in Chapter 7. In the present model, two groups of factors influence market supply: the number of suppliers and the factors that influence individual supplier behavior. Given the supply schedules for each supplier, the market supply schedule can be obtained once we know the number of suppliers. This is shown in Figure 6–4. Here the market is assumed to consist of three suppliers: ABC Labs, XYZ Labs, and GHI Labs. Each has a given supply schedule as shown in the figure. XYZ Labs supplies 5 tests at $1, 10 tests at $1.50, 15 at $2, and so on. GHI Labs supplies 3, 6, and 9 tests at these prices,

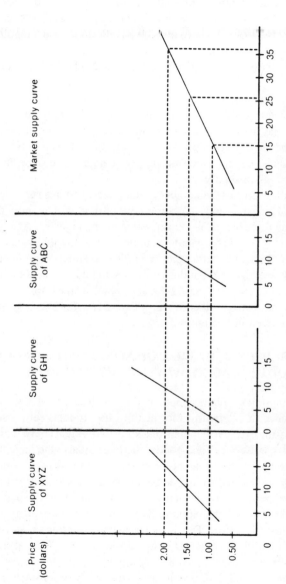

Figure 6-4 Derivation of market supply curve from individual supply curves. The market supply curve shows quantity supplied by all firms supplying the product to the market at each price. It is obtained by summing individual suppliers' quantities at each price.

respectively. And ABC Labs supplies 6, 9, and 12 tests. Given these schedules and the fact that these three labs are the only ones in the market, the market supply curve is the sum of these individual supply curves at each price. At $1, market supply is 14 (5 + 3 + 6) tests; at $1.50, 25 tests are supplied, and at $2, 36 tests are supplied. The market supply curve is shown as the horizontal sum of all individual supply curves. Given price, our model predicts the quantity that will be supplied in the market.

The market supply will shift outward (to the right) (1) if, given the number of producers, any factors cause the individual supply curves to shift outward, and (2) if the number of suppliers increases. In either or both cases, more will be supplied at any given price. Our model has enabled us to classify these influences and separate their effects on supply changes. The same analysis can be made for reductions in supply.

With regard to the number of suppliers, just as profits are the motivating force behind an expansion (or contraction) of output of an individual firm, so are they a driving force behind new firms entering the industry. At any particular time, there are a number of prospective suppliers who potentially can acquire the techniques and equipment to set up their own firm to supply a product (e.g., blood tests). If profits are high in the industry, they will be motivated to do so and thus will shift the supply curve to the right. Of course, it must not be discounted that existing firms, protective of their high profits, may act to keep potential suppliers out. This is discussed in Section 8.3.

6.4 SUPPLY BEHAVIOR OF NONPROFIT AGENCIES: THE OUTPUT MAXIMIZATION HYPOTHESIS

Nonprofit suppliers abound in the health care field. One reason appears to be the existence of externalities for health care products (discussed in Section 4.3). To satisfy the external demands that some individuals have for others' consumption of health care services and goods, the individuals who have these external demands may form nonprofit agencies whose purpose is to provide these services to the needy (as viewed by the demanders), usually on a less-than-cost basis. Health-related philanthropies, such as the American Heart Association, give away educational services that are financed by donors who have an external demand for others to consume them. The Red Cross blood program exists because there is a sufficiently large external demand on the part of blood donors for the health of those in need of transfusions. Voluntary hospitals were, until recently, providing free and subsidized hospital care to the needy in substantial amounts; this care was financed largely through philanthropic donations, which can be regarded as payments to satisfy the donors' external demands for the care of the needy. Public health departments represent services in which external demands for health care are satisfied through government rather than voluntary agencies.

There are, no doubt, other reasons for the formation of nonprofit agencies; for example, these agencies may be formed as "captive" agencies of other nonprofit groups. During the 1930s and 1940s, Blue Cross plans began under the auspices of nonprofit hospitals to ensure that hospitals were paid. The scope of our inquiry does not ask under what conditions health service agencies become organized on a voluntary basis (see Culyer, 1971). Rather, the existence of this type of organization is a given and we examine the supply behavior of these agencies once they are formed.

To ensure that the services offered by the nonprofit agency are provided in a reasonable manner, a board of trustees is formed. The members of such boards cannot gain direct financial benefits from the organization either in the form of appropriating profits or realizing the value from the sale of the enterprise; furthermore, they are frequently banned from indirect gains, such as having their law firm provide legal services to the organization. The board of trustees is primarily responsible for setting organizational policies, but many of their responsibilities are delegated to a full-time, salaried administrative staff. The actual responsibilities of each, the trustees and the staff, and thus the control of the supply decisions will vary from organization to organization.

Several approaches can be taken to form hypotheses about the supply behavior of nonprofit agencies. One approach is to regard the trustees as being in charge. Following this approach, we would hypothesize about the goals the trustees are likely to pursue and develop a model of the organization that incorporates these hypothesized goals. Another approach is to regard the salaried executives as the people who set the key policies, to make hypotheses about their behavior, and to develop a model of organizational supply based on their goals. No doubt a real nonprofit firm would contain some of each hypothesis. But to keep our analysis simple, we will examine each hypothesis separately. We begin with the trustee-dominance model. We will assume that the trustees' objective is to maximize the output of the agency, that is, to carry out their mandate to the fullest extent possible.

Now we will assume that our lab was initially financed by a public-spirited benefactor who had an external demand for others having their blood analyzed. Cost and revenue conditions are the same as in the previous example, with the exception that now the pathologist is under contract and receives an explicit payment of $5 per month for his or her services. From the point of view of the lab, once the contractual commitment is made, this is a fixed cost, and so total fixed costs of the laboratory are still $12. The quality of the product is the same as before and is constant. Revenues in our example are still $12 per test, but now the reimbursement may be made by a third party. (Reimbursements may be collected through individual donations or from a united agency.) The major difference in the operation of the lab is that now it seeks to maximize output rather than profits.

The conclusions of such a model are that, since revenues come only from reimbursements for services, output will be expanded to the point where the firm just breaks even, that is where $TR = TC$. In Table 6–1, given a price of \$12, output will be expanded to eight units. In Figure 6–1a the break-even point at eight units of output is shown in total terms. In Figure 6–1b the agency's operating point is where price per unit equals average total cost. The firm just covers costs for all units when it operates at this level.

Given our assumptions, output for a profit-making agency will be lower than that for a nonprofit agency that behaves as we have hypothesized (i.e., maximizing output). The supply curve for an output-maximizing agency is its ATC curve for prices above the minimum point on the ATC. If revenues do not meet at least this minimum point, the firm runs a deficit and must raise the funds from nonrevenue sources. For the moment we will assume that nonpatient revenues are zero and that the firm has no reserves to meet a deficit. If it does not meet *all* its liabilities, it will go out of business.

As long as price is above the minimum point on the ATC curve, the supply curve of the nonprofit agency that maximizes output is the ATC curve. As price rises, so will supply. Any factor that shifts the ATC curve *downward* (lower unit costs at any level of output) will cause output to increase at any price.

The response of a quantity-maximizing nonprofit firm to a fixed subsidy is very different from that of a profit-maximizing firm. Recall (Section 6.2.2) that a fixed subsidy will not influence a profit-maximizer's supply. Let us assume that our output-maximizing lab receives a \$25 subsidy from a donor, which is unrelated to output. Analytically, we can treat this as an overall increase in total revenues or as an overall reduction in total costs (and a reduction in average fixed costs of $\$25/Q$). In the former case, the analysis in Table 6–1 would be altered to show TR and profits higher at *every* level of output by \$25. Whereas, formerly, the output-maximizing output level was 8, with the subsidy output level 9 will show an *overall* (operating and nonoperating) profit of \$2.25 (\$25 − \$22.75). The lab would be in the red at output level 10, but it could now meet all its costs at level 9, and this is where it would maximize output (subject to the fact that it must break even).

Graphically, treating the fixed subsidy as a reduction in fixed costs, it would appear as a downward shift in AFC and also ATC (because AFC is part of ATC). This would thus appear as an outward shift in the firm's supply curve, ATC. The conclusion in either case is the same: a non-output-related grant *will* shift the supply curve of the output-maximizing firm and thus will lead to increased output. In this respect, the output-maximizing firm is very unlike the profit-maximizing firm.

The market supply analysis in the case of nonprofit organizations is somewhat more complicated than in the case of profit-seeking organizations. If we make the assumption that each separate nonprofit supplier has a vested interest in providing output to the needy population, the market supply curve will be made up of the sum of what all the individual suppliers would be willing to supply at each price or reimbursement rate. That is, the market supply curve is the sum of the individual producers' supply curves for prices above the minimum *ATC*. Individual nonprofit suppliers might develop vested interests in having their firms supply the output if trustees developed some sense of identification with separate organizations; the mission of each separate organization would then be their cause.

However, if this competitive sense did not develop among the nonprofit suppliers, trustees would not care which organization supplied the output to the needy, as long as it was supplied by someone. In this situation, market supply would consist of a far more complicated set of arrangements in which trustees would pull their organizations out of the market when other organizations supplying the same product appeared. We will assume that in the situation here organizational pride will develop to be the "appropriate" market supply model.

6.5 SUPPLY DECISIONS INVOLVING QUALITY

Until now we have assumed that quality of output was held constant and thus did not enter the supply decision. In fact, quality is an extremely important supply variable for suppliers. In particular, in the hospital field it has frequently been asserted that hospitals seek to supply output of the highest quality. In this section a model is developed to incorporate quality of care into the supply picture.

To understand the bias of hospitals toward high-quality supply, it is necessary to examine the unusual management structure of the nonprofit hospital. Like other nonprofit agencies, the nonprofit hospital includes a board of trustees and a group of salaried administrators. In the hospital, however, doctors have a special relation; they are in charge of the medical activities of the hospital and yet, for the most part, they are unsalaried staff members. Because their services are so crucial, indeed the hospital's activities revolve around them, doctors have enormous influence over hospital supply decisions. As a result of this influence, hospital supply policies are set by an informal arrangement between doctors and trustees. This type of arrangement has been termed a *management triangle*, and hospital activities are the result of directives (sometimes conflicting) of two lines of authority, medical and administrative. In particular, the medical influence in the decision-making process has been cited as being responsible for the bias toward quality in hospital objectives, since doctors benefit considerably from high-quality inputs.

A supply model that incorporates this quality bias can be derived from the previous analysis. Assume a given level of reimbursement, say $200 per patient day. This is shown in Figure 6–5. *ATC* curves are drawn for three different levels of quality of service; each higher level of quality is produced with more resources. ATC_1 represents an *ATC* curve for a specific level of output of a single quality. ATC_2 and ATC_3 are similar curves for successively higher output levels.

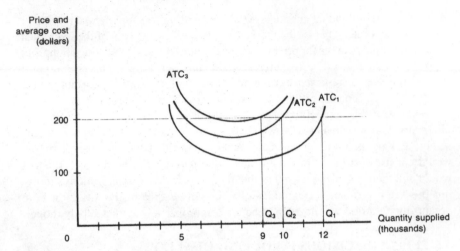

Figure 6–5 Representation of alternative quantities and qualities supplied by a nonprofit supplier. The *ATC* curves represent relations between *ATC* and output at various quality levels; ATC_3 represents the cost curve with the highest quality level, ATC_2 the intermediate level, and ATC_1 the lowest level. A nonprofit producer who maximizes quantity of output (given the quality level) will produce where the unit reimbursement rate or price equals *ATC*. At quality level 1, output will be 12. Higher quality levels will mean a reduction in the maximum output levels achievable, given the reimbursement rate.

An output-maximizing hospital will choose Q_1 (12,000) units of output if quality is given at level 1, Q_2 (10,000) units at quality level 2, and Q_3 (9,000) units at quality level 3. Indeed, a trade-off can be derived between quality and quantity of care. One can obtain more quality, but at the expense of quantity of output. This trade-off is shown in Figure 6–6, with quality of care shown on the vertical axis and quantity on the horizontal. Curve *XY* shows the maximum output that can be achieved for each quality of output, given the reimbursement rate of $200. Curve *XY* represents the constraints or the choices facing the hospital. The actual combination of quality and quantity supplied will depend on the hospital's policies. A highly quality oriented hospital will choose a quality level close to Qu_3, while an output-oriented hospital will choose a level closer to Qu_1. If the assertions about hospital goals being quality oriented are correct, it might be expected that Qu_3 would be more frequently observed. That is, of the various output combinations that the nonprofit hospital can choose, it will tend to supply higher-quality levels of care. The supply behavior of such a firm is heavily quality biased. By itself, however, this does not say that we will observe such high-quality care in the market. For it must be remembered that we are currently examining only the supply side of the market. The quality of care actually produced will be determined by what the suppliers are willing to supply and what the consumers are willing to take. Determining what output actually is produced and utilized requires that we

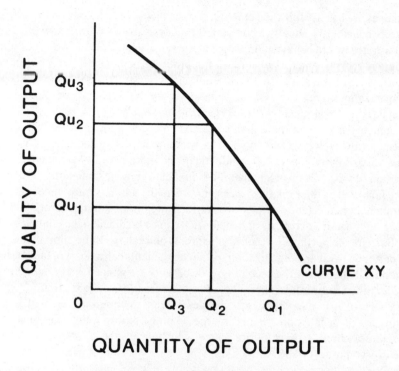

QUANTITY OF OUTPUT

Figure 6–6 Representation of trade-off between quality and quantity. Based on Figure 6–5, for any given reimbursement rate, a higher quality level can be achieved only with a lower quantity of output. The curve shows alternative levels of quantity and quality that can be achieved at a given reimbursement rate.

examine the market in its entirety. The following three chapters undertake this task.

6.6 SUPPLY BEHAVIOR OF NONPROFIT AGENCIES: THE EXECUTIVE-BENEFITS-MAXIMIZING MODEL

An alternative theory of resource allocation and product supply in nonprofit agencies focuses on the behavior of the executive or administrator of the organization, assuming that he or she has considerable control over the organization's resources. This is certainly a plausible way of looking at the resource-allocation decision-making process, considering that trustees of nonprofit agencies typically can devote only a small portion of their time to trustee-related activities, while the executives are usually full-time employees. The theory that focuses on the administrator's behavior is actually a comparative analysis that examines how the same administrator would behave if operating at the same agency under two conditions: as a profit-seeking enterprise and as a nonprofit agency. The differences in behavior, which are due solely to the different incentive structures that the two types of organizations create, cause different uses of the agencies' resources and differences in the products that the organizations supply.

The theory is nothing more than an extension of the basic demand hypothesis presented in Chapter 3. This hypothesis was that the lower the direct cost of a commodity or other benefit to an individual, the more it will be demanded. The extension of the analysis of Chapter 3 lies in identifying the commodities that are desired, as well as their relative prices or costs to the administrator under varying institutional circumstances. Since we are focusing on the administrator's behavior, we will identify two types of benefits that can be obtained in the context of the job. First are the pecuniary benefits in the form of a salary. If the administrator is part or full owner in the organization, pecuniary benefits can also be obtained from the profits that accrue. The second type of benefits are nonpecuniary, sometimes called on-the-job benefits. These include a high grade of office furniture, a work atmosphere that is nonharassing, "business" trips to exotic places, and so on. Both types of benefits are wanted by the administrator in either circumstance. Also, these sources of benefits are scarce, which means the administrator cannot have everything he or she would like.

Before developing the hypothesis about how much of each will be demanded, we will look at the implications for resource use of obtaining the two types of benefits. First, profits are greater when a small resource commitment is used to obtain a given output. Thus, in a profit-making enterprise, greater profits can be expected to result from a smaller commitment of resources to production. Nonpecuniary benefits, on the other hand, are obtained with the commitment of resources. Better office equipment, more liberal working conditions, and other on-the-job benefits are obtained from the expansion of the total resource commitment and result in an increase in costs. A use of resources in these *nonproductive* ways also results in a contraction of profits. In a nonprofit enterprise this reduction in profits does not detract from the manager's pecuniary benefits since he or she will not be rewarded on the basis of the profits the enterprise earns.

The hypothesis of comparative behavior stems from the constraints facing the same manager in the two different environments. In a nonprofit environment, since the manager cannot convert profits into pecuniary, take-home benefits, they must be converted into organizational resources, if any benefit is to be obtained. On the other hand, the use of these extra resources in a profit-making organization will detract from profits and hence from pecuniary or take-home benefits, assuming these are related. The personal costs of on-the-job benefits to the administrator of the nonprofit agency are lower, and we thus hypothesize that more will be demanded.

The implications of this hypothesis for nonprofit resource allocation are considerable. The hypothesis implies that the nonprofit agency will use more resources to get a given job done, because its costs will be higher. This absence of incentives for efficiency has been the target of criticism regarding their effects on nonprofit agency operating costs, particularly nonprofit health insurers (Frech, 1976), nursing homes (Frech, 1985; Borjas, Frech, and Ginsburg, 1983), and dialysis units (Lowrie and Hampers, 1981). Similar analyses regarding comparisons of nonprofit and for-profit hospital behavior have not been as conclusive for several reasons. First, if one is to compare operating costs between nonprofit and for-profit hospitals, variables such as case mix, case severity, and quality must be adjusted for. Assertions have been made that nonprofit hospitals have a more complex case mix because for-profit hospitals engage in "cream-skimming" by encouraging the admission of low-cost cases. Evidence on this score seems mixed (Renn et al., 1985; Bays, 1977; Schweitzer and Rafferty, 1976). Even more difficult to determine is whether quality differentials exist by ownership category. Nonprofit managers do have an incentive to produce quality care (which will show up in higher costs). The role of quality in higher costs has yet to be fully explored.

Another difference that has been uncovered when comparing nonprofit and for-profit hospital behavior lies in the pricing area. Two California studies found that for-profit hospitals had higher charges (relative to costs) for ancillary (lab, radiology, pharmacy) services; generally, mark-ups (charge to cost ratios) for ancillary services were found to be higher than basic room charges. For-profit hospitals also provided more (high profit) ancillary services per patient than nonprofits in the studies and were more profitable, although cost levels were similar (Eskoz and Peddecord, 1985; Pattison and Katz, 1983). An explanation of such a finding in terms of the property rights theory of this section would be that nonprofit managers (or trustees) gain nonpecuniary benefits from encouraging the *availability* of hospital care (see Section 4.3), and this goal can be achieved with a policy of lower patient charges (which may result in lower profits), as well as by providing more free care to indigents.

However, relying solely on the incentives identified in the executive-benefits model to explain cost and price differences between for-profit and nonprofit hospitals would be to rely on an incomplete explanation. The incentive differences incorporated in the model are but one factor operating to influence costs (and possible cost differences) in the two types of organizations. The reimbursement system is another major influence on cost and supply behavior. And, indeed, the *absence* of cost differences between nonprofit and for-profit hospitals that was uncovered by investigators in California may have been influenced by the reimbursement system, which, at the time of the studies, encouraged cost inflation in all types of hospitals. It is to this factor that we now turn.

6.7 PROVIDER REIMBURSEMENT

The effects of different types of reimbursement come into play when third parties are the providers of revenue to the firm. Once a third party undertakes to make part or total payment for the services that the provider offers the consumer, the issue of the basis under which these payments will be made becomes pertinent. This issue is explored in this section by looking at three types of reimbursement. Each is examined in terms of the supply analyses developed in this chapter. First, methods by which the physician is reimbursed and how these might affect the quantity supplied of physician services are examined. For the purposes of analyzing physician supply, the profit-maximizing model will be applied to the physician's practice. Second, the reimbursement of hospitals is presented in terms of the output-maximizing model of the nonprofit agency. Third, a joint form of reimbursement by which the consumer buys total (hospital and physician) medical care insurance from a single health care providing agency is discussed.

When reviewing this analysis, the reader should keep one qualification in mind. The supply analyses are primarily narrow ones about the reaction of a supplier to specific incentives. A complete analysis would examine how the relevant portions of the entire *system* are affected. To some degree, we will discuss the wider picture, although a discussion on how to conduct a more complete analysis will come later.

6.7.1 Physician Reimbursement

There are three major types of physician reimbursement: fee for service, per capita, and lump-sum payment. The fee-for-service method of reimbursement is similar to a piece-rate type of payment. The physician is paid a specific sum by a third party for each individual service he or she provides to the patient. The services are broken down into such entities as a complete physical exam, a follow-up visit, a tonsillectomy, and so on.

There are several ways in which the fees can be set by the third party. One, which most closely corresponds to the assumption in this chapter of an absence of control by the provider over the fee (i.e., a price taker), is the relative-value scale (Hsiao and Stason, 1979; Havighurst and Kissam, 1979). By this method, each category of service is assigned a relative value in accordance with some criterion (e.g., the number of minutes required to perform the procedure). For example, in the frequently used California Relative Value Scale (surgical component), a single coronary bypass operation would have an index number of 25. This relative value can be converted to fees by applying a conversion factor. If the conversion factor for surgery was $50 per point on the relative-value scale, the surgeon would be reimbursed $1,250 for the bypass operation. This system is used by a number of Medicaid agencies.

The second type of reimbursement does not really fit the criterion of fees being beyond the control of the individual provider. This method is referred to as the UCR (usual, customary, and reasonable) form of reimbursement. *Usual* refers to the usual or typical fee charged by the billing physician; *customary* refers to fees charged by all physicians in the community; and *reasonable* refers to particular circumstances (an allowance for exceptions because of difficult cases, for example). Suppose Dr. Welby performed 100 varicose vein injections with an average fee of $100; her usual fee for the procedure is $100. The customary fee is derived from two pieces of data. First is the frequency distribution of the fees charged by all doctors in the community for the procedure (e.g., the doctors in the tenth percentile charge $10, those in the twentieth percentile charge $20, and so on up to the one-hundredth percentile charging $100). The second piece of information is a decision rule on the part of the insurer as to which percentile to use to set an allowable maximum fee. If the reimburser used the seventieth percentile, then the associated charge in our example is $70. This is the maximum allowable set by the insurer. Dr. Welby will be reimbursed the lower of her usual or the customary fee. In this case it will be $70, not her fee of $100.

The reason why this method does not strictly conform to a "price taker" situation is that Dr. Welby's fee is part of the overall customary fee prevailing in the market. If all doctors raise their fees, the customary fee will increase as well. Each doctor has some control over the market's fees. When there are many doctors in the market, this control may be small, and for analytical purposes one might take the customary fee as a given fee.

Since the physician is paid a fixed rate per unit of service performed, the number of services produced will depend on what the reimbursement rate is and on the physician's marginal costs (applying the profit-maximizing model) for the specific procedure. If the marginal cost schedule slopes upward steeply, only a slight addition to supply will result from an increase in the fee (Phelps, 1976). As important as the level of reimbursement rates is the composition of fees. If surgical fees are high relative to general checkups such that surgical operations yield considerable profits relative to checkups, then the incentive will be for surgeons to operate more, but not for physicians to conduct checkups (which might be marginally profitable, if at all). Indeed, fee-for-service type of reimbursement is believed to encourage doctors to provide more medical care. As we have just seen, however, this will depend on the relation between the fee and the service's marginal cost. Some analysts have taken the argument one step further and claimed that fee-for-service encourages many unnecessary practices (Klarman, 1963). In the context of the present analysis, we can only say whether additional services are likely to be offered; we cannot determine from *this* analysis whether or not they would be necessary.

The fee schedule represents a potentially powerful tool for third parties to influence both the type of practices performed and where they are performed. For example, tonsillectomies are thought to be unnecessary in many instances; if a third party wanted to discourage this procedure, it could lower the reimbursed fee for it. Also, if a third party wanted to encourage certain procedures to be performed on an outpatient rather than an inpatient basis, it could reimburse physicians differentially for the same procedure. For example, the South Carolina Preferred Personal Care Plan reimburses physicians $675 for a colonoscopy performed in an outpatient setting and $515 on an inpatient basis.

A qualification to the profit-maximizing hypothesis can be made to take into account alternative possible behavior patterns of the physician–owners of the practices. A more complete analysis might change the assumption about physician objectives to recognize that physicians desire leisure as well as income. As their profits (incomes) rise, physicians may want to engage in activities that require more leisure time. They will then be forced to trade off some profits for additional leisure time. This will cause their supply curves to slope more positively (i.e., a smaller response to fee increase), and if the fee increase is sufficiently high, their supply curves may even become vertical and then slope backward. It should be stressed that this behavior is a generalization of profit-maximizing behavior. Although it is plausible, the evidence to date is mixed (Feldstein, 1970; Sloan, 1975).

As compared with fee-for-service practice, the incentives for physicians who are paid on a per capita basis or on a salary basis are decidedly different. In both these cases, there is no incentive for physicians to perform any more than the basic minimum level of services; indeed, some analysts might argue that the incentives exist to perform even less than that. In any event, considerable evidence exists about the impact that the payment system has on physician practices. Reference has been made to the large difference in surgical operations between the United States and England, pointing to the general payment patterns as one underlying influence: in England, surgeons are paid on a salary basis, while in the United States the usual payment basis is fee-for-service (Aaron and Schwartz, 1984). In the United States, several reimbursement experiments have been undertaken relating to physicians (Eisenberg and Williams, 1981; Myers and Schroeder, 1981). In one, primary care physicians were given financial responsibilities for the entire health care expenditures of their patients; they shared in any surpluses of premiums over total medical care costs (including hospitalization, lab and x-ray, etc.), as well as in any deficits. The incentive was for them to reduce the expenditures paid out so that their share of the surpluses would be greater. This experiment was based on the view of the physician as ''gatekeeper'' to the health care system, with the ability to control a good deal of the patient's cost. The results showed a considerable reduction in overall expenses relative to a fee-for-service comparison group (Moore, 1979). Additional evidence on incentives toward reduced utilization will be discussed in Section 6.7.4.

6.7.2 Hospital Reimbursement

Until the early 1980s, hospital reimbursement was made largely on a retrospective basis. That is, the third party reimbursed the hospital for the expenses it had already incurred (if reimbursement was on a cost basis) or the charges it had already made (if reimbursement was on a charge basis). There are numerous variations of retrospective reimbursement. The third party can pay on a *cost-plus* basis, which means it can reimburse the hospital for its allowable costs plus a specified amount (say 2 percent of costs). In another method of reimbursement, the third party pays the hospital whichever is lower, costs or charges. There can also be a considerable variation in how costs are defined. Allowable costs could exclude costs not directly related to the reimburser's patients' care (e.g., teaching costs). Whatever the variation, retrospective reimbursement had one overriding effect on supply and on costs: it encouraged an organization to expand. Increases in both the scope and quality of services are encouraged, and given the goals of a producer who is a maximizer of anything, retrospective reimbursement can lead to higher costs, more services, and higher-quality services.

In response to this recognized bias in retrospective reimbursement, a number of prospective reimbursement plans have been introduced. Prospective reimbursement involves setting the basis of reimbursement before the reimbursement period. There are many different ways in which this can be done and an infinite number of levels at which rates can be prospectively set. We will examine several of these variations and their hypothesized effects on cost and quantity supplied.

To help classify the effects of different reimbursement policies, we will break down total costs into components by the following formula:

$$\frac{\text{Total}}{\text{cost}} = \frac{\text{cost per}}{\text{service}} \times \frac{\text{services per}}{\text{patient}} \times \frac{\text{days of}}{\text{stay per}} \times \frac{\text{number of}}{\text{admissions}}$$
$$\text{per day} \qquad \text{admission}$$

Let us now hypothesize about the effect of different prospective reimbursement formulas on an output-maximizing hospital. We will compare three: a given per service rate, a given per diem or per day rate, and a given per admission rate. According to reimbursement on a service basis, the hospital will receive a given amount per service performed (e.g., operation, x-ray, or kidney dialysis). This given rate is set in advance, for example, $45 for a specific lab test, $300 for a complete computed tomography scan, and so on. In response to this type of reimbursement, an output-maximizing hospital will expand its services as long as the reimbursed rate at least covers the cost of provision. This may be done by increasing any or all of the number of services per patient per day, the number of days a patient stays (so more services can be provided), and the number of admissions (if this is feasible). Each of these components of output will be increased under per service reimbursement, according to our hypothesis.

If the second type of reimbursement, per patient day (referred to as per diem rate), is used, this will amount to setting a given rate for the cost per service times the number of services per patient day. There will be no incentive to expand the *number* of services per patient day because the hospital will receive no extra revenue for doing so. However, the hospital will receive added revenue from having more patient days. As long as the added reimbursement covers the added costs, the hospital will expand the number of patient days by increasing patient length of stay and, if possible, admissions. Since the cost to the hospital of adding an extra day to an admitted patient's stay is usually quite low (all the expensive services having been performed earlier in the patient's visit), the hospital will usually benefit considerably by increasing the length of stay of its patients under per diem reimbursement.

The third type of incentive payment, per admission, will reward the hospital only by adding more patients. Under these circumstances, we hypothesize that the hospital will cut back on length of stay and services per patient and attempt to draw in more patients, as long as it does not run a deficit by doing so. The hospital will also, according to this hypothesis, encourage the readmission of patients since this will mean an additional payment.

When evaluating hospital reimbursement formulas, several things have to be kept in mind. First, one must distinguish between an all-payor system and a multipayor system. In an all-payor system, each payor pays the same rate. For example, assume that Medicare, Blue Cross, and commercial insurers each have one-third of the overall caseload of 300 cases in a hospital, and that the case mixes and severities of the patient groups are identical (so there is no objective basis for differential payments). Assume, further, that the regulatory authority in the state has determined that the hospital's allowable revenues should be $900,000. This means that each insurer "should" pay $300,000. This is what they would pay in an all-payor system.

A multipayor system is more like a free-for-all, with each payor setting up its payment rules unilaterally or based on market principles. Let us say that, in the preceding example, the regulatory agency only regulates Medicare and Blue Cross rates and that it allows each to pay $270,000. The commercial group rates are unregulated. In this instance, the hospital must raise its charges to the commercials to cover its deficit. Whether or not it collects all of it is another issue. What is important here is that the hospital is no longer a price taker, and so a more complex model recognizing additional reactions by the hospital to the regulated rate is needed (see Section 8.2).

A second important factor is that other parts of the health care system may be affected by the reimbursement type and level. For example, if a system penalizes hospitals for keeping patients in the hospital for more than a specified time, this will most certainly reduce length of stay. It may have other effects as well. For instance, if home health care or nursing home care are reimbursed separately, the hospital may open up a nursing home or begin a home health care program and discharge the patients into these programs. (Of course, it could also simply refer the patients to others.) In this event, the early discharge incentive will have systemwide effects that must be recognized.

A considerable number of experiments with prospective reimbursements have been conducted at the state level (Bauer, 1977). Most of these have been in the context of multipayor systems, and so their predicted effects are more complicated than for an all-payor system. One such experiment, conducted by the New York State legislature, set per diem rates for Medicare and Blue Cross reimbursed patients according to a preset formula, beginning in 1970. In testing for the effect of this type of reimbursement, a comparison was made between length of stay and occupancy rates after 1970 in New York State and those in several comparison states where prospective per diem rates were not in force (Ohio and the New England states). Between 1970 and 1974, New York showed a slight increase in the average length of stay and no net change in the occupancy rate, that is, the average percent of all beds filled. Both of these indicators of hospital supply decreased considerably in the control states during the same period of time. The indication from this is that the reimbursement mechanism had its expected effect (Berry, 1976). (See Section 12.2.4 for a further discussion of prospective reimbursement.)

6.7.3 Diagnosis-Related Groups

In 1983 the federal government introduced a new prospective payment system (PPS) for Medicare hospital patients. According to this system, all Medicare discharges are reimbursed for on a per diagnosis basis, known as a diagnosis-related group (DRG) system. In this section, we review how diagnoses are grouped into separate DRGs and how rates are set for each DRG. We then discuss the use of the quantity-maximizing model to examine the effects of DRGs on the supply system.

The DRG grouping system is one of many possible ways of classifying patients according to common elements (Hornbrook, 1982). There is the presumption that, if the classification system is to be used for reimbursement purposes, all cases in each group will be similar with regard to resource use. Based on several patient characteristics (the major diagnostic group, patient age, the presence of comorbid conditions, the use of a surgical procedure, and discharge status), groups were formed that researchers determined to exhibit common resource-use tendencies (as measured in this case by length of stay) (Fetter et al., 1980). The component characteristics of one such set of DRGs is shown in Figure 6–7. As can be seen, DRGs for breast disorders were developed from criteria relating to whether surgery was performed, age, and the presence of other complications. The criteria were selected so that cases in each category would use similar amounts of re-sources and thus could be reimbursed with a single rate. There are 467 categories in the DRG classification system.

Based on cross-hospital studies, an average cost for each DRG was estimated; the components of these costs were the lengths of stay (within the DRG) in routine and special care, per diem costs in routine and special care, and estimated cost of ancillary services (laboratory, radiology, drugs, medical supplies, anesthesia, and other services) per case (Pettengill and Vertrees, 1982). From these studies, each DRG was assigned a relative weight that was to approximate the relative amount of resources used by one case in the group. For example, a cardiac arrest (DRG 129) was assigned a weight of 1.5506, while a coronary bypass (DRG 106) was assigned a weight of 3.9891. A reimbursement rate was set for each point. Originally, this rate had national, regional, and hospital-specific components. In 1988 there is slated to be one national rate, but this rate will vary by urban or rural area and will be adjusted for the number of residents per bed for teaching hospitals. For example, in 1985 the national rate per point for urban hospitals was $2,974.49

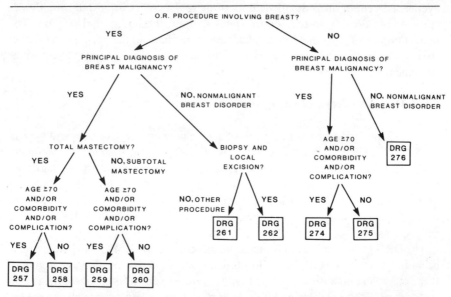

Figure 6–7 Derivation of diagnosis-related groups (DRGs) for breast disorders. Among the criteria used to separate the various DRGs are the use of operating room (OR) procedures, the principal diagnosis, the type of OR procedure (if used), age of patient, and complications and/or comorbidity.

($2,310.05 for the labor-related portion and $664.44 for the nonlabor portion). An urban hospital with no teaching facilities would be reimbursed $11,863.78 for a case in DRG 106 (i.e., 3.9891 points × $2,974.49 per point). If the hospital were a teaching hospital, it would receive an additional sum based on its resident per bed ratio (Lave, 1984). In addition, there is an adjustment for outlying cases, which use considerably more or less resources than the average, with use being measured by costs or length of stay.

We can use the output-maximizing model to predict the likely effects of DRGs. The DRG system replaces the old, inflationary-cost-based reimbursement system used by Medicare. Furthermore, this system reimburses hospitals on a per case basis. The simple one-product, output-maximizing model predicts that, to stretch its output as far as possible, the hospital will produce at minimum costs. Indeed, under the DRG system, the hospital is at risk for any expenses incurred above the given reimbursement rate. It will strive to reduce costs to an efficient level. This is unlike the behavior of a hospital that is reimbursed on a retrospective basis. Organizationally, to control costs administrators have to appeal to physicians, who are responsible for ordering lab tests, x-rays, and the like, and who determine length of stay (Young and Saltman, 1982). These appeals will lead to greater consultation with physicians than was undertaken in the past and may lead to additional collaboration. A reduction in quality of care is also fully consistent with the attempt to reduce services per case. While the extent to which this will happen is open to investigation, certainly the incentives run in that direction.

Overall, the model predicts a tendency for hospitals to maximize the number of cases admitted. Recognizing this, Medicare regulations make provision for professional review of admissions to determine necessity of care (see Section 12.2.3). However, the tendency remains. At the individual DRG level, those cases with the highest rates relative to costs will be "sought after" by hospitals. This has been claimed to be the surgical cases (Omenn and Conrad, 1984). How can hospitals influence their case mix? There appears to be a considerable amount of discretion in whether a case will be hospitalized, as indicated by large area-wide variations in hospitalizations by case (Wennberg, McPherson, and Caper, 1984). If specialists and facilities in certain areas are more readily available, patients are hospitalized to a greater degree in these specialties. By expanding in certain areas (e.g., ophthalmology) and "recruiting" physicians, hospitals can encourage a greater supply in these areas (Goldfarb, Hornbrook, and Rafferty, 1980).

The Medicare payment system is, of course, a system only for Medicare patients. Not being an all-payor system, there may be additional responses to the PPS rate level and structure by the hospital itself; that is, these rates may affect hospital policies with regard to non-Medicare patients. With low Medicare rates, hospitals may shift services toward non-Medicare patients, or they may shift costs to other patients (see Section 8.2).

DRGs also have systemwide ramifications. Shorter lengths of stay may not mean lower systemwide costs. If nursing home and home care product lines are financially viable, an output-maximizing hospital can expand into these areas and accept its own discharged patients. Since each form of care is separately reimbursed for, increased output in these other forms of care may be encouraged.

Finally, DRGs are not as clean-cut as one would like in a case-mix measure. A number of studies have shown substantial *within-group* variation in case severity and resource use (Horn and Sharkey, 1983). In this case, some hospitals might have a caseload that is comprised of more severe cases within the same DRGs than other hospitals; the system would not reward them for doing this. This has led some commentators to predict that some hospitals might try to avoid more costly cases (e.g., closing down specific services). While attempts are being made to modify DRGs for severity, the DRG system as it stands is quite complex. Additional modifications in the realm of complexity may make the system unwieldy.

6.7.4 Health Maintenance Organizations

There has been a considerable amount of interest in recent years in a combined insurance-provider type of organization known as a health maintenance organization (HMO). The major characteristics of an HMO from a supply standpoint are that it offers, simultaneously, two products—health insurance and health care. Health insurance coverage is sold to customers on a per capita basis. The medical care itself is provided, or contracted for, by the HMO directly. The HMO assumes all the financial risk for providing this care. At the same time, its physicians act as the patients' "gatekeepers" and therefore have some degree of control over the patients' utilization of care.

In discussing the supply incentives inherent in such an organization, we must recognize that an HMO can make a number of different types of arrangements with regard to the physicians that it contracts with and the hospitals to which it sends its patients. There are two primary ways that the HMO can contract with its physicians, on a salary basis or a fee-for-service basis. In the former case, the physicians will be employees of the HMO. In the latter case, the physicians maintain their own private practices in which they treat HMO patients; this form of practice plan is referred to as an Independent Practice Association (IPA). Frequently, the IPA will contract with a number of different physician groups, giving the patient a greater choice of physicians.

The incentives for supply behavior under the salary arrangements are quite clear. The HMO has an incentive to reduce costs, and this can be done by reducing patient use, especially hospital utilization. Since the HMO doctors are the gatekeepers of their patients into the system, the HMO has a considerable degree of control over its patients' hospital use.

The incentives in the IPA case are not so clear-cut. While the HMO wants to reduce its members' use, contract doctors are rewarded for providing more care, since they are being reimbursed on the fee-for-service system.

The majority of HMOs will contract with hospitals to provide care for their members when they are hospitalized. In the larger HMOs, the HMO itself may operate a hospital. In this case the HMO has control over the hospital product as well.

Evidence on HMO supply behavior is usually presented in the context of comparisons with fee-for-service patients. When making such comparisons, one must recognize that patient utilization is determined by both supplier and patient incentives. This is particularly true in the case of ambulatory visits. Patients with traditional insurance generally have very little insurance coverage for ambulatory visits such as checkups and so will demand less ambulatory care than will HMO members, who generally pay no direct price for these visits. If one observed fewer ambulatory visits in the data comparing fee-for-service with HMO practice, one could not conclude that it was differences in *supply* behavior that were being observed; indeed, the differences may be primarily due to demand behavior. This would not be generally true when making comparisons of *hospital* usage between HMO members and populations with traditional insurance. Under traditional insurance, hospitalization coverage is usually about the same as under HMO coverage. In this case, differences in the behavior of populations are more likely to be due to differences in supplier behavior.

In a similar vein, one must be sure that the comparison *population characteristics*, as well as their insurance coverage, are similar. As discussed in Section 4.7, it is possible that adverse selection will occur with regard to consumer choice of health plan; if, in fact, more healthy individuals join HMOs, then part of any difference in utilization between HMO and traditional plans may be due to the health status differences of the two populations.

Indeed, what has been observed in comparing populations with HMO coverage and traditional coverage is that the major utilization differences between populations lie in the hospitalization rates: hospital admission rates have generally been lower when comparing populations treated under traditional coverage (with fee-for-service reimbursement) with those covered in traditional HMOs (i.e., non-IPAs). The evidence when comparing IPA and traditional coverage is less clear (Luft, 1978a). Also, utilization of ambulatory care was found to be greater in HMOs. HMOs have less control over these visits, and insurance coverage and characteristic differences between populations create a demand effect, making it difficult to attribute differences in ambulatory visits to HMO *supply* behavior.

REFERENCES

Resource Availability and Supply

Goldfarb, M., Hornbrook, M., & Rafferty, J. (1980). Behavior of the multiproduct firm. *Medical Care, 19*(2), 185–201.

Hornbrook, M., & Goldfarb, M. (1983). A partial test of a hospital behavior model. *Social Science & Medicine, 17,* 667–680.

Nonprofit Organization Behavior

Culyer, A.J. (1971). Medical care and the economics of giving. *Economica, 38,* 295–303.

Harris, J.F. (1977). The internal organization of hospitals. *Bell Journal of Economics, 8,* 647–682.

Lee, M.L. (1971). A conspicuous production theory of hospital behavior. *Southern Economic Journal, 38,* 48–58.

McGuire, A. (1985). The theory of the hospital: A review of the models. *Social Science & Medicine, 20,* 1177–1184.

Pauly, M., & Redisch, M. (1973). The not-for-profit hospital as a physicians' cooperative. *American Economic Review, 63,* 87–100.

Supply Behavior and Incentives: Prepayment and HMOs

Ellwood, P. (1972). Models for organizing health services and implications for legislative proposals. *Milbank Memorial Fund Quarterly, 50,* 73–100.

Feldstein, P.J. (1968). A proposal for capitation reimbursement to medical groups for total medical care. In *Reimbursement incentives for hospital and medical care* (Research Report No. 26). Washington, DC: Social Security Administration, Office of Research and Statistics.

Hornbrook, M., & Berki, S.E. (1985). Practice mode and payment method. *Medical Care, 23,* 484–511.

Klarman, H.E. (1963)., The effect of prepaid group practice on hospital use. *Public Health Report, 78,* 955–965.

Luft, H.S. (1978). How do health-maintenance organizations achieve their "savings." *New England Journal of Medicine, 298,* 1336–1343.

——— (1978). Why do HMO's seem to provide more health maintenance services? *Milbank Memorial Fund Quarterly, 56,* 140–168.

——— (1981). *Health maintenance organizations.* New York: Wiley.

Reimbursement and Supply: Physicians

Aaron, H., and Schwartz, W.B. (1984). *The painful prescription.* Washington: The Brookings Institution.

Burney, I.L., Schreiber, G.J., Blaxall, M.O., et al. (1978). Geographic variation in physicians' fees. *Journal of the American Medical Association, 240,* 1368–1371.

Eisenberg, J.M., & Williams, S.V. (1981). Cost containment and changing physicians' practice behavior. *Journal of the American Medical Association, 246,* 2195–2201.

Feldstein, M. (1970). The rising price of physicians' services. *Reviews of Economic Statistics, 52,* 121–133.

Gabel, J.R., & Redisch, M.A. (1979). Alternative physician payment mechanisms. *Milbank Memorial Fund Quarterly, 57,* 38–59.

Havighurst, C.C., & Kissam, P. (1979). The antitrust implications of relative value studies in medicine. *Journal of Health Politics, Policy, and Law, 4,* 48.

Hornbrook, M.C. (1983). Allocative medicine: Efficiency, disease severity, and the payment mechanism. *Annals, AAPSS, 468,* 12–29.

Hsiao, W.C., & Stason, W.B. (1979). Toward developing a relative value scale for medical and surgical services. *Health Care Financing Review, 1*, 23–39.

Lowenstein, S.R., Iezzoni, L.I., & Moskowitz, M.A. (1985). Prospective payment for physician services. *Journal of the American Medical Association, 254*, 2632–2637.

Mitchell, J.B. (1985). Physician DRG's. *New England Journal of Medicine, 313*, 670–675.

Monsma, G. (1970). Marginal revenue and the demand for physicians' services. In H.F. Klarman (Ed.), *Empirical studies in health economics* (pp. 145–160). Baltimore, MD: Johns Hopkins University Press.

Moore, S. (1979). Cost containment through risk sharing of primary-care physicians. *New England Journal of Medicine, 300*, 1359–1362.

Myers, L.P., & Schroeder, S.A. (1981). Physician use of services for the hospitalized patient. *Milbank Memorial Fund Quarterly, 59*, 481–507.

Phelps, C.E. (1976). Public sector medicine. In C.M. Lindsay (Ed.), *New directions in public health care* (pp. 131–166). San Francisco: Institute for Contemporary Studies.

Scheffler, R.M. (1981). Reimbursement practices and the primary care physician. *Journal of Family Practice, 13*, 502–507.

Schreiber, G.I., Burney, I.L., Golden, J.B., et al. (1976). Physician fee patterns under medicare: A descriptive analysis. *New England Journal of Medicine, 294*, 1089–1093.

Showstack, J.A., Blumberg, B.D., Schwartz, J., et al. (1979). Fee-for-service payment; Analysis of current methods and their development. *Inquiry, 16*, 230–246.

Sloan, F.A. (1975). Physician supply behavior in the short run. *Industrial and Labor Relations Review, 28*, 549–569.

Stano, M., Cromwell, J., Velky, J., et al. (1983). Fee or use? What's responsible for rising health care costs? *Michigan Medicine, 82*, 228–234.

Reimbursement and Supply: Hospitals

Bauer, K. (1977). Hospital rate setting—This way to salvation? *Milbank Memorial Fund Quarterly, 55*, 117–118.

Berry, R.E. (1976). Prospective reimbursement and cost containment. *Inquiry, 13*, 288–301.

Dowling, W.L. (1974). Prospective reimbursement of hospitals. *Inquiry, 11*, 163–180.

Eby, C.L., & Cohodes, D.R. (1985). What do we know about rate setting. *Journal of Health Politics, Policy, and Law, 10*, 299–323.

Foster, R.W. (1982). Cost-based reimbursement and prospective payment: Reassessing the incentives. *Journal of Health Politics, Policy, and Law, 7*, 407–420.

Horn, S.D., & Sharkey, P.D. (1983). Measuring severity of illness to predict patient resource use within DRG's. *Inquiry, 20* (4), 314–321.

Hornbrook, M. (1982). Hospital case mix: Its definition, measurement, and use: Part I. *Medical Care Review, 39*, 1–43 and Part II: *Medical Care Review, 39*, 73–123.

Zuckerman, S., Becker, E.R., Adams, K., et al. (1984). Physician practice patterns under hospital rate-setting programs. *Journal of the American Medical Association, 252*, 2589–2592.

Diagnosis-Related Groups and Case-Mix Supply

Broyles, R.W., & Rosko, M.D. (1985). A qualitative assessment of the Medicare prospective payment system. *Social Science and Medicine, 20*, 1185–1190.

Fetter, R.B., Shin, Y., & Freeman, J.L. (1980). Case mix definition by diagnosis-related groups. *Medical Care 18* (Suppl. 2), 1–53.

Knoebel, S.B. (1985). The effect of cost containment on the practice of cardiology. *American Journal of Cardiology, 56*, 32C–34C.

Lave, J.R. (1984). Hospital reimbursement under Medicare. *Milbank Memorial Fund Quarterly, 62*, 251–268.

Omenn, G.S., & Conrad, D.A. (1984). Implications of DRG's for clinicians. *New England Journal of Medicine, 311*, 1314–1317.

Pettengill, J., & Vertrees, J. (1982). Reliability and validity in hospital case-mix measurement. *Health Care Financing Review, 4*, 101–128.

Vladeck, B.C. (1984). Medicare hospital payment by diagnosis-related group. *Annals of Internal Medicine, 100*, 576–591.

Wennberg, J.E., McPherson, K., & Caper, P. Will payment based on diagnosis-related groups control hospital costs? *New England Journal of Medicine, 311*, 295–300.

Young, D.W., & Saltman, R.B. (1982). Medical practice, case mix, and cost containment. *Journal of the American Medical Association, 247*, 801–805.

For-Profit, Nonprofit Comparisons

Bays, C. (1977). Case-mix differences between nonprofit and for-profit hospitals. *Inquiry, 14*, 17–21.

———— (1979). Cost comparisons of for-profit and nonprofit hospitals. *Social Science and Medicine, 13C*, 219–225.

Borjas, G.J., Frech, H.E., & Ginsburg, P.B. (1983). Property rights and wages: The case of nursing homes. *Journal of Human Resources, 17*, 231–246.

Clarkson, K.W. (1972). Some implications of property rights in hospital management. *Journal of Law and Economics, 15*, 363–384.

Eskoz, R., & Peddecord, K.M. (1985). The relationship of hospital ownership and service composition to hospital charges. *Health Care Financing Review, 6*, 51–58.

Frech, H.E. (1976). The property rights theory of the firm: Empirical results from a natural experiment. *Journal of Political Economy, 84*, 143–152.

———— (1985). The property rights theory of the firm: Some evidence from the US nursing home industry. *Zeitschrift fur die gestamte Staatswissenschaft, 141*, 146–166.

Lewin, L.S., Derzon, R.A., & Margulies, R. (1981, July 1). Investor-owneds and nonprofits differ in economic performance. *Hospitals*, 52–58.

Lowrie, E.G., & Hampers, C.L. (1981). The success of Medicare's end-stage renal disease program. *New England Journal of Medicine, 305*, 434–438.

Pattison, R.V., & Katz, H.M. (1983). Investor-owned and not-for-profit hospitals. *New England Journal of Medicine, 309*, 347–353.

Relman, A.S. (1980). The new medical–industrial complex. *New England Journal of Medicine, 303*, 963–970.

Renn, S.C., Schramm, C.J., Watt, J.M., et al. (1985). The effects of ownership and system affiliation on the economic performance of hospitals. *Inquiry, 22*, 219–236.

Ruchlin, H.S., Pointer, D.D., & Cannedy, L.L. (1976). A comparison of for profit investor owned chain and nonprofit hospitals. *Inquiry, 10*, 13–23.

Schweitzer, S.O., & Rafferty, J. (1976). Variations in hospital product: A comparative analysis of proprietary and voluntary hospitals. *Inquiry, 13*, 158–166.

Chapter 7

Competitive Markets

7.1 INTRODUCTION

In the previous four chapters a number of hypotheses relating to the behavior of demanding and supplying units were developed. These hypotheses were such that demand behavior and supply behavior were examined in isolation. As a result, although we could develop an explanation about what quantity would be demanded (supplied) at any price, our model did not incorporate the behavior of the supplying (demanding) units, and thus could not tell us whether the same quantity would be both demanded and supplied.

Beginning with this chapter, our focus shifts to models in which demanders and suppliers interact. The setting in which this interaction occurs is called a *market*. A market in economics should not be thought of as a physical location; rather, it is a term that denotes the web of interactions among those who potentially have commercial relationships with other buyers and sellers of similar commodities. We can think of a market for psychiatric services as consisting of a constellation of consumers and providers who may potentially have commercial relations with all members of the other group. Central to the analysis of the functioning of a market is the price that the buyer pays and the seller receives. In Chapters 3 and 6 this price was taken as given for both groups; variations in price were beyond the control of any one buyer or seller. Yet, as a consequence of the related interactions of these groups, prices are set; as a consequence of some change in demand or supply behavior, prices change.

The market analyses that we will examine consist of three categories of concepts. First are the phenomena we seek to explain. These are objective events, such as changes in the price or the quantity of medical care utilized. The phenomena with which we are concerned might be rising prices; our model would be used to explain why the phenomena have occurred. Second are the degrees of willingness of demanders to purchase at specific prices and the propensities of

147

providers to supply at specific prices, which have been referred to as *demand* and *supply,* respectively. These concepts may be referred to as *economic forces.* Third, the strength of these forces can be increased or decreased by individual factors, such as incomes and tastes on the demand side and input prices on the supply side. The force of demand can be increased by higher consumer incomes, for example; the force of supply can be decreased by higher input costs. As a consequence of such changes in causal factors, the demand or supply force will change, and price and quantity will change as well. Our models should be able to predict this cause–effect chain of events.

In this chapter, one particular market model is developed and used to explain the outcome of price and quantity in the medical care market. This is the *competitive market model,* which treats the market as an interactive mechanism with many suppliers competing for consumer business. Such a model is extremely rich in the range of events it can explain. It offers hypotheses to explain rising prices, increasing or decreasing utilization, shortages in commodities such as doctors' services, nursing services, and blood, and surpluses in areas such as hospital beds. Thus it is a valuable starting point for any analysis of markets. The competitive market model is presented in Section 7.2, and the predictions of the model are discussed in Section 7.3. Although the competitive model might be rich in the number of events it can predict, in no way should this be taken to mean that these predictions are borne out of actual events. Indeed, several events are either at odds or do not necessarily corroborate the predictions of the competitive model. Since accurate prediction is the bottom line of explanatory economics, we devote Section 7.4 to a discussion of corroborating evidence relating to the competitive hypothesis. In Section 7.5 we discuss a recent application of the competitive hypothesis in the health care field, that of selective contracting.

7.2 THE COMPETITIVE MODEL: ASSUMPTIONS

In our exposition of the competitive model, we will use a market for physician services as our example. The product is physician visits, which we will assume to be of a constant quality, each involving the same accuracy of diagnosis, effectiveness of treatment, and personal attentiveness.

Our initial demand assumptions are that each consumer has a normal demand curve, as set out in Chapter 3. This includes the stipulation that consumers are fully informed about the nature of the services they require and the benefits that they can obtain. Physicians cannot *directly* influence consumer demand for medical care. We further assume that there are many consumers in the market and that they are competing for physician services. This assumption rules out the possibility that individual buyers are large enough or can join together to have any influence over price.

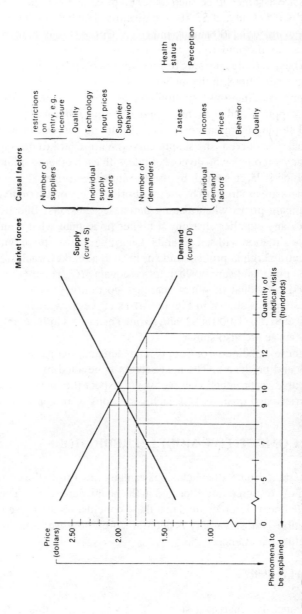

Figure 7–1 Representation of interaction of market forces. The phenomena, price and quantity, are influenced by the forces of supply and demand. These forces, in turn, are affected by a number of individual causal factors (listed in the diagram). The positions of the supply and demand curves assume that the causal factors are at given levels. Changes in the magnitude of any of the causal factors will cause a shift in supply or demand (or both).

The market demand curve (D) in our model is shown in Figure 7–1. Here conditions are assumed to be such that, at a price of $2.50 per visit, the quantity demanded is 500 visits; at $2.40, the quantity demanded is 600 units; at $2 the quantity demanded is 1,000 units; and so on. Curve D traces out this relationship. Any change in the underlying causal factors (tastes, for example) will shift demand. These causal factors are listed in the diagram for purposes of recalling the underlying assumptions in the model.

Our supply assumptions can similarly be broken up into assumptions about individual suppliers and about the supplier group. Individually, each supplier has an upward sloping marginal cost curve. Assuming supplier profit maximization, the marginal cost curve is the supply curve. With regard to the supply group, we assume many suppliers who do not collude with each other to influence prices and none of which is large enough by itself to influence price.

Consumers are assumed to be aware of price offers of alternative suppliers and so can compare prices when making purchase decisions. Because of consumer knowledge, any supplier charging a higher price than what would prevail in a competitive situation will sell no units. Charging a lower price will mean foregoing some intramarginal profits. And so, in such a market, each supplier will take the price as given and supply where price equals MC. The market supply will be the summed individual suppliers' marginal cost curves.

Market supply is shown in Figure 7–1 as curve S, with 700 units supplied at $1.70, 800 at $1.80, 1,000 at $2, and so on. The factors influencing the position of the supply curve are also shown.

Under these conditions of supply and demand, bargaining occurs between consumers and producers. The next section is devoted to the predictions of the model. That is, it presents what we would expect the market outcome to be (in terms of prices and quantities) if such conditions were approximated by reality.

7.3 THE COMPETITIVE MODEL: PREDICTIONS

Six important groups of conclusions can be drawn from the competitive model regarding how resources are allocated in the health care sector. These conclusions are presented next. Keep in mind that these conclusions are presented in the spirit of explanations whose validity is determined by how well the propositions conform to actual experience.

7.3.1 Market Price

In a competitive market a single price will emerge that clears the market. Competitive bidding will lower the price if a surplus of output exists (i.e., if there is unsold output or excess capacity) and will raise the price in the case of a shortage. Only when buyers are satisfied with the quantities they purchase at the established price and sellers are making maximum profits will market equilibrium be established, such that quantity supplied equals quantity demanded. In our example, equilibrium will be reached at a price of $2 with 1,000 visits supplied

If the price is higher, say $2.10, 900 units of service will be demanded while the suppliers will be prepared to supply 1,100. To eliminate this excess capacity at $2.10, physicians will lower prices and the amounts supplied. Quantity demanded will increase at the same time. The process goes on until both groups are simultaneously satisfied. The quantity supplied will just equal that which consumers demand. The same process will occur in reverse if the price is below $2, and prices will be driven up to the equilibrium point.

It can be shown that the end result of this process is a single price charged by all producers. If any single physician charged more than the equilibrium price per visit, the patients, assumed to possess full knowledge of prices charged by other physicians, would obtain medical care elsewhere. The physician would be forced to bring his or her price down to the price other doctors are charging. But if a doctor cuts his or her fees below the equilibrium level, patients will flock to this physician, and he or she will have an overload of work. Given a rising *MC* schedule for this physician, his or her profits on each additional unit sold will decline. The physician with such an *MC* schedule would have been better off, profitwise, to accept the highest price, which is the market price. The emergence of a single market-clearing price is thus a conclusion of the competitive model.

7.3.2 Price and Quantity Movements Caused by Demand Shifts

A second set of conclusions based on the competitive model can be drawn regarding price and quantity movements when there is a change in any of the factors that influence demand, causing the demand curve to shift upward or downward. This set of conclusions is illustrated in Figure 7–2. Assume D_1 to be the demand curve consistent with given initial values of underlying causal factors of demand. Let S be the supply curve, which remains stable because all supply shift factors are assumed constant. The equilibrium price for these conditions is P_1 ($2), and the equilibrium quantity for the market is Q_1 (1,000 visits). If any of the initial conditions that influence demand change, causing an increase in demand to D_2, for example, there will be a new equilibrium price and quantity at P_2 ($2.10) and Q_2 (1,200 units), respectively, such that the market price will rise. This is caused by the willingness of consumers to buy more at each price; the producers increase profits by producing more output, up to 1,200 units. Such a shift in demand can be caused by higher consumer incomes or a greater degree of illness in the population (see Chapter 3). Or it can be caused by an increase in the amount of health insurance purchased, which also causes demand to shift out (see Section 3.6). In either case the result is the same—higher prices and quantities. The

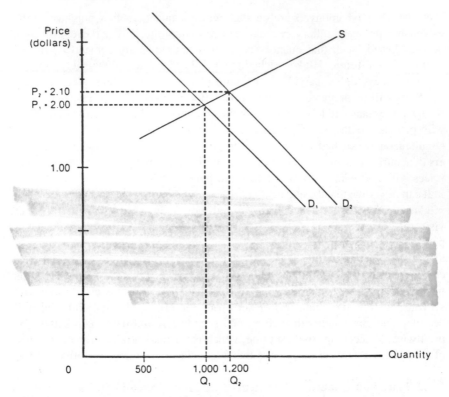

Figure 7–2 Representation of shifting demand with stable supply. An initial set of supply and demand forces characterized by D_1 and S will produce a given price and output level. An increase in demand to D_2 with a stable S will cause price and output to increase.

opposite predictions, lower prices and quantities, would be the consequence of factors changing to shift demand inward.

Concerning the term utilization, if quantity utilized is to increase, this increased quantity must be available. Thus *utilization* refers to the actual quantity traded in the market. This should not be confused with the amount demanded, because when there is disequilibrium, more or less might be demanded than supplied; nor should it be confused with the quantity offered by the supplier, because at any one price more or less may be supplied than consumers are willing to take at that price. These last situations, referring to disequilibrium, will occur when the price does not adjust so that quantity demanded and quantity supplied will equalize. Such situations are discussed in Section 7.3.5.

7.3.3 Price and Quantity Movements Caused by Supply Shifts

The third set of conclusions based on the model refers to changes in factors that cause supply to shift. The case for an increase in supply is shown in Figure 7–3. In

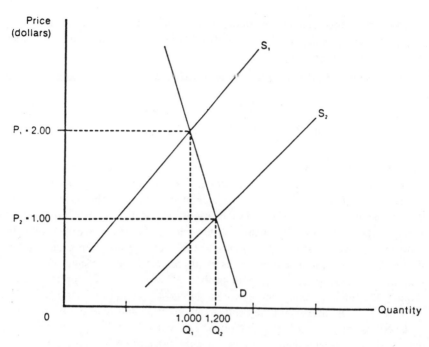

Figure 7–3 Representation of shifting supply with stable demand. Beginning with an initial demand and supply level *D* and *S*₁ and a resulting price and output level, an increase in supply to *S*₂ will cause output to increase and price to fall from their initial levels.

this example the service becomes less scarce and supply shifts from S_1 to S_2. If demand remains the same, supply becomes less scarce in relation to demand and the price falls. As a result, a new lower price ($1.00 or level P_2) and a higher level of utilization (1,200 units or level Q_2) are predicted. Of course, a factor that causes a reduction in supply will have the opposite effects on price and quantity utilized.

Changes in supply can occur because of changes in circumstances that are beyond the control of supplying firms and to which they react, or because of changes that the present or potential suppliers themselves initiate. The former situation might occur when the price that the physicians pay for paramedics increases because of a basic change in the market for paramedics. For example, if hospitals or public health departments decided to hire paramedics, they would enter the market and bid for the existing supply of paramedics. This would raise the price of paramedics that all market participants had to pay, because the supply remains relatively stable while the demand increases. An increase in the price of paramedics' services (or for that matter of any input) will shift the supply curve of all producers who use this input inward to the left. Thus the market supply curve will shift inward as well, and the price of physicians' services will increase.

Provider-initiated changes in supply will be undertaken by profit-seeking suppliers when these changes will potentially add to profits. Three types of situations are presented here:

1. a change in input combinations brought about by existing suppliers;
2. increases in the capital stock of existing suppliers;
3. entry into the market by new suppliers.

An example of the first situation, a change in input combinations, might occur when physicians hire paramedics or nurse practitioners to use partial, low-cost substitutes for their own services. Such a change might occur because of a change in a law that previously disallowed such practices to occur. The effect is to shift the average total cost curve downward and the marginal cost curve to the right. In a competitive market, one supplier making such a change would not cause a large shift in the market supply curve; prices would remain about the same and that one supplier would reap an increase in profits. However, if all suppliers made a change, the market supply curve would shift to the right considerably, and the price of medical care would then fall. Consumers would reap the benefits from such actions. The net profit position of each provider after all suppliers have acted may not be any greater than before because the price of output has fallen; but it is important to note that the competitive model is such that providers make their decisions to undertake cost reducing activities based on preexisting prices. Providers do not collude with their cosuppliers, and they do not always anticipate that prices will fall as a consequence of their concerted actions. The end result of their actions, however, is lower prices and greater utilization.

The same situation occurs with investment in plant and equipment made by existing suppliers. Additions to capital are often made in anticipation of additions to profits because of lower unit costs. If these investments cut costs, and if they are sufficiently widespread in the industry, the net effect will be to lower prices and raise utilization. As a result, after these effects have worked themselves out, profits may be no greater than before (they may even be less). These effects are presented in a before–after manner here. In actuality, they take a considerable time to occur. The potential for profits must first be realized, planning for the additions and financing them must occur, and the additional capital equipment and plant must then be constructed and put into use. As a result, the increase in supply and the fall in price may take months and even years. For this reason, the analysis of provider behavior involving capital additions, with resulting shifts in average and marginal cost curves, has been referred to as a long-run analysis, although it is a fine line to decide when a change in supply conditions is long run and when it is short run. The short run usually refers to changes in quantity supplied with existing capital equipment.

The third situation regarding changes in supply refers to the movement of new suppliers into the industry or market in response to high profits (in the case of profit-making providers). Such a movement results in an increase in supply and a consequent fall in price and increase in utilization. In this instance, since the cost conditions of existing suppliers remain the same, the profit levels must fall for all existing suppliers.

The ease with which potential providers can actually enter the industry and place their products on the market is referred to as *conditions of entry*. These conditions depend on existing productive techniques, as well as on legal impediments. In some industries, extensive capital requirements preclude many firms from entering because of the large financial commitment necessary to undertake the capital investment and to commence production. Such conditions may exist for some types of medical care, such as intensive surgery, although these financial impediments are not nearly as great as they are, for example, in the automobile industry. For many types of medical care, this sort of impediment is not relevant to entry conditions. More relevant are the legal impediments that are instituted in the licensing of medical personnel and facilities under legislative jurisdiction. Such procedures frequently amount to severe restrictions placed on potential entrants into an industry. Chapter 8 discusses entry conditions, and Chapter 12 discusses restrictions in the context of the political process through which they are generated.

7.3.4 Simultaneous Demand and Supply Shifts

In addition to creating movements in either demand or supply forces alone, whose effects are readily predictable, underlying factors may cause shifts in both demand and supply forces at the same time. We must be careful at this stage of the analysis to specify that we are referring to separate factors causing changes in demand and supply. That is, an increase in the number of ill people occurring at the same time as an influx of physicians into the market will cause both demand and supply curves to shift; the increase in the illness level will cause demand to increase, and the increase in the number of physicians will cause supply to increase. In Figure 7–4, this is shown as a shift in demand from D_1 to D_2 and, at the same time, a shift in supply from S_1 to S_2. While quantity increases, the net effect on price is ambiguous and will depend on how much each curve shifts, that is, on the change in the value of the causal variables and the degree to which they cause demand and supply to shift. In the specific case of Figure 7–4, price will fall. But if we do not know the extent to which both curves are shifted, our model fails us as a predictive device and thus fails in its prime purpose.

A second type of simultaneous shift may occur when the same factor that causes demand to shift also causes supply to shift independently. Quality is a factor that causes supply to decrease as quality increases; at the same time it has an effect of

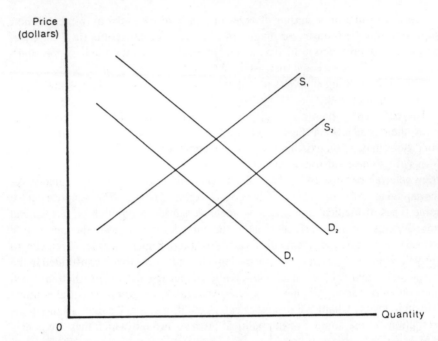

Figure 7–4 Representation of simultaneous shifting of demand and supply curves. Beginning with an initial demand and supply level D_1 and S_1 and a resulting price and output level, a simultaneous shift in demand and supply curves such that demand is increased to D_2 and supply to S_2 will have an ambiguous effect on price and will increase output. The extent of both shifts determines the effects on price and quantity. Some directional shifts, such as a simultaneous decrease in demand and increase in supply, will lower the price but have an ambiguous effect on quantity traded.

increasing demand. In such a case, when demand increases and supply decreases, price will increase, but quantity will increase, fall, or remain the same depending on the extent of the shifts. Another type of simultaneous shift that does not belong in this category is when supply and demand forces are not independent, such as when physicians can induce consumer demand. This phenomenon is discussed in Chapter 9.

7.3.5 Shortages

Our predictions so far have been concerned with what happens to equilibrium price when one or several factors change. Not all situations we observe are such that quantity demanded is the amount that is supplied. In many instances in the medical care market, we observe shortages. A *shortage* occurs when quantity demanded exceeds quantity supplied at the current price. Our model shows that in a competitive market with free bidding a shortage will cause the price to rise, with suppliers offering more at higher prices and consumers reducing their quantities demanded at the new price level. The shortage will disappear. Yet persistent shortages have been observed in the blood market, the market for nurses, the physicians' services market, and, in some countries, the hospital market. A slightly altered view of the competitive model allows us to predict why these shortages occur and how they can be eliminated.

Refer to our example in Figure 7–1. Assume that by some government regulation the price cannot rise above $1.70 per visit. Perhaps such a regulation is enforced to help lower-income consumers who may go without medical services if the price is $2. The consequences of such a regulation can be determined from the competitive model. At $1.70, consumers will be more anxious to visit their physicians, and according to our figures 1,300 will call for appointments. But at this price it would be unprofitable for physicians to see 1,300 patients. Indeed, they will reduce quantity supplied and will see only 700 patients. A queue will form of untreated patients; in this case, 600 patients who want treatment will be untreated. Shortages may be explained as a result of such price ceilings. In a competitive market, a shortage can only persist if the price is somehow administered to remain below the market-clearing price. This will usually be done by an official or semiofficial agency that can overrule the price market forces set.

A shortage can also occur when insurance is purchased or when a government program "guaranteeing" medical care is instituted. In such situations the consumers may face a zero money price, which will mean a high quantity demanded, for example, 10,000 units, as shown in Figure 7–5. The reimbursed price to the provider may be only $20 per unit, and at this price 7,000 units are provided. In our example, it would take a price of $100 to bring forth 10,000 units supplied. At the administered reimbursement rate of $20, there is a shortage of 3,000 units.

Such a situation requires a mechanism to ration the 7,000 available units, assuming that quality produced remains the same. One such mechanism is to make the prospective patients wait in line; those who are willing to pay the "time costs" will receive the service (Buchanan, 1965; Culyer and Cullis, 1976; Sloan and Lorant, 1976). Another possibility is for the providers to lower the quality of their product, for example, by reducing the time it takes per examination. Such an action would shift demand inward, since the commodity would not have the same worth as before, and it would shift supply out; the shortage would be reduced and perhaps even eliminated.

7.3.6 Surpluses

The usual definition of a *surplus* is one of an excess of quantity supplied over quantity demanded at a given price. For a surplus to persist, some factor must keep quantity supplied above that demanded. If the price in the market were kept

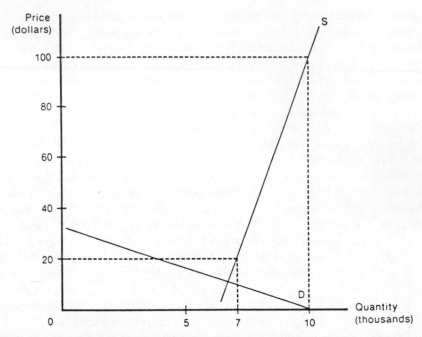

Figure 7–5 Representation of supply and demand forces using the example of full service coverage by a third party. Full service (zero direct price) coverage with a reimbursement rate of $20 will lead to a quantity demanded of 10 and a quantity supplied of 7. To reach a quantity supplied of 10, the reimbursement rate would have to be 100 (curve S).

permanently above the equilibrium price, a surplus would persist: suppliers would be willing to provide more units than consumers would be willing to purchase. In Figure 7–1, if both the suppliers' reimbursed price *and* the consumers' direct price were at $2.10 and could not be lowered, a surplus would appear. In this case suppliers would be willing to supply more units *at that price* than demanders would want: the suppliers would find themselves with excess capacity.

For a surplus to persist, something must prevent the market price from falling, because in a normal competitive situation an excess supply situation would induce suppliers to lower their prices to induce demanders to buy more. If the government pegged or supported an above-equilibrium price in the market, a surplus would occur. In the case of health care, where insurance exists, a surplus can occur if the reimbursement rate to the suppliers induces a greater quantity supplied than the quantity demanded by consumers at their direct price. In Figure 7–1, if the reimbursement rate to suppliers was $2.50 and the direct price to consumers was $1.90, a surplus would exist.

In recent years there has been much talk of a ''physician surplus.'' Accompanying the discussion of such a surplus, one hears talk of falling physicians' fees and incomes. To the extent that the fees and incomes of doctors are falling, this situation does not represent a surplus in the technical sense. Falling fees are characteristic of prices responding to (say) shifting supply en route to a new equilibrium point. For a surplus to develop, the market cannot be allowed to move to a new equilibrium: it must remain in disequilibrium.

The case of a surplus of hospital beds is more likely one of permanent disequilibrium. High hospital reimbursement rates have induced a large quantity supplied; at given direct prices, there has not been enough quantity demanded to clear the market.

7.3.7 Multimarket Analyses

The competitive model is well suited to making predictions about the effect of supply and/or demand changes in one market on price and quantity in a related market. Let us take an example of two substitute services, inpatient and outpatient surgical care. Because of the development of shorter-acting anesthetics, outpatient surgery has become more feasible. The total cost of outpatient surgery is much less than inpatient surgery for most cases, but until recently outpatient surgery was rarely covered in insurance policies. However, outpatient surgery for many procedures is now covered.

Analytically, the impact of moving from no outpatient coverage of a procedure (e.g., tonsillectomy) to outpatient coverage can be shown in Figure 7–6. The preoutpatient coverage market for inpatient procedures is characterized in Figure 7–6a. Here S is the inpatient supply curve and D_{n+i} is the market demand curve (inpatient). In Figure 7–6b, D_n is the demand curve for outpatient tonsillectomies (without insurance) and S is the supply curve. Note that the demand function for *inpatient* care is dependent on the *direct* price for *outpatient surgery* because the two are substitutes.

An increase in outpatient coverage will shift the market curve for outpatient care outward (to D_{n+i} in Figure 7–6b) and simultaneously lower the direct price of outpatient care. This will result in an inward shift in the D_{n+i} curve for inpatient care to D^1_{n+i}. Inpatient price will fall and the quantity of inpatient procedures will be reduced. Note also that the outpatient procedures are increased.

Similar types of analyses can be conducted for other types of substitute procedures or for complements, such as inpatient surgery and surgeons' services. In some cases it is not always clear whether two services are substitutes or complements. For example, it is not clear whether nursing home care replaces hospital care or is used in conjunction with it. The same holds for home health care and hospital care. In these instances the model cannot provide unambiguous conclusions.

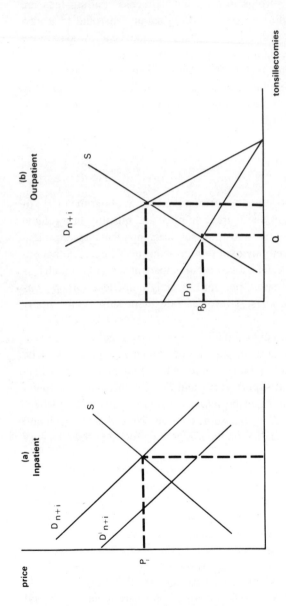

Figure 7-6 Representation of multimarket analysis. Demand curves in inpatient and outpatient markets are related (the services are substitutes). When the direct price in the outpatient market falls (because of an increase in insurance coverage), the demand curve in the inpatient market shifts inward; price and quantity fall in the inpatient market.

7.4 EVIDENCE ABOUT THE COMPETITIVE MODEL

There has been some use of the competitive model in explaining resource-allocation trends in medical care markets. In the physicians' services market, the phenomena of rapidly rising physicians' fees, both before and after the watershed year of 1966 when Medicare and Medicaid were instituted (see Chapter 11), were explained with the competitive model by hypothesizing that the rapid increase in medical care insurance caused demand shifts (see Section 4.4) and consequent rising prices. In this market, in particular, the length of time required to train new physicians means a slow supply response, even in a competitive market, and prices are thus predicted to rise (Garbarino, 1959; Newhouse and Phelps, 1977). In the hospital care market the same type of explanation can be made for rising hospital costs, with one addition. While insurance was increasing during this time period, hospital input prices, notably employee wages, were also rapidly rising. This latter phenomenon would shift the supply curve inward. Coupled with a rapidly outward shifting demand curve for hospital care, the net effect would be a larger price increase. Whether utilization would increase or decrease would depend on the magnitude of both shifts. As seen in Chapter 2, hospital utilization increased. Our "after-the-fact" explanation would state that the supply and demand shifts were such that this turned out to be the case. (An application of the competitive model to the hospital field is found in Ro, 1977.)

The competitive model has also been used in its disequilibrium form to explain the large queues and unmet demands that have resulted and persisted in England following the institution of the National Health Service (NHS) in 1946. The NHS can be characterized by a zero money price paid by consumers, a per capita remuneration to general practitioners, and a salaried remuneration to surgeons. The application of the competitive model to this situation would predict large increases in quantity demanded following the lowering of the price to zero. Supply decisions passed into the hands of the central government following the institution of socialized medicine, and large increases in supply did not materialize. As a result, persistent shortages, particularly in hospital care, were evidenced (Culyer and Cullis, 1976).

Although the competitive model is a useful device in explaining price and quantity movements, as well as the causes of shortages of medical care, much attention has focused on the shortcomings of the model. Evidence of the competitive model's shortcomings is of three sorts. Evidence can involve examining data on market outcomes, such as profits and prices. If such outcomes are not what we would expect in a competitive market (i.e., not what the competitive model predicts would happen), we can infer that the model does not explain well and seek alternative models to better explain the data. Second, we might observe some preconditions, such as consumer ignorance or product quality level differences, that are so much at odds with the competitive model's assumptions that we seek a different model that incorporates these. Third, we might observe direct actions on the part of providers that imply noncompetitive practices. These might include constraints on certain activities usually thought of as competitive. Free entry is an example. We turn to some of this evidence.

7.4.1 Excessive Profits

Studies made of the profits accruing from medical practice have shown these profits to be persistent and considerable. These profits, which are the net incomes of the physicians operating the practices, must be adjusted for the costs incurred in medical training, including fees paid and earnings foregone while practicing medicine or engaging in internship and residency. Adjusting for these costs, the net present value (see Chapter 11) of medical practice has indicated persistent economic profits (i.e., earnings in excess of normal returns) to medical practitioners (Lindsay, 1976; Sloan, 1976). Generally, the competitive model predicts that such excess profits would eventually be bid away by new providers entering the industry to take advantage of the high returns in this field. This has not occurred in medical practice.

7.4.2 Fee Differences among Patients

The competitive model predicts that one price will prevail in the market for all suppliers and demanders. Before the spread of health insurance, physician pricing was characterized by a sliding scale of fees, with higher-income patients paying higher prices than lower-income patients. These phenomena have led economists to reject the competitive model as being applicable to the physician services market in favor of a monopoly model (Kessell, 1958; Newhouse, 1970; Ruffin and Leigh, 1973; Wu and Masson, 1974; see Chapter 8).

7.4.3 Quality of Care

The competitive model assumes a homogeneous service is being bought and sold and that competition is based on price. Yet product quality is a major element of a hospital's output, and health insurance companies often offer different types of policies in terms of coverage (viewed as differences in the quality of the policy as well as differences in service).

When a supplier can vary its quality, it can attract consumers on the basis of its quality. It follows that some "brand loyalty" may ensue, and buyers will not switch brands easily (i.e., at a slight increase in price). Each supplier then faces a downward sloping demand curve, not a horizontal one (as is the case in perfect competition), and can choose to supply both quality and quantity of output. Providers can compete with each other on the basis of price and product quality.

The competitive model is not equipped to handle this eventuality, which requires a somewhat more complex model (Chapter 8).

7.4.4 Restricting Competitive Behavior

Additional evidence on anticompetitive control mechanisms is found by examining the behavior of physicians when confronted with potentially competitive colleagues. Two practices have been restricted by physician associations, the advertising of physician fees and the participation by physicians in prepayment group practices. In an ideal world, such as that set out in the model in Section 7.2, advertising is unnecessary because consumers know all about physicians' fees. But as seen in Section 4.11, considerable consumer ignorance exists in the medical care industry and advertising would reduce such ignorance about alternative physician prices (and perhaps qualifications). Coupled with fee cutting (price reductions), advertising would result in more business for the fee-cutting advertiser, but in generally lower prices and profits in the industry.

Advertising bans have been enforced by state medical societies (Kessell, 1958), and although such bans are no longer legally enforceable, their existence in the past was evidence that physicians were able to intervene in the market on behalf of themselves and eliminate some degree of competition in the market. Bans on advertising (and other competitive practices) have been used as evidence of the availability of mechanisms to restrict competition (see Chapters 8 and 12).

7.4.5 Consumer Ignorance and Supplier-Induced Demand

The competitive model operates under the assumption that consumers possess a considerable degree of information about their condition, the product they need, and the outcome of using the product. In fact, consumers appear to operate under a considerable degree of ignorance in this area, which has led some commentators to view the physician as behaving as an "agent" on behalf of the consumer (Feldstein, 1974). To the extent that physicians do behave as agents for their patients, the implicit assumption of independence between suppliers and demanders is broken: demanders are subject to direct supplier influence.

Nor can one assume that, if they do act as the agent for the patient, physicians will always behave in the patients' own interests. Once the patients are prone to manipulation, the possibility exists that physicians can use this influence to further their own interests. Consumer demands can be shifted by the suppliers providing different information.

Such a demand-shifting phenomenon can be detected in market outcome statistics under some circumstances. According to the competitive theory, an increase in the per capita supply of physicians results in an increase in market supply. With everything else held constant, this should bring down the price. Yet it has been alleged that the relationship between physician per capita supply and price is the exact opposite to that predicted by the model; that is, the more physicians in an area (on a per capita basis), the higher the observed price is (Evans, 1974; Fuchs and Kramer, 1972; Kushman, 1976). The reason why these phenomena are alleged rather than demonstrated is that a number of intervening factors exist that may cause demand to rise at the same time as physician supply increases.

Let us make a simple comparison of two hypothetical medical markets, one in a small town and one in a large metropolitan center with several medical schools. The large city may have more doctors per capita than the small town, and the price for a visit to a physician may be greater. This "raw" relationship, by itself, does not mean that the higher supply has caused the higher price. Many other intervening variables must also be accounted for, among them being insurance, the health status of the two populations, and the quality of care provided. The third factor, the quality of care, is especially important in making comparisons, mainly because it is such a difficult variable to measure and thus may be ignored. It may well be that the quality of care in the city is higher than in the town. If all factors other than the quality of care were adjusted for, we might still observe a positive relationship between physician density and price. Until quality has been adjusted, however, we cannot be certain that the higher price is not due to a payment for better-quality service.

This type of confounding relationship has caused the observed relationship between price and physician density to be controversial (Sloan and Feldman, 1978). Nevertheless, some commentators have proceeded "as if" it were true and have constructed alternative models to explain these phenomena (see Section 9.2).

7.5 COMPETITIVE BIDDING

The competitive market has often been held up as an ideal, a standard in the light of which other allocative arrangements might be judged (see Chapter 10). One set of arrangements that has been put forward as potentially providing a competitive-style outcome is competitive bidding in a public program. Competitive bidding occurs when a purchaser (e.g., a government) requests bids from alternative competing providers and allocates the right to treat patients based on the bids. The objective of this practice is to have the patients treated in a least-cost manner.

One approach to modeling the competitive bidding process is to examine the behavior of the individual supplier who is facing a single paying agency and who is competing with other providers for the right to provide the service. An essential feature of such a model involves the recognition that the bids are made under conditions of risk. When they submit their bids, the bidders do not know for certain whether or not they will be selected as providers. Their behavior can be modeled in a manner similar to that of consumers who are faced with risky medical expenses (Section 4.4).

The bidder faces two alternative states: (1) the successful alternative, when the bid is accepted, and (2) the unsuccessful alternative, when the bid is rejected. To simplify matters, let us assume that no losses are associated with an unsuccessful bid (i.e., the bidder is no worse off than if he or she did not bid). What the bidder must do is compare the outcomes of the various bids to assess which will prove the most satisfactory.

Our simplified model is presented in numerical form in Table 7–1. We make the following assumptions. First, a request is put out calling for providers to bid for the right to serve a given number of patients in a public program. The bids are to be expressed in per capita terms for a certain set of services (physician care, hospital care, and drugs). Second, five options are open to the bidder; these options, labeled A through E, consist of bids of $100, $95, and so on, through $80. Third, as the bidder lowers his or her bid, the probability of being a successful bidder (having the bid accepted) increases. At a bid of $100, there is a 20 percent chance ($= 0.2$) of the bid being accepted. This rises to 90 percent with a bid of $80. Third, the bidder's profits, *if the bid is accepted,* are equal to the revenues less costs of serving the given number of patients. Given the number of patients (Q) and the costs per patient (C), the higher the *accepted* bid, the higher will be the profits [equal to $(B \times Q) - (C \times Q)$]. Fourth, we translate the postprofit situation of the bidder into a wealth level. We assume that, under a no contract situation, wealth would be $200. A successful bid thus adds to the successful bidder's wealth level by the level of the bidder's profits.

The bidder is thus faced with a trade-off between profits (and hence wealth) and the probability of a successful bid. The individual bidder can increase the likelihood of success, but only by lowering his or her bid, and thus lowering his or her profits. Given the range of alternatives, which option will the bidder choose? As

Table 7–1 Hypothetical Data Relating to Alternative Bids by a Provider

(1)	(2)	(3)	(4)	(5)	(6)	(7)
				Wealth	Utility Levels	
			Profits	Level	for:	
		Probability	(if bid	(if bid	Risk	Risk
Option	Bid Price	of Acceptance	accepted)	accepted)	Averter	Taker
A	$100	0.2	800	1,000	126	2,000
B	95	0.4	400	600	122	800
C	90	0.6	200	400	118	400
D	85	0.8	100	300	110	200
E	80	0.9	50	250	100	100

set up now, our model is incomplete: it does not incorporate the objectives of the bidders, nor does it discuss the bidding rules set up by the contracting agency.

With regard to bidders' objectives, let us assume first that the bidder is extremely *risk averse*. He or she puts a high personal value on small gains and successively lower additional values on larger gains (i.e., he or she exhibits a diminishing marginal utility of wealth). This assumption is shown in column (6) of Table 7–1. Under these assumptions, the bidder will choose the option that maximizes his or her *expected* utility, measured as the product of the probability of success (P_s) and the utility associated with the wealth level of that option. In our example, the risk averter will choose option E, which yields an expected utility of 90. Option D, for example, would yield an expected utility of 88. The high probability of being successful, coupled with the importance to the bidder of having at least *some* profits, results in the bidder selecting a very safe, but relatively unprofitable, outcome.

The *risk taker*, whose tastes are summarized in column 7, demonstrates the all importance to such individuals of high wealth levels by having a schedule with sharply increasing utilities of wealth. To this bidder, high wealth levels are so important that they overshadow the very small chances of attaining those levels. To the risk taker, option E has an expected utility of 90, whereas option A has one of 400. Option A is the one to be selected by the risk-taking bidder.

As can be seen, competitive bidding does not automatically lead to a low price bid. Much of the outcome depends on bidders' costs and goals. But there are several other factors as well. First, an increase in the number of bidders will reduce the probability of any single bidder being successful. Depending on their utility schedules, a larger number of competitive bidders may cause each bidder to reduce his or her bid. Second, there are a number of alternative types of selection and reimbursement arrangements that a contracting agency can resort to. These may influence the bidding strategies of the bidders (Christianson, Smith, and Hillman, 1984). One possible set of arrangements is to reimburse each winning bidder (more than one provider in an area may be chosen as a winner) at the level of the bid that they submit. Thus, if bidder I submits a bid of $95, bidder II, $90, and bidder III, $85, and if II and III are selected as providers, then II would be reimbursed at $90 and III at $85. A set of rules such as these tends to encourage bidding providers to gamble and seek a higher price, since there is a potential reward to them for doing so (they are reimbursed at the price they bid if their bid is accepted). An alternative set of selection and reimbursement arrangements might check this tendency. If the set of rules were such that all winning bidders would be reimbursed at the rate bid by the *lowest* winning bidder, there would be no benefit to a winner making a higher bid if he or she deems that some other winner will bid lower. Indeed, raising the bid merely reduces the chances of being successful.

Competitive bidding *may* lead to an outcome resembling that of a competitive market. But this will depend on a number of factors, including the number of bidders, their attitudes toward risk, and the bidding rules set up by the agency. There has been little experience with such arrangements in the health care field. Both California and Arizona Medicaid programs have developed such practices, but it will be several years before it is clear whether such arrangements yield any better results than straight rate setting by the contracting out agencies (Christianson, 1985; Christianson, Hillman, and Smith, 1983; Kirkman-Liff, Christianson, and Hillman, 1985; McCall, 1985).

REFERENCES

Competitive Market Model

Buchanan, J.M. (1965). *The inconsistencies of the National Health Service.* Occasional Paper 7. Institute of Economic Affairs, London.

Christianson, J.B., & McClure, W. (1979). Competition in the delivery of medical care. *New England Journal of Medicine, 301,* 812–818.

Culyer, A.J., & Cullis, J.G. (1976). Some economics of hospital waiting lists in the N.H.S. *Social Policy 5,* 239–264.

Evans, R.G. (1974). Supplier induced demand. In M. Perlman (Ed.), *The Economics of Health and Medical Care* (pp. 162–173). London: The MacMillan Co.

Feldstein, M.S. (1970). The rising price of physicians' services. *Review of Economics and Statistics, 52,* 121–133.

———— (1974). Econometric studies in health economics. In M. Intriligator and D. Kendrick (Eds.), *Frontiers in quantitative economics* (pp 377–434). Amsterdam: North Holland Publishing Co.

Frank, R.G., & Welch, W.P. (1985). The competitive effects of HMO's: A review of the evidence. *Inquiry, 22,* 148–161.

Friedman, M. (1962). *Capitalism and Freedom.* Chicago: University of Chicago Press.

Fuchs, U.R., & Kramer, M. (1972). Determinants of expenditures for physicians' services in the United States 1948-1968 (Publication No. HSM 73-3013). Washington, D.C.: National Center for Health Services Research, U.S. Department of Health, Education and Welfare.

Gabarino, J.W. (1959). Price behavior and productivity in the medical market. *Industrial and Labor Relations Review, 13,* 3–15.

Hay, J.W., & Leahy, M.J. (1984). Competition among health plans: Some preliminary evidence. *Southern Economic Journal, 50,* 831–846.

Kelly, E.T., Rodowskas, C.A., & Gagnon, P.J. (1975). An examination of the effect of market demographic and competitive characteristics on gross margins of prescription drugs. *Medical Care, 13,* 956–965.

Kessell, R. (1958). Price discrimination in medicine. *Journal of Law and Economics, 1,* 20–53.

Kushman, J.E. (1976). Market structure, health capital production, and physician behavior. *Atlantic Economic Journal, 4,* 39–47.

Lindsay, C.M. (1976). More real returns to medical education. *Journal of Human Resources, 11,* 127–129.

Newhouse, J.P. (1970). A model of physician pricing. *Southern Economic Journal, 37,* 147–183.

———— , & Phelps, C.E. (1977). Policy options and the impact of national health insurance revisited. *International Journal of Health Services, 7,* 503–509.

Pauly, M.V., & Langwell, K.M. (1983). Research on competition in the market for health services. *Inquiry, 20,* 142–161.

Ro, K.K. (1977). Anatomy of hospital cost inflation. *Hospitals and Health Services Administration, 22,* 78–88.

Ruffin, R.E., & Leigh, D.E. (1983). Charity, competition, and the pricing of doctors' services. *Journal of Human Resources, 8,* 212–222.

Salkever, D. (1975). Hospital wage inflation. *Quarterly Review of Economics and Business, 15,* 33–84.

―――― (1978). Competition among hospitals. In W. Greenberg (Ed.), *Competition in the health care sector* (pp. 191–206). Washington, D.C.: Federal Trade Commission.

Sloan, F.A. (1976). Real returns to medical education. *Journal of Human Resources, 11,* 118–126.

―――― , & Feldman, R. (1978). Competition among physicians. In W. Greenberg (Ed.), *Competition in the health care sector* (pp. 57–120). Washington, D.C.: Bureau of Economics, Federal Trade Commission.

―――― , & Lorant, J.H. (1976). The allocation of physicians' services: Evidence of length of visit. *Quarterly Review of Economics and Business, 16,* 86–103.

Wu, S., & Masson, R. (1974). Price discrimination for physicians' services. *Journal of Human Resources, 9,* 63–79.

Competitive Bidding

Brown, E.R., Cousineau, M.R., & Price, W.T. (1985). Competing for medical business. *Inquiry 22,* 237–250.

Christianson, J.B. (1984). Provider participation in competitive bidding for indigent patients. *Inquiry, 21,* 161–177.

―――― (1985). The challenge of competitive bidding. *Health Care Management Review, 10*(2), 39–54.

――――, Hillman, D.G., & Smith, K.R. (1983). The Arizona experiment: Competitive bidding for indigent medical care. *Health Affairs, 2,* 87–103.

――――, Smith, K.R., & Hillman, D.G. (1984). A comparison of existing and alternative competitive bidding systems for indigent medical care. *Social Science & Medicine, 18,* 599–604.

Kirkman-Liff, B.L., Christianson, J.B., & Hillman, D.G. (1985). An analysis of competitive bidding by providers for indigent medical care contracts. *Health Services Research, 20,* 549–577.

McCall, N., Henton, D., Crane, M., et al. (1985). Evaluation of the Arizona health care cost-containment system. *Health Care Financing Review, 7,* 77–88.

Melia, E.P., Aucoin, L.M., Duhl, P.J., et al. (1983). Competition in the health-care marketplace: A beginning in California. *New England Journal of Medicine, 308,* 788–792.

Chapter 8

Market Power in Health Care

8.1 INTRODUCTION

Market power refers to the ability of one participant in a market to influence the terms on which he or she makes an exchange. Market power can be wielded by both buyers and sellers. For example, a heart surgeon can be in a position to influence the fee that patients or insurers pay. Similarly, an insurance company or government health insurance program can be in a position to influence the rate at which it reimburses providers for supplying services to its members.

Essential ingredients of market power are the availability of viable substitutes for the service and the ease with which buyers and sellers can weigh these alternatives. A hospital may be the only hospital for hundreds of miles, in which case it possesses some degree of market power; that is, it has some leeway to set price and other terms in which it provides the service. On the other hand, a large number of HMOs may be vying to become providers for a firm's employees; in this case, the HMOs have little or no market power, although the firm may possess some.

Market power is important because, if buyers or sellers possess it, it might allow them to wield influence over the use of resources to the benefit of the demander or supplier and to the detriment of the other bargaining parties. Discussion of the desirability (or lack of it) of market power must wait until we discuss yardsticks with which to gauge actual market conduct; in this chapter we develop the analysis of how market power influences the market outcome (i.e., prices, quantities, and quality). In Chapters 10 to 12, we discuss the evaluation of the performance of market power.

We will examine several models that explain resource allocation when either buyers or sellers possess some degree of market power. In Section 8.2 we discuss two models of the behavior of the ultimate wielder of market power—the monopolist—that offer predictions about how monopolistic suppliers and demanders set price and quantity. All suppliers and demanders would benefit from market power, and a pertinent question is, how does one obtain it? In Section 8.3 we present a discussion of the determinants of market power. In Section 8.3.1 we present a general discussion, particularly with regard to insurance companies; in Section 8.3.2 we present some institutional details about how providers in one market that possesses many of the preconditions of a competitive market, the physicians' services market, were nevertheless able to develop and maintain a considerable degree of market power and use it to bolster their incomes.

The monopolistic model and the competitive model are, in fact, two polar extremes of models of market power. In many (perhaps most) markets, market power and competition are mixed to varying degrees. In Section 8.4 we present several models of incomplete market power that explain how product quality can be an important outcome in provider competition.

8.2 MONOPOLISTIC MARKETS

8.2.1 Simple Monopoly

A *monopoly* is a supplier that is the sole source of supply in a market. In such a market, the demanders do not have any *close* substitutes for the service. They may indeed have *some* degree of substitutability. This is especially true when one remembers that in most health care instances an alternative to treatment usually exists, even if that alternative is to do nothing.

We will develop the monopoly model in the context of a supposed monopolistic market, that for pediatric ambulatory services. In this market there is assumed a single physician's practice servicing a captive market. The product is defined as quality-constant pediatric visits. The simple monopolistic model consists of demand, cost, and behavioral assumptions.

With regard to demand, we assume that the pediatric group faces a single *market* demand curve such as that given in Table 8–1 and, graphically, in Figure 8–1. Note that there is a price, $10, at which patients will abstain from making any visits. As discussed in Section 3.5, as one moves down the demand curve, one moves through elastic, unit elastic, and inelastic portions of the demand curve; and total revenue will increase, level off, and decrease. Marginal revenue is falling throughout, although it is positive when it is associated with the elastic portion of the demand curve and zero relative to the unit elastic point on the demand curve. For the provider, marginal revenue represents the additional total revenue that it will receive by lowering the price enough to sell one more visit. Note that as the provider lowers its price it sells more units, but *all of them* at the new, lower price. The marginal revenue *(MR)* is the *net* change in total revenue *(TR)* and is the difference in the two *TR*s at the two quantity levels.

Table 8–1 Revenue and Cost in a Hypothetical Monopolistic Market

(1)	(2)	(3)	(4)	(5)	(6)	(7)
		Total	Marginal	Total	Marginal	
	Units of	Revenue	Revenue	Cost	Cost	Profits
Price	Output	(TR)	(MR)	(TC)	(MC)	(TR − TC)
10	0	0		3		−3
9	1	9	9	4	1	5
8	2	16	7	6	2	10
7	3	21	5	9	3	12
6	4	24	3	13	4	11
5	5	25	1	18	5	7
4	6	24	−1	24	6	−0
3	7	21	−3	31	7	−10

The monopolist has the ability to set price at any level it wishes. This ability represents the ultimate degree in market power. Of course, the price it sets will influence buyer's demand, but the monopolist has control over a number of alternative prices that it can set.

Our cost assumptions are that total fixed cost *(TFC)* is $3, and total variable cost *(TVC)* is increasing in such a way that marginal cost *(MC)* is increasing as output expands (see Table 8–1, column 6). Total cost *(TC)* is the sum of *TVC* and *TFC*.

Profits (column 7) are equal to *TR* − *TC* and initially increase and then decrease as output expands. But we cannot tell what price will be charged and what the output level will be until we know what objectives the provider is pursuing. Let us assume that the provider's objective is to maximize profits (equal to *TR* − *TC*). Then the price will be set at the appropriate level and consumers will demand the corresponding quantity of output.

The workings of our model can now be set out. First, the price will be set at that point on the demand curve at which *MR* comes closest to (or equals) *MC* (without *MC* exceeding *MR*). In Table 8–1, let us assume that the monopolist initially set its price at $10 per visit. It would have no buyers at such a price; its losses would be confined to its fixed costs since it would have no variable costs at zero output. If, now, price were lowered to $9, one visit would be sold and the *MR* would be $9. One additional visit would cost only $1 extra *(MC = $1)* and would add $8 to the previous output level's profits. Total profit would therefore be $5. This is certainly better than not operating at all, but not as good as lowering the price to $8, selling two units in total, and deriving an additional $7 in revenue in the process *(MR =* $7). For then it would cost the pediatricians only $2 more to provide this added visit, and they would be adding another $5 (= *MR* − *MC*) to the previous profit level, making profits $10 in total. Indeed, the practice would lower its price to $7,

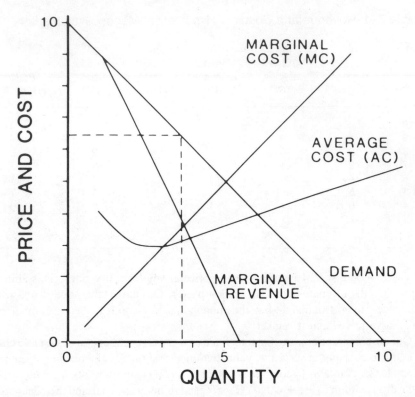

Figure 8–1 Equilibrium price and output in a monopolistic (single seller) market. The monopolist faces a given demand curve for the service from which is derived its marginal revenue curve. The monopolist's cost conditions are presented in marginal *(MC)* and average *(AC)* terms. The profit-maximizing monopolist will set price and quantity such that its *MR* = *MC*. Equilibrium price is between $6 and $7, and equilibrium quantity is between $3 and $4. Based on data in Table 8–1.

selling three visits. It would stop there, because beyond this level of output *MC* is beginning to rise steeply; *TC* increases more than *TR* is increasing, and as a result *MR* − *MC* becomes negative. Any further increase in output would detract from total profits.

Our analysis is shown graphically in Figure 8–1 with smoothed out revenue and cost functions. Here we see that *MR* and *MC* intersect (are equal) at a quantity of between 3 and 4 (because of our smoothed out values), which corresponds to a price on the demand curve of between $6 and $7. Profitability cannot be increased by raising or lowering price.

Let us now see what the model implies. First, the provider will set price at that point on the demand curve above which the *MR* and *MC* curves intersect. Because *MC* is positive, *MR* must also be positive (since *MR* = *MC*) at the profit-maximizing point. As discussed later and in Section 3.5, *MR* is positive only at those quantities where its related demand curve is on its *elastic* portion. Therefore, a monopolist will set price only on the elastic portion of its demand curve. Indeed, if price were set on the inelastic portion of the curve, say at $3, *MR* would be negative, meaning that a reduction in output coming from a price increase would raise total revenues. At the same time a reduction in output would reduce *TC*. Profits would therefore always be greater at a higher price (one on the elastic portion of the demand curve).

An additional conclusion is that, since the most profitable level of output is determined by *MR* and *MC* alone, and since *MC* is unaffected by fixed costs, the profit-maximizing price will similarly be unaffected by changes in fixed costs. Let us say that fixed costs in our example increase to $5. Profits would be lower by $2 at *every* level of output. But the maximum profit level would still be the same (at $Q = 3$), only now the provider would be earning less profits. This important result implies that if the provider's fixed costs increase (say because of an increase in mortgage rates) it cannot do anything about it. If it tries to pass on these added fixed costs to the consumer by raising the price, it will only be moving away from the profit-maximizing position: in raising price it will sell less, and *MR* will decrease more than *MC*. This, of course, is not true for an increase in variable costs (i.e., *MC*).

In a similar vein, if the profit-maximizing monopolist received a fixed subsidy (i.e., one unrelated to output) of, say, $2 to treat poor patients, *TR* would be increased at every level of output by $2, but *MR* would not be affected. Its profit-maximizing price will not change, and unless the granting agency enforces the terms of the subsidy, nothing will change. That is, the *profit-maximizing* monopolist will not lower the price to induce people to demand more.

The outcome of the monopoly model is such that the firm could be persistently earning excess profits. Since the *AC* curve incorporates all the monopolist's costs, including opportunity costs (see Section 5.3), the monopolist's profits in this analysis are equal to $TR - TC$ or, using average terms, the product of the unit margin $(P - AC)$ and output (Q). These profits are true *economic profits*. That is, they are profits over and above all the costs required to operate the enterprise, including a normal return for the owner's efforts and capital. Furthermore, nothing in the model will allow the monopolist's profits to be bid away. There are no potential entrants into the market who can charge a lower price (see Section 8.3.1 for a discussion of the conditions under which this might occur). As a result, the monopolist can earn above-normal profits that persist over time. Recall that, in the competitive market model, entry is inexpensive and any excess profits will attract new entrants, who will expand supply and lower price and profits.

8.2.2 Buyer's Market Power

Market power can also exist on the buyer's side. Let us assume that there is a single buyer of nursing services, a hospital in a small city. A number of nurses are available to be hired by the hospital, and their supply curve is drawn in Figure 8–2. At a wage of $2 weekly, two nurses will supply their services; if the wage is increased to $3, three nurses will supply their services; and so on. The successive marginal values that the single hospital places on nurses is also shown in Figure 8–2. Let us assume that additional nurses allow the hospital to treat more patients, but the marginal productivity of these extra nurses is declining; the price received for the extra patient by the hospital is constant. The hospital's value curve has been derived from the estimated additional revenue that the hospital estimates the additional nurses will bring in. The *marginal revenue product,* the additional value of one more nurse to the hospital, is $9 for the first, $8 for the second, $7 for

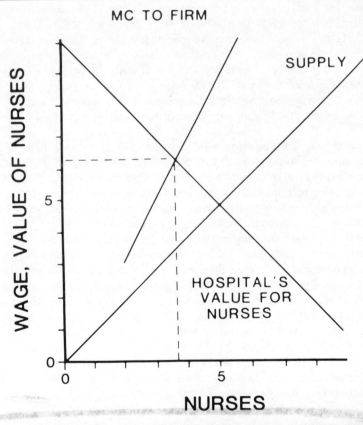

Figure 8–2 Equilibrium wage and number of nurses hired, in a monopsonistic (single buyer) market. The firm's marginal cost for hiring additional nurses is derived from the supply schedule of nurses in the market. The value of an additional nurse is based on the amount of output the nurses can produce (their productivity) and the price of output, in short, the amount of revenue brought in by hiring additional nurses. The profit-maximizing firm will hire that number of nurses where the *MC* equals the additional revenue from hiring another nurse.

the third, and so on. Note that the total value to the hospital of three nurses is $24 (= $9 + $8 + $7). We will assume that the hospital wishes to maximize profits.

The profit-maximizing hospital will hire additional nurses as long as the marginal cost of doing so is less than the additional revenues. But the *MC* of nurses to the hospital is not the nurses' supply curve, *S*. Since *S* is sloped up, each successive nurse wants an extra dollar to be attracted to work. Assuming that the hospital must pay *all* nurses the same wage, by hiring the second nurse it must pay a higher wage to the first as well. In this light, the *MC* to the hospital is more steeply sloped than the supply curve. In this case, the *MC* of the second nurse is $3 and of the third nurse is $5 (= $9 − $4). This curve is shown as *MC* in Figure 8–2. The profit-maximizing hospital will then hire three nurses (between 3 and 4 in Figure 8–2), for then the hospital's added revenues will equal its *MC* for hiring nurses. At such a level of hiring, it will pay a wage of $3, since that is the wage at which three nurses will supply their services.

In such a market, fewer nurses would be hired than in a competitive market. In a competitive market, competitive forces would drive the wage up to the level where supply equals demand: more nurses would be hired and wages would be driven up. However, a single *monopsonistic* buyer can prevent this from happening, thus maintaining its profits. At the same time as it depresses wages, it causes a restricted supply. Such buying power may be characteristic of buyers of health insurance, for example, if there is one or several large businesses in an area, and potentially a large number of HMOs and traditional insurance companies. It might also be characteristic of some preferred provider organizations. An insurer, for example, can offer lower premiums if it can get its enrollees to agree to go to designated lower-cost providers. The insurer would then negotiate with the providers for lower rates. If the insurer had a substantial enrollment, it could wield monopsonistic power.

8.2.3 Price Discrimination

Under some conditions a monopolist can further increase its profits by charging different prices to different buyers. This is called *price discrimination*. Price discrimination can be practiced only when the product or service in the lower-price market cannot be resold in the higher-price market. In addition, the demand elasticities in the two markets have to be different to make the practice worthwhile.

Let us assume that a pediatric practice can separate its patients into two distinct markets according to patient income. Assume further that demand elasticity is influenced by income, so that each market will have different demand curves. Thus one of the preconditions for price discrimination is met. The product sold is patient visits: these can hardly be resold from one market to the other, and so the other precondition is met as well. The demand curves for the two separate markets, "rich" and "poor," are shown in Figure 8–3a and b. Our cost assumption is that

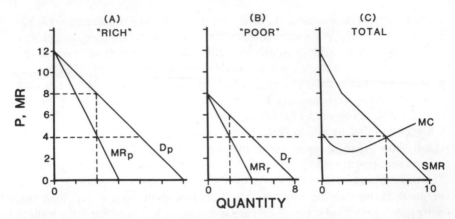

Figure 8–3 Price setting by a discriminating monopolist. The monopolist can separate its markets into two submarkets, "rich" and "poor." The price charged in each market is derived from firm level conditions and occurs where the marginal revenue in each market equals the overall marginal cost to the firm. The curve *SMR* in part (c) shows the total quantity in all markets at each level of *MR*. Note the equality of *MR* in each submarket.

MC is eventually rising, as shown in Figure 8–3c. Note that there is one *MC* for the entire operation; production is not separated. Our behavioral assumption is that the pediatric practice seeks to maximize its profits.

Given these assumptions, our monopolistic model can be used to illustrate the monopolist's pricing policy. To do so, we must rely on the equimarginal principle of maximization. To maximize profits, the provider will set price (and therefore quantity) in each market such that (1) the *MR* earned by lowering (raising) the price in all markets is the same, and (2) overall the *MR* in each market is equal to the *MC* of producing that level of output.

The derivation of the profit-maximizing prices is shown in Figure 8–3. *MC* is the provider's marginal cost for all units provided (it does not have a separate cost for each market), and the curve *SMR* shows the quantity that would be supplied overall when the firm allocated output to each market according to the specific level of *MR*. *SMR* is thus the sum of quantities in both markets at a given level of *MR*. Given the *MR* curves for the poor and the rich as MR_p and MR_r, at a given level of *MR* in both markets of 4, the corresponding quantities in these markets are 4 and 2, respectively. The *SMR* curve for those quantities will be at a quantity of 6, where $Q_m = Q_p + Q_r$.

The firm's maximum profit position will be determined by equating *MC* with the *MR* in *each* market. Overall, this occurs where $MC = SMR$ (at quantity 6). The corresponding outputs in each market are 4 and 2, and the prices in the two markets that equate the *MR*'s are 8 and 6, respectively. Profits, which are equal to the sum of *TR* in each market less *TC*, will be greater than if the same price were set in all markets.

Price discrimination such as this cannot exist in a competitive market, and this is one reason why physician pricing has been characterized as monopolistic. For many years physicians, particularly specialists, resorted to a sliding scale of fees when setting prices, charging the richer patients more than the poorer ones (Kessell, 1958). In recent years, physician services have become more highly insured and the sliding scale has all but disappeared (Newhouse, 1970).

8.2.4 Physician Pricing and Supply in Public Programs

The two-part monopoly model of Section 8.2.3 has been used to explain physician pricing and supply decisions under multipayor systems related to reimbursement policies of Blue Shield (Sloan and Steinwald, 1978), Medicare (Paringer, 1980; Rice, 1984), and Medicaid (Kushman, 1977; Hadley, 1979; Cromwell and Mitchell, 1984), and under the price limitations of the Economic Stabilization Program from 1972 to 1975 (Hadley and Lee, 1978–1979).

The Medicare studies examined the effect of Medicare reimbursement levels (80 percent of the physicians' reasonable charges) on the assignment decision, the decision of physicians to accept the Medicare-determined fee as full payment for their services. On an individual-case basis, physicians can accept Medicare assignment of their patients. Those physicians who accept the reasonable fee in full (i.e., who accept assignment) for specific patients receive 80 percent of the fee direct from Medicare and can bill those patients for the copayment. When physicians do not accept assignment, they can bill the patients for whatever fee they choose; in this case Medicare will reimburse the patients directly for 80 percent of its reasonable fee for that service or procedure, and the physicians must collect the entire bill from the patients. The acceptance by physicians of assignment relieves patients from the financial risks associated with higher physician fees.

The analysis is set out graphically in Figure 8–4. The physician is assumed to be a monopolist facing two submarkets: one with private patients and one with patients in a public program. (We ignore the "extra billing" in this analysis.) The output is defined as patients served. D_p is the demand curve for private patients, and MR_p is the related MR curve. The public agency reimburses the physicians for its patients at a fee level F_m; since the fee level is fixed, F_m is also the physician's MR for public patients. Assume that the physician's MC curve is at MC_1. Finally, assume that the physician is a profit maximizer.

According to the equimarginal principle, the physician will supply services to Q_1 private and $Q_3 - Q_1$ public patients, since at this output $MR_p = F_m$ and both are equal to MC_1. The private patients will be charged a price of P_m. To attract any additional private patients, the physician would have to lower the price to private patients below P_m, which would imply an MR for private patients below that for public patients. A profit maximizer will thus prefer to serve additional public

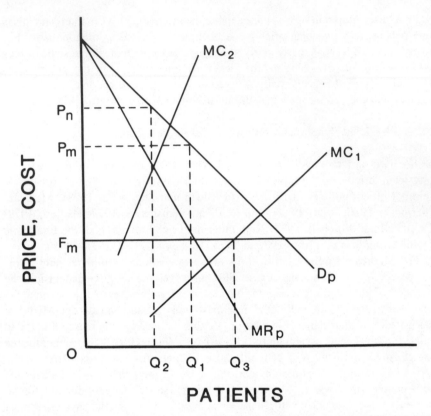

Figure 8–4 Representation of price setting by a monopolist facing a private market (with demand represented by D_p and marginal revenue by MR_p) and a publicly financed market (with a set fee, and therefore a marginal revenue of F_m). With a marginal cost of MC_1, the monopolist will set price to equate MR in each market; in this case, price in the private market is set at P_m. The marginal revenue for public and private patients will be the same, MC_1. Total output supplied is Q_3, with $Q_3 - Q_1$ going to the public patients. With an MC such as MC_2, the monopolist would not supply any output to the public patients; the price and output levels in the private market would be P_n and Q_2.

patients where the MR is constant at a level F_m, rather than lower his price and have an MR below F_m.

A lower public fee would lower the supply to the public patients (it would also cause the physician to lower his or her private fee since the physician will now move down the MR_p curve.) A physician facing the same demand curve but with a higher MC (say MC_2) will not supply any services to public patients and will set a private fee of P_n.

This analysis demonstrates that the public and private sectors are interdependent. A public program that lowers fees will reduce the supply to the public market and will also affect the private market. A similar model has also been used to explain hospital *cost shifting,* a phenomenon by which hospitals were purported to raise fees on self-pay and commercially insured patients in response to low reimbursement levels by Medicare, Medicaid, and in some instances Blue Cross (Danzon, 1982; Sloan, 1984; Sloan and Ginsburg, 1984).

8.3 DETERMINANTS OF MARKET STRUCTURE

8.3.1 Determinants of Structure

Market structure refers to one of the major preconditions for market power. Structure is usually presented in terms of an index or percent, representing the size of the largest firm (or four firms or eight firms) relative to the overall market's output, or else measuring the distribution of firm size in the market. A four (eight)-firm concentration ratio represents the percent of the total market (in terms of sales, assets, or some other indicator of firm size) represented by the largest four (eight) firms. For example, a completely monopolized market has a concentration ratio of 100 percent; a market with 20 firms, total sales of \$1 billion, and the sum of sales of the largest four firms of a half-billion dollars, would have a four-firm concentration ratio of 50 percent. The choice of four or eight firms is arbitrary, and does not indicate the concentration of the remainder of the market. A more general measure of concentration, which incorporates all firms in the market, is the *Herfindahl (H) index.* According to this index, concentration is measured as

$$H = \Sigma \left(\frac{S}{M}\right)^2 \times 10{,}000$$

where S is the size of each firm and M is the size of the total market. The 10,000 is because H is usually presented as a sum of percentages, expressed in absolute terms. The summation sign (Σ) refers to the sum over all firms. Thus a monopolist with sales of \$200 is the only firm in the market; its H index is (200/200) $\times$ 10,000, or 10,000. If there were three hospitals, each with sales of \$100, the H index for that market would be 3,300, which is

$$\Sigma \left(\frac{100}{300}\right)^2 \times 10{,}000$$

There is no true cutoff point for a concentrated versus a nonconcentrated market, although a figure of about 1,800 is sometimes used (Wilder and Jacobs, 1986). Generally, it is thought that the greater the degree of concentration, the greater will be the leading firm's (or firms') ability to influence price, quantity, and other characteristics of output.

Market structure can be thought of as having market and governmentally imposed (regulatory) determinants. Let us examine these in the context of the health insurance market. In the United States, the health insurance market is largely a localized market, in part because each state requires operating licenses for any insurance company operating within the state and also because of unique relations between local providers and some insurers (primarily the Blues). Aside from government insurance, health insurance has been broken down into two categories of operators, the Blues and the commercial insurance companies. The Blues are made up of Blue Cross for hospitalization insurance and Blue Shield for medical and other insurance. In some states the two plans are combined. The Blues are nonprofit in terms of organization. Commercial insurers are made up of a large number of mutual (member owned) and commercial (for profit) firms, none of whom has a substantial share of the health care market. Blue Cross and Blue Shield collect about one-half of the total health insurance premiums nationally; their share of the private insurance market varies considerably by state.

Among the most important market determinants of market power are economies of scale. Let us assume that the market demand for private health insurance is D_m in Figure 8–5, and that the technology of health insurance provision is such that the long-run average cost curve for a state-of-the-art insurance company is LAC. Two things should be noted in our example. First, LAC incorporates capital and other fixed setup costs as well as current operating costs; if there are high start-up costs for the industry, the LAC at low output levels will be quite high. Second, the LAC in our example includes insurance administration costs *and* the amount the insurance company reimburses the providers. The shape of the LAC in our example is such that the minimum cost is reached at a large scale of output (about 12 million subscribers in our example).

Given cost conditions such as LAC, one firm can capture a considerable portion of the market. To do so, it must resort to a second, and related, market share determinant: pricing policy. If the insurance company sets a very low price (relative to costs), say $80 per subscriber, market demand would be quite large, 20 million subscribers. In such a case the insurance company would have considerable discretion in choosing its own output level; the level chosen would depend, of course, on its objectives. If it provided services for 13 million subscribers at this price, there would be an excess demand of 7 million potential subscribers. If the technology of insurance provision was known to other potential entrants, a second firm could provide insurance on a cost basis like that of LAC. However, to reach a unit cost of $80, it would need to operate at a scale of 8 million subscribers; since the potential entrant could not obtain such a volume, it might simply produce at a higher cost, charge a higher price, and obtain a smaller share of the residual market.

The final distribution of market shares will thus depend on the extent to which there are scale economies relative to potential market size and the pricing policies

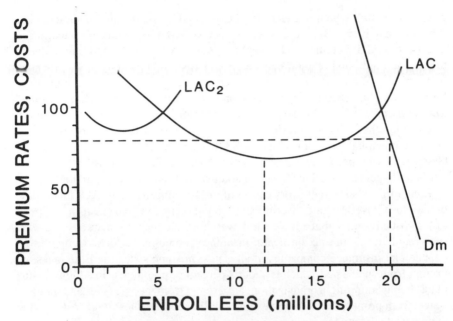

Figure 8–5 Representation of output in an insurance market, with alternative cost conditions. D_m represents total p and market demand for insurance coverage. If the cost conditions are represented by cost curve *LAC*, one firm can capture a substantial portion of the market by virtue of its scale economies and pricing policies. A producer with cost conditions of *LAC* could set a price of $80; if it did so and chose to supply 13 million policies, another producer (with the same cost conditions) could not reach a large enough scale of output to match the first producer's costs (and price). If cost conditions were represented by LAC_2, no producer could dominate the market in this way.

of the larger firms (if there are significant scale economies). As seen in Figure 8–5, if the initial insurance company charged a higher price, say $90 or $100, potential entrants would have less problems in gaining an entry to the market.

If, on the other hand, the state-of-the-art cost curve were like LAC_2 (with no substantial scale economies), no firm could obtain a substantial share of the market, and a concentration of firms would be unlikely. There is some evidence of economies of scale in health insurance operations, but these economies are not of the magnitude that would permit a single firm to dominate the health insurance market (Blair, Jackson, and Vogel, 1975).

A third cause of market concentration relates not to the cost–*scale* relation, but to the potentially different *levels* of cost curves for different providers. If, for example, one provider could obtain its inputs (workers, materials, etc.) at a lower cost than could a second provider, its cost curve would be lower at all scales of output than for the second provider. The first firm could capture a larger share of the market by turning its cost advantage into a price differential. One such input price differential, which relates to Blue Cross and hospitalization insurance, is a *discount* that many Blue Cross plans receive from hospitals (Goldberg and Greenberg, 1985; Feldman and Greenberg, 1981), which is perhaps partly due to the special traditional relation between Blue Cross and hospitals (it was founded by hospitals). While commercial insurance companies typically have reimbursed hospitals for close to full charges, about half of the Blue Cross plans have received a discount ranging from 2 to 30 percent and averaging from 8 to 15 percent. Such a discount has the effect of lowering the *LAC* curve of the Blue Cross plans relative to the commercial ones. Blue Cross could then gain an increased market share by charging lower premium rates than the commercials. One recent estimate attributed 7 percent of Blue Cross's market share to this cost differential.

There might also be regulatory causes of market concentration. As with the case of the Blue Cross discount, discriminatory regulations can give one firm or type of firm a cost advantage that allows it to lower price and increase market share. One such regulation is the tax on health insurance premiums, which is imposed on commercial insurance companies in all states; in some states the Blue plans are exempt from such a tax, which is about 2 percent of premiums. In addition, Blue plans, being nonprofit in organization, are exempt from income taxes and, in some states, from property taxes. Such exemptions lower the Blues' total costs, giving them a cost advantage.

However, these advantages need not always result in a larger market share. As shown in Section 6.6, nonprofit agencies can incur costs for on-the-job sources of benefits for management; this is particularly true for nonprofit firms, whose profits cannot be of direct benefit to management. Thus any cost advantage to a nonprofit firm can be appropriated by the management rather than passing it on to consumers in the form of lower premiums. The nonprofit's costs would then appear to be higher, but in fact would incorporate expenses for the on-the-job amenities. This has been shown to be a factor in the behavior of Blue Shield plans that were not "controlled" by physicians. Blue Shield plans that were deemed physician controlled were found to have lower operating costs; this relation has been explained as being due to the physician-controlled plans passing on any potential surpluses to the physicians in the form of reimbursements. Non-physician-controlled plans could appropriate these potential surpluses and in the process generate higher operating costs (Eisenstadt and Kennedy, 1981).

8.3.2 Market Power in the Market for Physicians' Services

Market structure and market power are not always synonymous. In the physician services market there are a number of manifestations of market power, and yet the market structure does not have a high degree of provider concentration. With regard to evidence of market power, for many years physicians were able to maintain a sliding scale of fees, indicating price discrimination. Also, their incomes have been well above normal, even allowing for the high costs of medical training. Yet significant economies of scale in medical practice are not present, and there is a very low degree of market concentration.

The explanation of this paradox lay in a mechanism of control developed by the medical profession to police its members so that certain elements would not engage in competitive practices such as price cutting (Kessell, 1958, Rayack, 1970). The control of such a mechanism lay in the hands of organized medical associations at the county, state, and national levels.

The key players in this control mechanism were the teaching hospitals, the American Medical Association, the local medical associations, and practicing physicians, especially specialists (see Figure 8–6). The operation of the mechanism relied on its benefits to several of the key groups: (1) interns were a key (and low cost) input in the operation of a teaching hospital; (2) physicians, especially specialists, needed membership on hospital medical staffs to have viable practices.

The functioning of the mechanism lay in a convention developed by the American Medical Association (AMA) with regard to the certification of teaching hospitals. According to this convention, known as the Mundt Resolution, hospitals that were certified as teaching hospitals were advised that their medical staffs

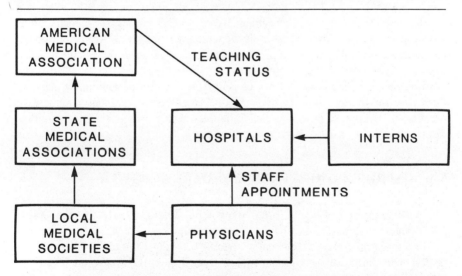

Figure 8–6 Representation of control mechanism in the medical profession. Key players include hospitals with teaching programs that needed accreditation from the Council on Teaching Hospitals (AMA associated) and physicians (who benefitted from staff appointments in hospitals). Membership in local medical societies was required for a staff appointment to a hospital, a resolution enforced by the AMA by virtue of its control over hospital accreditation. Local medical societies could enforce regulations (regarding pricing policies, for example) by virtue of their control over membership.

should be composed only of physicians who were members of local medical societies. Since the AMA certified hospital teaching status, the resolution carried great weight with the hospitals.

With this resolution in effect, it was up to the local medical societies to enforce one of the preconditions for physician membership on a hospital teaching staff, and that was membership in the local medical society. Doctors, and particularly specialists, requiring hospital staff positions, thus needed to gain membership in their local medical societies.

Herein lay the mechanism to limit competitive practices. County medical association members generally disapproved of price cutting and other competitive practices. One such practice was the development of prepaid group medicine (now known as health maintenance organizations; see Section 7.7.4). Prepaid practices charged a single fee for all members, thus undermining the price discrimination system which had become common practice. The expulsion of physicians who joined prepaid group practice staffs from county medical societies occurred in several instances (Kessell, 1958) and the threat of expulsion was sufficient to make physician recruitment difficult for these organizations. In addition, other competitive activities, such as advertising, were also discouraged by the organized medical profession.

The control of competitive practices by the medical profession at large has not relied solely on such formal mechanisms. With the growth of specialization, physicians have become increasingly dependent on referrals from colleagues. Physicians who engaged in competitive practices could be "controlled" to some degree if they lost referrals from colleagues (Havighurst, 1978).

In recent years there has been a considerable amount of regulatory activity, especially on the part of the federal government, to contain anticompetitive practices on the part of physicians and other health care providers. This activity is discussed in Section 12.4.2.

8.4 NONPRICE COMPETITION AND MARKET POWER

The vast majority of health care markets will be neither perfectly competitive nor completely monopolistic: there will be some elements of each. Consumers will develop some loyalty or attachment to specific providers, but this loyalty will not be complete. Furthermore, product quality or attributes other than price play a key role in the output of most health care providers; therefore, quality has a key role to play in the competitive process as well. In this section we discuss this area of market power and the role that nonprice competition has to play in it.

In addition to competing on price, there are many product attributes that providers can provide that might potentially attract patients. They can increase patient convenience by having excess capacity or longer hours in order to cut down on patient and physician (in the case of staff physicians) waiting time. They can build satellite facilities and clinics to cut down on patient travel time. Pharmacists can initiate delivery services, emergency service, family prescription monitoring records, and prescription waiting areas. Providers can have more attending staff. Insurance companies and HMOs have a wide variety of services that might be covered and can also vary the degree to which these can be covered (e.g., copayments, deductibles, and treatment limitations). Note, however, that in all such instances additional quality is costly to provide.

There are three relevant variations in terms of price–quality competition: (1) when producers compete in terms of both, (2) when producers compete only in terms of quality, and (3) when producers compete only in terms of price. We have already considered (3) in Chapter 7 when quality was held constant.

8.4.1 Monopolistic Competition

Vigorous competition on price *and* quality is called *monopolistic competition*. In such a market model we assume that there are many competitors and potential competitors (i.e., low-cost entry). Each firm can vary product quality (e.g., location of facilities, operating hours, etc.) and in the process will develop some consumer loyalty (and hence market power); that is, consumers will not be as willing to change suppliers as in the quality–constant perfect competition case.

Let us develop our model in terms of an HMO example. We will assume that Palmedico HMO is one among a number of alternative providers (some of whom might offer more traditional insurance and fee-for-service options). The HMO will be assumed to be a provider of average efficiency. We can characterize the partial loyalty toward Palmedico by its subscribers with a downward sloping demand curve D in Figure 8–7a. Associated with this demand curve is an MR curve. Palmedico's cost curve will depend on the product characteristics offered: the extent of coverage, the credentials of its staff, its operating hours, the number of satellite clinics it operates, and so on. Initially, let us assume that Palmedico is a profit-maximizing institution. Given these conditions, it will set its price at the quantity where $MR = MC$; price will be just above \$600 per subscriber and enrollment will be 5,000.

At this price Palmedico is earning excess profits, and since it is a representative firm in the industry, presumably others are earning excess profits as well. Since entry is inexpensive, other potential entrants will be attracted by the scent of high profits. To gain enrollees, they may lower price, and they may also offer potential enrollees a higher-quality product (longer hours, for example). Palmedico's demand curve will shift to the left unless it responds with a higher quality and lower price of its own. In the process its costs will increase (because of the higher quality). The same forces will be affecting all firms in the market.

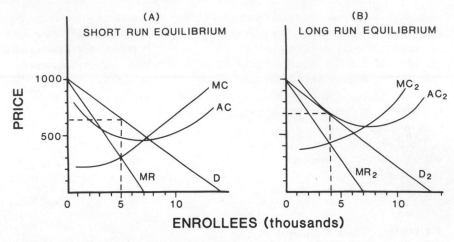

Figure 8–7 Representation of equilibrium in monopolistic competition. In the short run (a), equilibrium price and quantity of a provider are set where $MR = MC$ (at 5,000 enrollees and a price just above 600). In the long run (b), competitive responses, including increasing quality, lead to an equilibrium where no excess profits are made (price just equals average cost).

As long as there are any excess profits to be made, this process will continue. Quality for each firm will continue to rise. Demand for each firm will shift outward in response to its higher quality and then inward in response to competitors' quality and price responses. Price margins (the excesses of price over average cost) will continually be lowered as a result of this competitive process. For any firm, we cannot predict whether price will ultimately increase or decrease (i.e., we cannot predict the net result of the competitive process) because demand has shifted in both directions. For the same reason, we cannot predict the direction in which enrollment changes. However, the final equilibrium will appear as in Figure 8–7b, where AC_2 just touches the firm's demand curve D_2. Equilibrium quantity is that at the point where $MC = MR$ (i.e., it is the most profitable position Palmedico can have); in this case, Palmedico is just breaking even. All that we can say for certain about this equilibrium is that AC_2 represents a higher quality level; we cannot say for certain whether price and enrollments are higher or lower. For this reason, the monopolistic competition model has been criticized as being incomplete: it fails to make predictions on the direction of some key variables—price and quantity.

Competition between nonprofit firms would have a similar outcome. If our behavioral assumption were that the firm wants to maximize enrollees, for example, quality and price competition would still prevail and the final result would be that each provider breaks even.

Models similar to the monopolistic competition model in this section have been used to explain resource-allocation decisions in markets where a number of HMOs (Christianson and McClure, 1979; Goldberg and Greenberg, 1980) and retail drugstores operate (Cady, 1976). The importance of nonprice (including quality) factors in these markets has been stressed. Similar models have also been used to explain the diffusion of (high quality) technological developments in the hospital industry, such as the use of radioisotopes and intensive-care units (Rapoport, 1978; Lee and Waldman, 1985).

8.4.2 Increased Concentration

When concentration increases and providers are fewer in number, the possibility of price collusion increases. Price collusion refers to explicit agreements *or implicit understandings* among competitors in a market to limit price competition. With only a few suppliers in a market, and with each understanding that the ultimate outcome of price competition is lower price and profits *for all,* the likelihood of suppliers refraining from price competition increases.

Explicit agreements to restrict price competition are illegal (see Chapter 12), but cautious pricing behavior involving the avoidance of conflicts in pricing policies among competitors is not illegal. Such cautious behavior is more likely to be found when a market contains a small number of competitors because, as the number of competitors increases, the ''cheating'' factor is more likely. With fewer suppliers it is easier to detect cheating. Also, the impact of one supplier's price cuts is less dispersed; that is, each supplier's demand curve is shifted inward more when there are only a few suppliers.

Markets with a small number of suppliers and a significant degree of provider interdependence are referred to as *oligopolistic*. While vigorous price competition is not usually a characteristic of an oligopolistic market, quality competition is. In providing higher quality to attract and retain patients, the costs of oligopolistic competitors increase and profits are reduced.

Oligopolistic competition might occur when there are a few HMOs and traditional insurers in a market competing for the business of a large number of enrollees. In such an instance, we would expect to see rising quality but not much price competition (Hay and Leahy, 1984). However, this may not generally characterize markets where HMOs enter. For oligopoly to persist, entry by new competitors must be difficult (either because of natural means such as scale economies or because existing providers set prices low enough to discourage entry). The start-up costs for an HMO may not be great. Also, buying power may discourage providers from engaging in oligopolistic behavior. In many such markets, businesses play a considerable role in selecting which insurers (including HMOs) will insure its employees. If the buyer's side of the market is dominated by one or a few large businesses, price competition may become important.

8.4.3 Nonprice Competition

Price competition is sometimes not relevant. When patients are fully or substantially insured for a service and they have free choice of supplier, they will choose suppliers based strictly on nonprice or quality considerations. Quality competition then becomes the only form of competition; and if the supply side of the market is competitive, costs will increase in response to higher quality until the suppliers reach break-even, or else until the limits placed by third-party reimbursers are reached. Such a competitive process has been characterized for hospital markets (Joskow, 1980; Farley, 1985) and dialysis markets (Held and Pauly, 1983).

REFERENCES

Monopoly and Physicians

Havighurst, C.C. (1978). Professional restraints on innovation in health care financing. *Duke Law Journal, 1978* (2), 303–388.

Kessell, R. (1958). Price discrimination in medicine. *Journal of Law and Economics, 1*, 20–53.

Leffler, K.B. (1978). Physician licensure: Competition and monopoly in American medicine. *Journal of Law and Economics, 21*(1), 165–186.

Newhouse, J.P. (1970). A model of physician pricing. *Southern Economic Journal, 37*, 147–183.

Rayack, E. (1964). The supply of physicians' services. *Industrial and Labor Relations Review, 17*, 221–237.

———— (1970). *Professional power and American medicine.* Cleveland, OH: World Publishing Co.

Profits in Medicine

Lindsay, C.M. (1973). Real returns to medical education. *Journal of Human Resources, 8*, 331–348.

———— (1976). More real returns to medical education. *Journal of Human Resources, 11*, 127–129.

Sloan, F.A. (1976). Real returns to medical education. *Journal of Human Resources, 11*, 118–126.

Price Discrimination and Physician Reimbursement

Cromwell, J., & Mitchell, J. (1984). An economic model of large Medicaid practices. *Health Services Research, 19*, 197–218.

Gabel, J.R., & Rice, T.H. (1985). Reducing public expenditures for physician services. *Journal of Health Politics, Policy, and Law, 9*, 595–609.

Hadley, J. (1979). Physician participation in Medicaid: Evidence from California. *Health Services Research, 14*, 266–280.

————, & Lee, R. (1978-1979). Toward a physician payment policy: Evidence from the economic stabilization program. *Policy Sciences, 10*, 105–120.

Kushman, J.E. (1977). Physician participation in Medicaid. *Western Journal of Agricultural Economics, 2*, 22–33.

Muller, C., & Ostelberg, J. (1979). Carrier discretionary practices and physician payment under Medicare Part B. *Medical Care, 17*, 650–666.

Paringer, L. (1980). Medicare assignment rates of physicians: Their responses to changes in reimbursement policy. *Health Care Financing Review, 1*, 75–89.

Rice, T. (1984). Determinants of physician assignment rates by type of service. *Health Care Financing Review, 5*, 33–42.

Sloan, F.A., & Steinwald, B. (1978). Physician participation in health insurance plans. *Journal of Human Resources, 13*, 237–263.

Hospital and Nonprofit Agency Pricing

Bauerschmidt, A.D., & Jacobs, P. (1985). Pricing objectives in non-profit hospitals. *Health Services Research, 20*, 153–161.

Danzon, P.M. (1982). Hospital "profits." *Journal of Health Economics, 1*(1), 29–52.

Hay, J.W. (1983). The impact of public health care financing policies on private sector hospital costs. *Journal of Health Politics, Policy, and Law, 7*, 945–952.

Jacobs, P., & Wilder, R.P. (1984) Pricing behavior of non-profit agencies. *Journal of Health Economics, 3*, 49–61.

Johnston, W.P., Jacobs, P., & Dickson, W.M. (1985). Interhospital variations in hospital pharmacy mark-ups. *American Journal of Hospital Pharmacy, 42*, 2492–2495.

Sloan, F.A., & Becker, E. (1984). Cross subsidies and payment for hospital care. *Journal of Health Politics, Policy, and Law, 8,*660–685.

———, & Ginsburg, P.B., (1984). Hospital cost shifting. *New England Journal of Medicine, 310*, 893–898.

Wilder, R.P., & Jacobs P. (1986). Antitrust considerations for hospital mergers: Market definition and market concentration. *Advances in Health Economics, 7.*

Market Power and Health Insurance

Adamache, K.W., & Sloan, F.A. (1983). Competition between non-profit and for-profit health insurers. *Journal of Health Economics, 2*, 225–244.

Blair, R.D., Jackson, J.R., & Vogel, R.J. (1975). Economies of scale in the administration of health insurance. *Review of Economic Statistics, 57*, 185–189.

Eisenstadt, D., & Kennedy, T.E. (1981). Control and behavior of nonprofit firms: The case of Blue Shield. *Southern Economic Journal, 48*, 26–36.

Feldman, R., & Greenberg, W. (1981a). Blue Cross market share, economies of scale and cost containment efforts. *Health Services Research, 16*, 175–183.

——— (1981b). The relation between Blue Cross market share and the Blue Cross "discount" on hospital charges. *Journal of Risk and Insurance, 48*, 235–246.

Frank, R.G., & Welch, W.P. (1985). The competitive effects of HMO's: A review of the evidence. *Inquiry, 22*, 148–161.

Frech, H.E., & Ginsburg, P.B. (1978, March). Competition among health insurers. In W. Greenberg (Ed.), *Competition in the health care sector*. Washington, DC: Federal Trade Commission.

Goldberg, L.G., & Greenberg, W. (1977). The effect of physician-controlled health insurance. *Journal of Health Politics, Policy, and Law, 2*, 48–78.

——— (1985). The dominant firm in health insurance. *Social Science and Medicine, 20*, 719–724.

Lynk, W.J. (1981). Regulatory control of the membership of corporate boards of directors: The Blue Shield case. *Journal of Law and Economics, 24*, 159–174.

Imperfect Competition

Cady, J.F. (1976). *Restricted advertising and competition*. Washington, DC: American Enterprise Institute.

Christianson, J.B., & McClure, W. (1979). Competition in the delivery of medical care. *New England Journal of Medicine, 301*, 812–818.

Farley, D.E. (1985). *Competition among hospitals: Market structure and its relation to utilization, costs and financial position.* Hospital Studies Program, Research Note 7. (DHHS Publication No. PHS 85-3353). Washington, DC: U.S. Department of Health and Human Services, National Center for Health Services Research and Health Care Technology Assessment.

Getzen, T.E. (1984). A "brand name" theory of medical group practice. *Journal of Industrial Economics, 33*, 199–217.

Goldberg, L.G., & Greenberg, W. (1980). The competitive response of Blue Cross to the health maintenance organization. *Economic Inquiry, 18*, 55–68.

——— (1979). The competitive response of Blue Cross and Blue Shield to the health maintenance organization in northern California and Hawaii. *Medical Care, 17*, 1019–1028.

Hay, J.W., & Leahy, M.J. (1984). Competition among health plans: Some preliminary evidence. *Southern Economic Journal, 50*, 831–846.

Held, P.J., & Pauly, M.V. (1983). Competition and efficiency in the end stage renal disease program. *Journal of Health Economics, 2*, 95–118.

Joskow, P.L. (1980). The effects of competition and regulation on hospital bed supply and the reservation quality of the hospital. *Bell Journal of Economics, 11*, 421–447.

Kelly, E.T., Rodowskas, C.A., & Gagnon, J.P. (1975). An examination of the effect of market demographic and competitive characteristics on gross margins and prescription drugs. *Medical Care, 12*, 956–965.

Lee, R.H., & Waldman, D.M. (1985). The diffusion of innovations in hospitals. *Journal of Health Economics, 4*, 374–380.

Morrisey, M.A., & Ashby, C.S. (1982). An empirical analysis of HMO market share. *Inquiry, 19*, 136–149.

Rapoport, J. (1978). Diffusion of technological innovations among non-profit firms. *Journal of Economics and Business, 30*, 108–118.

Chapter 9

Models Specific to the Medical Care Market

9.1 INTRODUCTION

In Chapters 7 and 8, several standard market models were developed and applied to the medical care market. When presenting these models, we assumed that, even though medical care possessed some characteristics that might influence the nature of the market in which it is provided, these special characteristics could be handled by standard textbook models of competition or monopoly. We also pointed out that the bottom line of any theory is how well it explains what is actually occurring in a market. Two alleged facts, in particular, have led to the development of models specially tailored to medical care markets because either the more traditional models cannot predict the occurrence of these facts or they present incomplete explanations of the workings of these markets.

The first of these facts is the alleged positive relation between price and supply; as the number of physicians per capita has increased, it is alleged that the price of physicians' services has increased in response. It was pointed out in Section 7.4.5 why such a fact has not been categorically established as being a true relation. Nevertheless, its possible (and some would say likely) existence has led some analysts to develop models that can explain this occurrence. In these models, suppliers are assumed to have some direct influence in manipulating demanders' perceptions of health status and the efficacy of medical care, and hence in shifting demand. Such models are discussed in Section 9.2. In Section 9.3 we discuss the hospital variant of the *availability effect,* known as Roemer's law.

The second set of facts concerns the simultaneous rise over time (until the early 1980s) of medical care costs, of utilization, of the number of individuals who possess medical insurance, and of the average amount of coverage. The first two facts, rising unit costs and rising utilization, can be explained by increasing insurance coverage. However, increasing insurance coverage is not an exogenous (i.e., independently determined) phenomenon: as shown in Chapter 4, insurance demand increases with medical care costs, and so there is a feedback effect that, unchecked, could lead to an inflationary spiral. In fact, the two markets, health care and health insurance, are so closely related that for some purposes they might better be considered as a single complex market. Indeed, some health care firms, HMOs, both sell health insurance and provide medical care. To further complicate matters, the role of business firms in the participation of the insurance demand decision has been growing. This participation has been credited with playing a major role in putting a brake on the medical care cost inflationary spiral. In recognition of these interactions, we present a discussion of the interrelations among the various participants in these markets in Section 9.4.

9.2 SUPPLY-GENERATED DEMAND MODELS

The type of fact that lies behind the rejection of the competitive model can be shown with the use of an example, illustrated in Figure 9–1. Let us say, initially, that in a certain region A the number of surgical services performed per 100,000 population is 5,000 per year and that the price is $80 per operation. In another region, B, services are priced at $90 and 6,000 operations are performed. Let us further say that all factors that might cause demand to be greater in region B, such as the characteristics and health status of the population or the level of insurance, are the same in both regions, so demand should also be the same in both regions. Also, assume that the only factor that differs between the two regions on the supply side of the market is the number of surgeons per 100,000 population; in region A this number is 30, and in region B it is 40.

The price–utilization situation in region A is in Figure 9–1 at the intersection of the D_1 demand curve and the S_1 supply curve. With reference to this situation, since region B has more surgeons, its supply curve would be expected to shift outward, say to S_2. With the same demand, price would be expected to be lower in region B, according to the competitive model, and utilization would be expected to increase as a result. The equilibrium in region B would be at the intersection of the D_1 and S_2 curves. We have just stated that there is no reason to believe that demand is greater in region B than in region A. If, however, utilization and price are greater in B than in A, one way of rationalizing this would be to say that the surgeons were able to influence demand; the extra surgeons in region B, in the context of our example, were able to shift demand to a level shown by D_2. If, in fact, price in region B is $90 and the number of operations per 100,000 population is 6,000, our demand-generation hypothesis is indeed consistent with the facts. The competitive model is not.

It is theoretically possible for surgeons to be able to shift demand, while the price still falls. If D_2 was only slightly greater than D_1, even though demand shifted, it would not shift enough to cause prices to rise in response to the increased

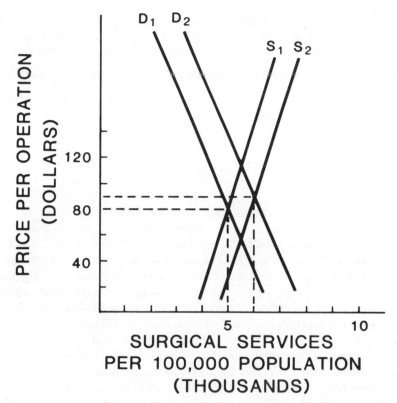

Figure 9–1 Demand and supply conditions with physician-induced demand. Given an initial demand D_1 and supply position S_1, an increase in the number of surgeons will lead to an increase in the supply of surgical services to S_2. To maintain their income and workload levels, surgeons create a shift in demand to D_2, with a resulting increase in price and utilization rate.

supply. We could then not distinguish between the physician-induced demand shift and the standard competitive situation with no demand shift. However, if price does rise, the physician-induced demand-shift hypothesis is the one that is consistent with the facts of rising price and increased supply (Reinhardt, 1978).

The rationale for physician-induced demand creation was presented in Section 4.9. There it was shown that consumers may shift out their demand for medical care if the *perceived* levels of their health status and/or the effectiveness of medical care in improving health change. Doctors potentially can influence patient perceptions of these variables and thus can shift out the demand curve for their services. (Williams, 1985, also hypothesizes that physicians can influence consumer tastes for health.) However, this ability to generate demand is limited by the amount of information that the patients possess (or can obtain) about the values of these variables. Furthermore, the degree to which physicians generate demand within the given limits will depend on their own behavioral goals, that is, on the degree to which they are willing to deviate from being perfect agents on behalf of their patients. A complete analysis thus must incorporate the physicians and their behavior.

Perhaps the simplest supplier-induced demand models are based on the *target-income* hypothesis (Evans, 1974). We begin our exposition with a breakdown of physician income into fee levels, visit rates, and physician density. The overall relation can be expressed as

$$\frac{\text{Income}}{\text{per physician}} = \frac{\text{fee per}}{\text{visit}} \times \frac{\text{visits per}}{\text{population}} \times \frac{\text{population}}{\text{per physician}}$$

Using this equation as a framework, two assumptions are then posited: (1) doctors' goals involve a *target* income and a maximum workload; and (2) doctors can cause shifts in consumer demand by stipulating that patients "need" more care.

To see how such a model works, let us take some initial values for our variables. In region I each physician has a target income of $10,000 and a maximum annual workload of 2,000 patient visits. The population per physician in this region is 500. The physicians choose to set a price of $5 per visit and to have each member of the population visit the physician four times per year. The physicians in region I thus achieve their target incomes and do not exceed their self-imposed maximum workloads. The physicians in region II have the same goals as those in region I. In region II, however, the physician supply is more dense than in region I; there are 400 persons per physician. With fewer people per physician, the physicians in region II must generate sufficient demand to bring their incomes up to their target levels. Many options are open to them in doing this. One would be to increase the average number of visits per person to 4.5 and raise the fees to $5.50 per visit. This would allow the physicians to meet their target incomes and not exceed the maximum workload. In this case, with an increase in supply, price rises as well.

Such a model does not tell us by how much fees and per capita visits will each rise. It merely states that the two together will increase to achieve the physician's target income. But the model does not provide any guidelines to enable us to predict the composition of the increase in expenditures between prices and quantity supplied. This is a major problem with the model (Evans, 1974).

There are several other problems with such a model. First, there is no mention of how target levels of income and maximum case load become formulated and how they might change. Presumably, these desired levels are set with reference to the levels of income and maximum workload that exists in the community at large. However, the presence of a desired income level is at odds with the economic tradition that states that people have unlimited wants. Certainly, if the physician can get more income just for the asking (or, in this case, by the generation of demand), why would he or she not do so? The reply to this objection might be that the physician is sincerely concerned with the well-being of the patient. That is, a physician's pricing and demand-generating activities are made with reference to their effects on the patient's total welfare (including income), and not merely on the wealth of the physician. If this is so, the model leaves out a very important component of the picture: the level of willingness of the physician to generate demand. Without a specification of this moral constraint on the physician, the model leaves many questions unanswered.

A second objection to the model is that the physician may not be able to generate an unlimited amount of demand for his or her services. The factors that might influence the patient's change in tastes for medical services include information received from sources other than the attending physician. This was discussed in Chapter 8.

In response to these criticisms, a number of models have been formulated that attempt to predict a positive relation between price (physician fee levels) and the physician–population ratio. To avoid the criticisms leveled at the fixed target income "satisficing" models, these models have attempted to incorporate more sophisticated maximizing goals. The gist of many of these models is that physicians' goals incorporate several entities: one desired entity is income (Y), which has a falling marginal utility or value (the more one has, the less an *additional* unit is worth; see Chapter 4); a second is workload, (W), and a third is excessive care produced (D), both of which have an increasing marginal *dis*utility (Anderson, House, and Ormiston, 1981; Hay and Leahy, 1982; Rossiter and Welensky, 1984; Sloan and Ginsburg, 1978). Given prices, time per procedure, and total time available to the doctor, output will be expanded to the utility-maximizing point, which is where the marginal utility of income equals the marginal disutility of D and W combined. Given an increase in the population–physician ratio, some of the existing patients will go to the added doctors. Income of existing doctors (Y) will fall, and so the marginal utility of income will increase. To maximize utility, the physician will generate further demand until utility is once again maximized. Thus the model predicts that a higher physician–population ratio is associated with higher utilization, while prices remain unchanged. Variations on such a model could also cause prices to increase.

Another type of model has been developed that seeks to explain the positive relation between prices and the number of physicians in the area without resorting to demand creation. Such a model posits that information costs (the costs of seeking appropriate physicians) increase with the *number* of physicians in a market area, because the larger the number of physicians, the more diffuse the information on the appropriate physician becomes. As a result, the degree of monopoly increases with the greater number of physicians. As shown in Chapter 8, prices increase with the degree of monopoly power. This model thus predicts higher prices in areas with more physicians (not more physicians per capita) (Pauly and Satterthwaite, 1980).

A number of studies have sought to test for the demand generation relation by refining the variables in statistical analyses or by developing novel ways to identify the phenomena. Most of these studies have examined how *per capita* use of services varies with physician availability. Strictly speaking, an increase in per capita use of services is consistent with *both* the competitive model and the supplier-induced demand model. In the competitive model, an increase in supply lowers price and causes an increase in utilization. The theory does not say that *per capita* utilization will remain the same; indeed, a lower price may well induce the average consumer to demand more.

These studies have been conducted with respect to utilization rates for populations in given areas and to variations in physician treatment patterns. Stano (1985) drew a distinction between the proportion of a population that seeks care and the average intensity per treated patient of that care. It is the latter that is in the spirit of demand inducement. Stano's statistical study of Michigan data failed to identify an availability effect on intensity. Other studies have found availability effects for specific services such as medical and surgical services and lab tests (Rice, 1983; Wilensky and Rossiter, 1983). Epidemiological studies based on small-area analyses, hypothesizing *physician* uncertainty about appropriate treatments, have uncovered wide variations among small areas in the rates of specific procedures such as tonsillectomies, hysterectomies, and prostatectomies (Wennberg, Barnes, and Zubkoff, 1982). And controlling for patient characteristics using actual (Rosenblatt and Moscovice, 1984) and hypothetical data (Hemenway and Fallon, 1985), wide variations in treatment patterns suggest a considerable degree of physician discretion does exist, which can translate into more or less intensively provided care, depending on the caseload.

9.3 THE HOSPITAL AVAILABILITY EFFECT

The hospital equivalent to the physician-induced demand hypothesis is known as *Roemer's law* (Roemer and Shain, 1959), which states that an increase in the number of hospital beds in an area will create additional hospital use. Unlike physicians, however, who are their patients' agents, hospitals cannot fill themselves; they need doctors to refer patients and discharge them. For such a law to work, some other mechanism must be in operation.

One such mechanism may relate to time costs of patients (see Chapter 4). As hospitals create excess capacity, waiting time of patients for services may fall. Patient demands may increase in response to the reduced waiting time, thus filling the empty beds. One study, using 1974 data, estimated that a 10 percent increase in the number of beds would raise days of hospitalization of Medicare patients by 4 percent. If indeed, the mechanism by which Roemer's law operates is by affecting time costs, then if hospital occupancy rates fall, time costs will fall with the existing number of beds. Additional beds may not then have such an inducement effect (Ginsburg and Koretz, 1983). Thus the ''law'' really relates to occupancy rates rather than actual bed numbers.

9.4 INTERRELATED MARKETS

During the 1970s and early 1980s, the economic performance of the U.S. health care sector was characterized by inflationary tendencies. Increases in unit costs and utilization could be explained by shifts in the demand curve *resulting from* continued increases in insurance coverage. But in such a model a critical element, insurance coverage, is treated as exogenous, that is, as unaffected by the workings of the model. In fact, higher medical costs feed back to influence insurance premiums, and so what we have is a potential spiral, with the medical care and insurance markets so closely intertwined that we lose a critical portion of our understanding of the medical care inflation process when we exclude the insurance market from our model.

In addition to the traditional view of the participants of the medical care market as consisting of suppliers (hospitals, doctors) and demanders (consumers, patients), two other groups play a major role in the workings of the market. First, insurance intermediaries (Blue Cross, commercial insurance companies, etc.) can potentially play a role other than as a conduit of funds. Insurance companies can involve themselves in utilization review, performing the function of ensuring that hospitalization is appropriate and that hospital stays are not excessive. In addition, insurers can establish reimbursement systems; for example, they can reimburse hospitals on a retrospective or prospective basis. Which reimbursement system they choose will have an effect on hospital prices and total reimbursement.

Second, because so much health insurance is employer financed, business firms can play a major role in the purchase of health insurance. In recent years, employers have played an active role in the design of health insurance benefits, thus ending a long period of passivity.

If these groups are incorporated into our model, we lose the simplicity of the two-group supply–demand model and must resort to a more complicated explanation. In this section a complex market model of the hospital care sector is presented.

The flow of funds and services on which this model is based is shown in Figure 9–2. The role of government as a financing agent is excluded so that a simpler view of the market can be presented. This view still captures the essential role of the third party in the market. In the flow diagram in Figure 9–2 we see that consumers and employers pay premiums to an insurance intermediary to obtain insurance coverage for hospital expenses.

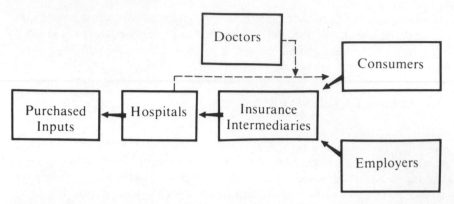

Figure 9–2 Flow of funds and services in the hospital care market. Consumers and employees pay for insurance policies to insurance intermediaries, who reimburse hospitals, who, in turn, pay inputs. Doctors control much of the flow of services, for which hospitals are reimbursed. In the traditional system, incentives worked to increase the size of the flow.

9.4.1 Consumers

Because the onset of illness is a risky event, the consumer of medical services is faced with two choices: (1) how much insurance to buy and (2) how much medical care to consume in the event of illness. In Section 4.4 it was shown that the higher the cost of medical care and the lower the direct cost of insurance are, the more insurance coverage that will be demanded.

One factor that affects the direct price of health insurance premiums is the income-tax treatment of health insurance premiums. For income-tax purposes such premiums, if paid by the employer, are considered nontaxable benefits. This gives health insurance benefits an edge over additional monetary compensation from the employee's viewpoint. If the employee pays a tax of 40 cents on each additional dollar of wages, he or she gets 60 cents in consumption benefits. On the other hand, if the employer purchases for the employee an extra dollar in health insurance benefits, the employee receives the full dollar's worth of benefits. For employment-related health insurance, the relative price of health insurance benefits is thus distorted by the tax law, and it favors a higher demand for benefits (and a lower demand for other goods purchased with after-tax dollars).

An additional consideration in the model is that, when one insures, the direct cost of medical care at the time of utilization will fall, and the quantity demanded will be greater than if there were no insurance. This proposition was developed under the conditions that the consumer behaved independently of physician influence. However, if the physician is a perfect agent (see Section 4.11), there can still be a downward sloping demand curve: physicians will order fewer discretionary tests and will perform fewer discretionary procedures when their patients must pay higher direct prices.

9.4.2 Employers

Theoretically, employers are indifferent between offering a dollar's worth of wages and providing an extra dollar in health insurance premiums. Both add a dollar to the company's expenses. Thus, the choice as to how much of each form of compensation to provide is the employee's decision. In this sense, the employer is a neutral force in the market, with the exception that the very fact that it provides health insurance coverage gives the employee a subsidized (tax free) benefit.

9.4.3 Hospitals

Hospital costs per admission are equal to the product of average input prices, inputs used per service, and the number of services per admission. If we assume input prices (e.g., wages and prices of supplies) to be constant, all increases in costs per admission consist of increases in inputs used per service performed and in the number of services performed per admission. We will consider quality of hospital care to be consonant with more inputs per service and/or more services per admission. The number of admissions will be referred to as the quantity of care.

In Chapter 6 we developed several hypotheses about the behavior of nonprofit suppliers. The one used here is that hospitals are joint quality–quantity maximizers (see Section 6.5). The more that they can have of either, the better off they will be. Assumptions must also be made about the hospitals' cost–output relations, revenue conditions, and the degree of competition among hospitals for patients. Concerning the cost–output relation, no unique level of costs is associated with any given level of output. The nature of the product is such that a number of qualities can be produced at any given level of admissions. If the hospital can be reimbursed for providing care at a level of quality higher than the one at which it is currently operating (and thus at a higher unit cost), it will be better off. Regarding hospital revenue, the constraining conditions placed on the hospital will depend on the nature of the reimbursement by the insurance company.

Regarding competitive conditions among hospitals, it will be assumed that there are a number of hospitals competing for patients. Since doctors have considerable say as to whether and where patients are hospitalized, we can regard the competition among hospitals as working itself out in the form of bargaining between hospitals and staff doctors. To attract and retain the services of a doctor, a hospital must offer the physician favorable working conditions. Since most hospitals do not directly pay doctors, the price hospitals must "pay" for the services of the doctors takes the form of quality and quantity of equipment, supplies, and complementary personnel (nurses, therapists, technicians, etc.). The end result of such bargains is higher cost levels for the hospitals. The degree to which hospitals must compete for the services of doctors will depend on how competitive the conditions are, and this will be determined by the number of doctors and the number of hospital posts available.

9.4.4 Insurance Companies

The final group in this market consists of insurance companies. We will assume a single insurance company in the market. Furthermore, we will assume that it is a nonprofit company. The company's revenues consist of its premiums. Its costs consist of reimbursement to hospitals and administrative expenses. The objectives of the organization will be the maximization of the number and size of policies sold; that is, the greater the number of enrollees and the larger the premiums, the better off the company will be. The rationale for this assumption is that, to satisfy its special status as a nonprofit organization, the plan must enroll as many people as possible.

9.4.5 The Market Mechanism

We can now develop a picture of the entire process by which resources are allocated in the market. Let us begin with an initial level of insurance held by the public and a certain level of quality of care provided by the hospitals. Let the hospitals raise the quality of care by hiring more inputs. As a result, costs per admission rise. Higher costs will lead to more policies sold and increased coverage for existing policies. In turn, this has the effect of lowering the direct price of hospital services to the previously uninsured (who are now insured) and increasing the demand for admissions. Hospitals are better off as a result.

For the market to continue this inflationary cycle, the third party must somehow ratify this process. Given its goals, the nonprofit insurer will surely do so, since it will become better off. The way in which an insurer can further the inflationary process lies in the types of contracts it provides to consumers and hospitals. As seen in Section 3.6, a full-service policy will encourage the demand of insured patients more than a policy with copayments or deductibles. As seen in Section 6.7.2, full-cost reimbursement will enable the hospital to expand quality with fewer impediments. The conclusion of our model, then, is that both of these inflation-encouraging policies will be followed by the third party. Indeed, both such policies have been in wide evidence in recent years. In the process, premiums will have to be raised in order for the insurer to meet its administrative and reimbursement expenses. But, since the cost of hospitalization is continually on the increase, consumers facing larger risks will be more willing to pay these higher premiums.

The physicians, in their roles as negotiators for "better working conditions," reinforce these inflationary tendencies. With hospitals continually facing a loss of staff doctors, the prospect of empty beds encourages them to continue in the bidding process. With permissive third-party reimbursement policies, such bidding practices become affordable to the hospitals.

According to the model just described, with all groups pursuing their own interests—hospitals attempting to increase output, insurance intermediaries increasing enrollments or premiums, consumers obtaining "free" (at time of consumption) medical care at their doctors' prescriptions—the system will expand to a limitless degree. The cost–insurance spiral, according to this model, can continue to increase until it eats up the entire resources of the economy!

In fact, such a model is a caricature, exaggerating certain inflationary tendencies, which were prevalent during several decades prior to the early 1980s, of the professionally dominated marketplace. The way the incentive structure was set up allowed doctors to practice medicine with a miminum of economic impediments; in the process, the costs of consumers' actions were (partly or fully) shifted on to some other party. Employees sought insurance and employers provided it at rates subsidized by the tax system. Doctors prescribed care and hospitals provided it to patients who had little concern for what the care cost. Insurance companies, who were caught in the middle, did not seek more economical insurance packages for their clients, primarily because they had no incentives to do so. Lying at the heart of this open-ended system were taxpayers, whose contributions to the process were well hidden in a system of tax-free benefits and tax deductions.

It should not be thought that this state of affairs was arrived at accidentally. From the 1940s on the dominant ethic with regard to health care was to increase its access as much as possible. Capital subsidies were developed to increase hospital facilities and medical personnel (see Section 2.3), and consumer access to these increasingly available services was encouraged through subsidies on insurance, as well as through public programs such as Medicare and Medicaid. The net result of these subsidies has been a highly inflationary medical economy, as caricaturized in the model in this section.

Recently, there has been a growing policy emphasis on the expenditure side of the picture and de-emphasis of the access side. Federal policies, such as the implementation of DRGs and increasing the flexibility of states to redesign their Medicaid programs, have already been implemented, and others, such as limitations placed on tax-free health insurance premium benefits, have been proposed. Employers have also awakened to the possibilities of cost-containment in medical care with regard to their own employees' health care benefits. This awakening was brought about with the recession of 1981 and the growing threat to American industry of foreign competition. Business began to realize that a potential for economizing on health care benefits existed through changes in benefit structures (e.g., increased copayments and deductibles) and self-insuring.

Perhaps the lesson that can be learned from the model presented in this section is that no system is neutral with regard to incentives. Each health care system has a constellation of incentives built into it, which pushes resource allocation in one direction or another. The incentives in the American system were to hide the true cost of resources from the users. This meant lower *direct* costs and more use of the system. Of course, at the end of the day, someone had to pick up the tab for the system's costs; but given the active role played by the tax system, it was never clear who paid what.

In recent years a number of policy prescriptions have been put forward to make the health care system behave more like the competitive system of Chapter 7. These prescriptions attack the market on the supply side (through reducing professional dominance) and the demand side (through restructured incentives). They are presented, in a policy framework, in Chapter 13.

REFERENCES

Interrelated Markets

Frech, H.E. (1979). Market power in health insurance, effects on insurance and medical markets. *Journal of Industrial Economics, 28*, 55–72.

Supplier-induced Demand: Physicians

Anderson, R.K., House, D., & Ormiston, M.B. (1981). A theory of physician behavior with supplier-induced demand. *Southern Economic Journal, 48*, 124–133.

Auster, R.D., & Oaxaca, R.L. (1981). Identification of supplier induced demand in the health care sector. *Journal of Human Resources, 16*, 327–342.

Blackstone, E.A. (1980). Market power and resource misallocation in medicine: The case of neurosurgery. *Journal of Health Politics, Policy, and Law, 3*(3), 345–360.

Evans, R.G. (1974). Supplier induced demand. In M. Perlman (Ed.), *The economics of health and medical care* (pp. 162–173). London: McMillan Co.

Fuchs, V. (1978). The supply of surgeons and the demand for operations. *Journal of Human Resources, 13* (Supplement), 35–55.

Hay, J., & Leahy, M.J. (1982). Physician induced demand: An empirical analysis of the consumer information gap. *Journal of Health Economics, 1*, 231–244.

Hemenway, D., & Fallon, D. (1985). Testing for physician-induced demand with hypothetical cases. *Medical Care, 23*, 344–349.

Pauly, M.V. (1979). What is unnecessary surgery. *Milbank Memorial Fund Quarterly, 57*, 95–117.

——— (1980). *Doctors and their workshops*. Chicago: University of Chicago Press.

———, & Satterthwaite, M.A. (1980). The pricing of primary care physicians' services: A test of the role of consumer information. *Bell Journal of Economics, 12*, 488–506.

Ramsey, J.B. (1980). An analysis of competing hypotheses of the demand for and supply of physician services. In J.S. Hixson (Ed.), *The target income hypothesis* (DHEW Publication No. HRA-80-27). Washington, DC: Department of Health, Education, and Welfare, Bureau of Health Manpower.

Reinhardt, U. (1978). Comment. In W. Greenberg (Ed.), *Competition in the health care sector* (pp. 156–190). Washington, DC: Federal Trade Commission.

Rice, T.H. (1983). The impact of changing Medicare reimbursement rates on physician-induced demand. *Medical Care, 21,* 803–815.

Rosenblatt, R.A., & Moscovice, I.S. (1984). The physician as gatekeeper. *Medical Care, 22,* 150–159.

Rossiter, L.F., & Wilensky, G.R. (1984). Identification of physician-induced demand. *Journal of Human Resources, 19,* 232–244.

Sloan, F., & Feldman, R. (1978). Competition among physicians. In W. Greenberg (Ed.), *Competition in the health care sector* (pp. 57–131). Washington, DC: Federal Trade Commission.

Stano, M. (1985). An analysis of the evidence on competition in the physician services markets. *Journal of Health Economics, 4,* 197–211.

Sweeney, G.H. (1982). The market for physicians' services: Theoretical implications and an empirical test of the target income hypothesis. *Southern Economic Journal, 48,* 594–613.

Wennberg, J.E., Barnes, B.A., & Zubkoff, M. (1982). Professional uncertainty and the problem of supplier-induced demand. *Social Science and Medicine, 16,* 811–824.

Wilensky, G.R., & Rossiter, L. (1983). The relative importance of physician-induced demand in the demand for medical care. *Milbank Memorial Fund Quarterly, 61,* 252–277.

Williams, A. (1985). The nature, meaning, and measurement of health and illness. *Social Science and Medicine, 20,* 1023–1027.

Hospital Availability Effect

Ginsburg, P.B., & Koretz, D.M. (1983). Bed availability and hospital utilization: Estimates of the "Roemer effect." *Health Care Financing Review, 5,* 87–92.

Roemer, M., & Shain, M. (1959). *Hospital utilization under insurance.* Chicago: American Hospital Association.

Part III

Evaluative Economics

Chapter 10

Value Judgments and Economic Evaluation

10.1 INTRODUCTION

In this chapter we begin a different level of inquiry. In Part II we were concerned with what would be the actual allocation of resources devoted to medical care. We were interested in explaining only the various allocations that might occur under different circumstances. We did not concern ourselves with whether any particular allocation was "good" or "acceptable" or "equitable," to use only a few of the terms with which we might label an allocation. In this chapter we begin the task of evaluating alternative possible allocations of resources. This task will lead us to inquire whether totally free care can be judged "better" than a simple market provision of medical care, for example. Or whether and in what sense a regulated system is preferable to an unregulated one.

First, we must lay the ground rules for conducting an evaluation. That is the task of this chapter. In Section 10.2 the importance of having a standard that is both recognizable and unvaried in terms of which we can gauge alternative possible allocations is discussed. Individual valuations for particular commodities that can be used to build a social evaluation based on these individual valuations are then discussed in Section 10.3. One particular standard of resource use is developed, which employs the individual valuations. This standard, used frequently by economists, is referred to as efficiency criterion. Such a standard takes individuals' starting situations as given and therefore bypasses questions relating to equity and need. Policy goals emanating from this analysis are presented in Section 10.4. Other standards relating to fairness are discussed in Section 10.5; these include the concepts of right, equity, and need.

10.2 VALUES AND STANDARDS IN ECONOMIC EVALUATION

Suppose we are faced with a situation in which Mr. A has cancer, but is receiving no medical care, and Mrs. B is quite well, but is spending $4,000 on surgical services for a facial lift. Would this be an acceptable allocation of our medical resources? Many would say it is unfair, without bringing into play the basic standard they were using to judge the situation. Suppose, instead, that it was necessary heart surgery Mrs. B was receiving. Would this change one's evaluation of the situation? Would it change the standard being used to gauge the situation?

In our example, the resources are being allocated differently in the two situations. However, unless we had a standard that did not itself vary from situation to situation, we really could not compare the two situations. That is, without an independent scale of fairness or acceptability, we could not have an acceptable measure by which to gauge alternative allocations. This section presents a classification of available standards systems. That is, it concentrates on the bases with which standards may be formed.

For the purposes of economic evaluation, there are two ways in which we can derive systems of values for use in the development of a ranking of alternative uses of resources. The first method is called *delegatory,* by which we mean that the choosing of a value system has been delegated, willfully or otherwise, by the members of society to some ultimate source. This delegation can come from several directions, and the value system that arises from the delegation can take any number of forms. The delegation can be imposed from a higher being, such as a deity, be it God or Jupiter or Apollo. In each such case the value system will come from this deity (see arrow 1 in Figure 10–1). Sometimes the delegation can be from an interpreter of the ultimate word, such as Moses or Mohammed (arrows 2 and 3). Another form of delegation can be imposed by a dictator, who settles on some value system based on his or her values (arrow 1). Or the value interpreter can actually consider himself or herself a spokesman for society (arrows 3 and 4). That is, he or she can say, "Society wants a decent standard of health for all," or some such statement. Such a statement, while shrouded in democratic terms, is really an observer's own interpretation of what society wants. Any commentator who chooses to speak for society without a unanimous mandate is really stamping his or her own interpretation on what society wants. The method of value formation is still delegatory.

Once the source of the values has been determined, we can turn our focus to the system of values itself from which the standards can be derived. These value systems vary immensely. They can range from being very specific to being very vague. They can take the form of the laws given from God to Moses or of the Christian principle of agape. Or the ultimate value chosen can be somewhat more folksy, such as "with fairness to all."

In the field of health services analysis, we have many examples of writers proposing value systems on delegatory grounds. Since no established ground rules exist by which to select a true value system, a wide variety of delegatory value systems has been proposed for society to follow.

For example, writers (who have taken on the roles of value interpreters) have posited a "right" to health or health care coming from different directions. One

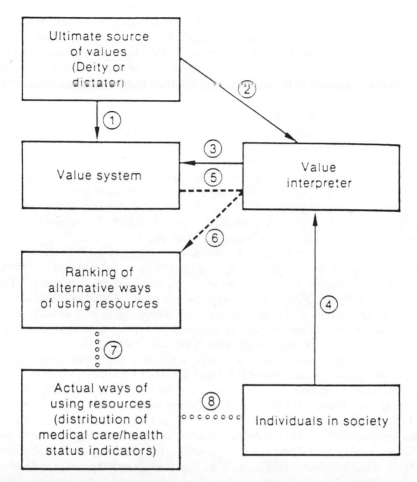

Figure 10–1 Representation of the transmission and translation of value systems into standards. Flows of information required in the process of evaluating resource use: (a) Deriving a value system: flows 1, or 2 and 3, or 3 and 4. (b) Deriving a ranking system from the value system: flows 5 and 6. (c) Developing measures of how resources were used: flow 8. (d) Comparing resource use measures with ranking of alternatives: flow 7.

commentator summoned the God-given principle of agape to derive this right (Outka, 1974). In terms of Figure 10–1, this writer was undertaking steps 2 and 3. Another writer appealed to a "strong sense in the population" to invoke this right to health care (Mechanic, 1976); in terms of Figure 10–1, steps 3 and 4 were taken. Both writers ended at the same point—the positing of a "right to health care."

Assuming that our problems in choosing a value system have been settled, we then face the problem of translating the chosen value system into gauges with which we can measure alternative ways of using resources. The gauge is called a *ranking* of alternative ways of using resources. In this case, when we are adhering to a delegatory system, the translation is done by a value interpreter. In Figure 10–1, we show the translation process by the dashed lines numbered 5 and 6. This translation step can sometimes be controversial; it is often the case that the same system of values, being at times somewhat vague, can be translated into several or even many ranking schemes that have very different implications regarding what is a good use of resources. When this is the case, we run into the problem of which value interpreter to listen to. Having decided on a ranking system, we then compare it with indicators of actual or proposed states of resource use (e.g., distributions of health care or levels of health; dotted line number 7) to determine their desirability from a policy standpoint.

It should be stressed that delegatory systems are not necessarily evil. They may stem from a highly respected and loved authority. They may contain laudatory ideals and may lead to ranking schemes that seem totally reasonable and compassionate. Nevertheless, they are not built up from the values of "the masses" and therefore retain some degree of nonrepresentativeness.

As probably anticipated, the second method by which a system of values can be derived is through total participation by the members of the community. These value systems require the consensus of all members of the community. The authority question is dispensed with, as is the interpreter. The ultimate values are left to the individuals. As a result, our yardstick is based on individual well-being. Two assumptions can immediately be specified concerning a participatory value information system. The first condition such a system must meet is that everyone's values must be taken into account in ranking alternative ways of using resources. The second is that each individual is the best judge of his or her own welfare. This second condition ensures that individuals' best interest will not be interpreted by someone else; if this were the case, we would revert to a delegatory system.

In Section 10.3 and 10.4, a participatory system of evaluation is developed. This system, well known in economic circles as the Paretean system after the famous sociologist Vilfredo Pareto, examines what improvements could potentially be made in resource allocations if we start from an initial position and allows us to arrive at a unique optimum position. This optimum holds *only* with reference to some initial starting point (i.e., the initial endowments each member of society is given). We do not judge the starting point, which may or may not be fair, a consideration to which we return in Section 10.5. In Section 10.3, we develop the economic interpretation of individual valuations with respect to different commodities. In Section 10.4, we build a social ranking based on these individual valuations.

10.3 EFFICIENT OUTPUT LEVELS

10.3.1 Individual Valuations of Commodities or Activities

If we accept individuals' own valuations as the best indicators of their own welfare, we must then determine, at least in principle, what these valuations might be. Since our analysis is concerned with specific commodities, our task is simplified somewhat. We need only determine what individuals' valuations are like with respect to those commodities with which we are concerned.

As seen in Chapter 3, economists have developed a hypothesis regarding an individual's valuation of units of a specific commodity. The hypothesis, which is based on our demand analysis, states that the more of any good the individual has, the less will successive units of the commodity be worth to him or her in terms of other commodities. The entire analysis can be recast using money as the basic unit of the individual's value. To recast this analysis in this way, we must assume that money, being used as the measure of individual value, is itself of constant value. That is, if one gives up $2, that $2 will always represent the same loss to the individual, however much income he or she has. This assumption will hold at least partially true if the outlay for the commodity in question is a reasonably small portion of the individual's total budget.

Whether an individual spends $100 or $150 on a commodity, if his or her income is $10,000, it is unlikely to cause the valuation of each dollar to change for the individual. However, as the amount that must be given up to obtain a commodity becomes very large relative to income (as explained in the analysis in Chapter 4 on risk and insurance), the utility of or the subjective valuation placed on the marginal dollar will change. We are making the explicit assumption that it does not.

With the assumption of money income having a constant value to the individual for all relevant ranges of expenditures, we can now specify individual valuations of successive units of a commodity in terms of money. These valuations, we must stress, are the individuals' own evaluations of specific units of the commodities; they qualify for insertion into our overall social evaluation.

10.3.2 Values in a Selfish Market

To simplify our analysis, let us assume initially that there are two individuals in our market, Mr. A and Mrs. B. Each has a specific schedule of valuations that he or she places on his or her own consumption of medical care. Let us refer to these valuations as *marginal valuation* (*MV*), which is defined as the extra amount of money an individual would be willing to pay for each additional unit of the commodity. Thus the *MV* is a measure of what an extra unit of the commodity is worth to the individual in money terms. Note that quality does not enter into our simplified analysis: all units of medical care are taken to be of the same quality level.

In our initial analysis, both A and B derive satisfaction or value from their own consumption of the service, and this is the only satisfaction that anyone in society gets from their consumption. Mr. A places a marginal value of $80 on his first unit consumed, $70 on his second, and so on, as seen in columns (1) and (2) in

Table 10–1 Values and Costs of Medical Care

(1) Quantity Consumed by Mr. A (Q_A)	(2) Quantity Consumed by Mrs. B. (Q_B)	(3) Quantity Consumed by A and B $(Q_A + Q_B)$	(4) Marginal Value of Consumption (MV)	(5) Marginal Cost of Output at Output Level of $Q_A + Q_B$
1	0	1	80	5
2	0	2	70	10
3	0	3	60	15
4	1	5	50	25
5	2	7	40	35
6	3	9	30	45
7	4	11	20	55
8	5	13	10	65
9	6	15	0	75

Table 10–1. It can be seen that we make the assumption of declining marginal valuations placed by each individual on successive additions to his or her own consumption of medical care. Recall from Chapter 3 that all other factors, such as health status, income, and wealth, are held constant (i.e., the initial values of these variables are held constant). For purposes of social evaluation, then, we have a measure of the social worth of Mr. A's consumption of medical care (since no one else values this care other than A himself).

This assumed relation between marginal value and quantity consumed can be presented geometrically. Referring to Figure 10–2, the curve MV_a represents A's marginal valuation of successive units of medical care. It is assumed, for ease of geometric exposition, that the units of medical care can be made very small so that the MV curve becomes smooth. Mr. A's valuation of his own consumption is referred to as the private, or internal, valuation of his consumption. Under the present assumptions (no one else cares), the private valuation is the same as the social valuation (the total value placed on Mr. A's consumption by all of society).

Similarly, we present the private valuations of a second individual, Mrs. B, in Table 10–1 and, geometrically, as MV_b in Figure 10–2. For whatever reason (she is poorer, or more healthy, or less well educated), Mrs. B places a lower value on each unit of health care than does A. Indeed, her first unit has an MV of $50, her second, $40, and so on. These valuations might seem low to us, but since she is the ultimate judge of her own welfare, we cannot question these evaluations; they are simply part of the data.

In our assumption, A and B are the only members of society who participate in the medical care market. The marginal social values of medical care coincide with

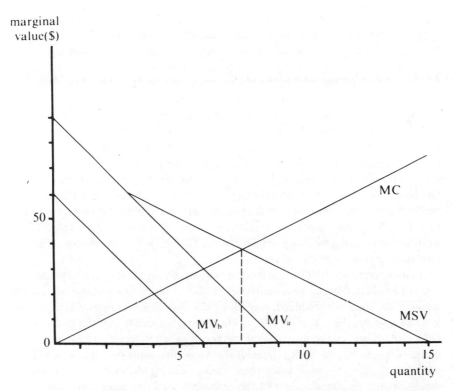

Figure 10–2 Representation of efficient output level. Individuals A and B have private marginal valuations for medical care (MV_a and MV_b, respectively). Using these, we calculate the marginal social value (MSV) curve, which relates aggregate quantity to each individual's valuation. MC is the marginal social cost of medical care. The efficient level of output is that quantity at which the MSV equals the MC.

the marginal private values. In column (4) of Table 10–1, we present the aggregated quantities that correspond to each level of MV. For example, at an aggregate quantity of five units of medical care (four by A and one by B), each consumer's marginal value will be $50. If seven units were consumed (five by A and two by B), each individual's MV would be $40. We now have hypothesized how much each additional unit of medical care is worth to each participant. Furthermore, we have derived an aggregate level relationship between the quantity of medical care and the marginal value to each individual if he or she were consuming at the level of consumption indicated by the respective MV curve. This aggregate curve is called MSV (for marginal social value) and shows the value to *each* member of the market if all individuals are consuming at the respective levels indicated by the curve. Because B does not have an MV above $60, then for values above $60 the MSV curve coincides with A's MV curve.

An implicit assumption of our analysis is that consumer evaluations are expressed in terms of medical care. But medical care is not valued for its own sake; it is really health that is valued. In fact, each consumer's MV is made up of two components: an MV for *health* (termed *H*), and the *marginal productivity* of an additional unit of medical care (*M*) in producing health ($\Delta H/\Delta M$). Thus the valuation of medical care is derivative, stemming from the two components.

We come next to the cost of producing medical care. Our initial assumption here is that each level of output is being produced at the minimum cost. This assumption is sometimes referred to as the *technological efficiency* assumption. It implies that, given production conditions and input prices, the lowest cost combinations of inputs are used at any output level. In column (5) of Table 10–1 and in Figure 10–2, we show the minimum marginal cost at which providers can produce medical care. We assume that this minimum marginal cost rises as output increases. Note that the *MC* is the additional cost *per unit* of care; in Table 10–1, aggregate units jump by 2 (e.g., from 7 to 9). The *MC* is the cost of producing one more unit at those specific levels.

An interpretation of *MC* is that it is the amount of money that must be paid to the inputs to induce them to provide those additional quantities of medical care. If medical care were not produced, something else, of value to consumers, would be. We can assume, then, that the *MC* is the amount we had to pay the resources to induce them *not* to produce something (or somewhere) else. Thus the *MC* is marginally above (and approximates) the value that someone else would have placed on these resources in an alternative use. Viewing *MC* in this way means that the *MC* is the *opportunity cost* of the resources used (the alternative value that users of other commodities would have placed in them).

10.3.3 The Socially Optimum Quantity of Medicare Care

The next step in our analysis involves the definition and identification of desirable or optimum resource allocations. Since we are dealing with a participatory system, we are seeking to identify allocations of resources that would be judged superior by *all* members of the community. As will be seen presently, it is possible in a participatory system to rank some allocations as superior to others, although we cannot compare every conceivable situation. The criterion used is that of the maximum social value of the resources: that is, if the resources are used where consumers are willing to pay the most for them, then output will be at the "right" or economically efficient level.

Using the valuations of A and B and the *MC* of medical care, we will be at a socially optimal (or economically efficient) level of output if the *MV*s of each A and B equal the *MC* (i.e., $MV_a = MV_b = MC$). If output is at a level where the *MV*s are greater than *MC*, say at an aggregate quantity of 3 in Table 10–1, then an expansion of output to 5 (an increase of 1 for each A and B) would have an *MC per* *unit of output* of $25, but would yield $50 extra in value to each A and B. Similarly, if *MC* is rising and is greater than *MSV*, this is an indication that resources are worth more elsewhere than medical care, and so output should fall. In Figure 10–2, the optimal level of medical care is between 7 and 8. Given our assumptions, this is how much medical care *should* be produced.

In reality, a medical care market could produce too much or too little, as well as just enough. Too much could be produced if the government had a policy of financing medical care and giving it away for "free." At a zero price, demand will be at 15 units (where the *MV*s are zero); the *MC* of additional units will be well above this, if the government is willing to ensure that all that is demanded is provided. The financing of the program could be through taxes. However, by meeting all demands, the government is clearly providing too much.

On the other hand, the market may provide too little. If medical care were in the hands of a monopolist, the monopolist would set a price well above that where *MV* = *MC*. If this price were at $50, then three units in total would be demanded (all by A). Here the market would be producing too little care.

In addition, the optimum level of resource use could result in little, or even no, use of medical care by some individuals. The height of the *MV* curve, which is, in effect, a demand curve, will depend on health status, wealth, income, and so on. Poor people (e.g., Mrs. B) may have low *MV*s. Indeed, if *MC* were higher than in our example, a socially optimal quantity of output would be perfectly consistent with no consumption of medical care by B. (This is true, even though B may have a low income and poor health.) One might argue that this is unfair or inequitable, and, indeed, depending on the definition of equity one uses, this may very well be the case. But given our ground rules (initial wealth levels are given), the notion of economic efficiency is consistent with such unfairness. One should recognize, however, that the root cause of the inequitable distribution of *medical care* actually results from an inequitable distribution of wealth or income. A higher income for Mrs. B would mean higher demand and *MV* curves for medical care. But, as far as the notion of economic efficiency is concerned, initial wealth and income levels for each individual are given. If one redistributed income or wealth among individuals *involuntarily*, this might be fair to many observers, but it would not be evaluated within the bounds of the present notion of economic efficiency.

10.3.4 Optimal Output with Altruism

To preserve the present notion of economic efficiency, and indeed to extend it to cover some inequitable situations, an analysis has been developed to allow for some individuals' concern for the low medical care consumption levels of others. This analysis relates to the social demand for some goods discussed in Section 4.7. To cover this analysis, let us extend the previous example to allow for A's *external* demand for B's consumption of medical care.

From A's viewpoint, it may well be that B has a level of consumption of medical care that is too low. If this is the case, we must find some representation for A's valuations of B's medical care consumption. What is likely is that A's concern for B's medical care consumption is not unlimited. A is concerned, but only up to a point, for A has other private and public concerns as well. In fact, as seen in Section 4.3, A's valuation of B's medical care consumption can be treated as any other commodity: the more B consumes, the less the value of the marginal unit to A. In Table 10–2, A's MV for B's consumption is \$20 for the first unit, \$15 for the second, and so on. In Figure 10–3, this external MV curve is shown as $MV_a{}^b$.

It may seem strange that A's altruistic concern for B's welfare can be translated into such mercenary terms and therefore can be given a money measure. This rests on the assumption that commodities are scarce and A must simply make some choices at the margin. Even if A decided to give all his money away and use none of it for his family or own personal use, there would still be hard decisions to make. Should the money be donated to the cancer society or heart association? Should the money go toward the preservation of Newfoundland seals or bald-headed eagles? Depending on their tastes, even the most altruistic of people must make choices regarding scarcity, and our analysis is merely a formalization of this fact. Of course, most people will engage in private consumption as well as altruistic consumption; their values can be presented by marginal evaluation curves for both types of activities. The benefits to be obtained from others' consumption will be termed *external benefits*. The valuations that people place on these will be termed *external values*.

We can now arrive at a measure of what value society places on B's medical care. This value can be called the *social value* and is made up of the sum of all individuals' private and external values for the specific commodities. Thus the marginal social value, that of both A and B, for B's consumption of medical care

Table 10–2 Private and Social Values of B's Consumption of Medical Care

(1) Quantity Consumed by B	(2) Marginal Value of B for Own Consumption (MV_b)	(3) Marginal Value of A for B's Consumption $(MV_a{}^b)$	(4) Marginal Social Value of B's Consumption $(MV_b + MV_a{}^b)$
1	50	20	70
2	40	15	55
3	30	10	40
4	20	5	25
5	10	0	10

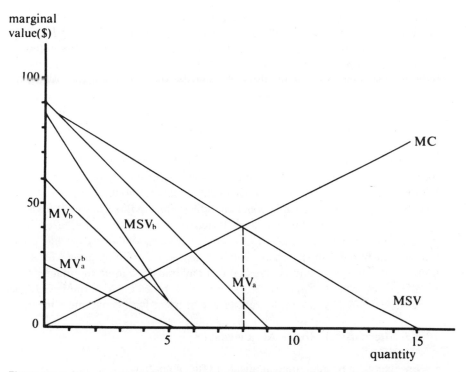

Figure 10–3 Representation of efficient output level. Individuals A and B have private marginal valuations for medical care (MV_a and MV_b, respectively); in addition, A places an external value on B's consumption. The marginal social value of B's consumption is the sum of the values placed on B's consumption by both A and B. The *MSV* of all medical care also reflects this externality. The *MC* is the marginal social cost of medical care. The efficient level of output is that quantity where *MSV* = *MC*.

can be obtained by adding up both individuals' valuations placed on each successive unit of medical care that B might consume. In Table 10–2, society has a marginal evaluation of $70 for the first unit of B's medical care (equal to the sum of $MV_b + MV_a^b$), $55 for the second, and so on. In geometric terms this can be shown in Figure 10–3 as MSV_b, which is the *vertical* sum of MV_b and MV_a. By vertical sum we mean that each unit of B's consumption has a value to society (A and B) greater than the value placed on it by B alone. Because of this public characteristic of the commodity, we sum all individuals' valuations placed on each unit of B's consumption.

The marginal valuation curve facing the market for medical care for A and B is *MSV*, which shows the quantity for all individuals at alternative *MSV*s for each individual. *MSV* is much like the *MSV* curve in the previous diagram, except it incorporates A's valuation of B's consumption along with the private *MV*s.

The socially optimum level of output is similarly interpreted: output is optimal at the quantity where the *MSV* for all individuals equals the *MC*. In Figure 10–3, the optimum level of output is at eight units of medical care. This optimum incorporates each individual's private valuations, as well as any external valuations for the poor, the needy, the sick, and the like. As compared with Figure 10–2, the optimum that incorporates the external concerns of A is greater than that in which only selfish concerns appear. However, these outcomes are results of the data, and it may well be that B's optimal consumption level is still at a low level.

The results of our extended analysis are consistent with some kind of transfer of funds from A to B for the purposes of increasing B's consumption of medical care. However, the analysis does not say what kind of transfer should take place. It may be voluntary, through charitable donations either direct to B or via some providing agency. Or it may be through taxes levied on A with the funds used by a government either to provide care directly to A or to finance it through some reimbursement mechanism. In either case, the optimal solution allows for some transfer, although it should be stressed that any transfer can be too much or too little. The government can over- or underprovide, based on A's criteria. All that our analysis shows is that *some* transfer is consistent with economic efficiency.

10.3.5 Alternative Delivery Arrangements

Now that we have identified an ideal or efficient output level, we can compare alternative delivery arrangements to see how they compare in relation to the ideal; that is, we can determine whether expected output under alternative delivery arrangements is too little, just enough, or too much (in relation to the ideal). First, assume that B is given all the medical care for free that she can consume. She would choose to consume six units of output. The social optimum is eight units for A and B, and the *MC* at this quantity is $40. Optimally, B should consume three (i.e., where $MSV_b = MC$). For every unit B consumes beyond three, the value of B's consumption is less than the cost to society (everyone). Since someone must bear the burden of this care, and since *MC* exceeds *MSV* for all units beyond three, there is a net social loss for these units. B gains handsomely; that is, her private benefits exceed her private costs. But the overall social evaluation of this type of arrangement may lead to a great deal of medical care being consumed with very little value attached to it.

Let us look at another arrangement, that of the competitive market with no philanthropy or government programs. Recall from Section 7.3 that the outcome of the competitive market will occur where marginal private cost equals price. In our example, we can show it to be where marginal value equals marginal cost. In this case, A will consume the right amount for himself, but B will not. B's consumption will be less than the socially efficient amount because all society would have been willing to pay more for the first four units than the marginal cost of medical care. A freely operating competitive market with no philanthropy will yield less than the optimal level of output when externalities would have justified a larger output. As for a monopolistic market, recall from Section 8.2.1 that the output of such a market will be less than that for the competitive market. We can conclude that the outcome for a monopolistic market will be even more suboptimal than that for a competitive market without philanthropy.

It has also been contended that even a competitive market with philanthropy will not produce the optimal amount of output. The basis for this contention arises when several or many donors of medical care exist, each of whom has a positive, external value for B's medical care. In this case some social arrangement must be found for ensuring that the values of these donors will be expressed in the market. If each of these potential donors offers to give what the output is worth to him or her, the social value will reflect the sum of the private values. However, if each donor feels that the others will also give, each donor might give less, hoping to gain a "free ride," that is, gain the benefit of the others' donations while giving less. It is in the interests of each private donor to initially offer less than the value he or she places on the output in the hope that someone else will pay the tab. If everyone behaves in this way, the total amount given in philanthropy will lead to less than the socially optimal amount being produced. Analysts who accept the efficiency criteria frequently justify compulsory government programs as a basis for making everyone pay what the program is worth; of course, if one accepts these grounds, it is difficult to decide how much the program would be worth to each taxpayer, since the individual still has an incentive to understate the value of the program.

Even accepting this justification for government programs, we still must determine an arrangement that will lead to the correct amount of medical care being utilized. As can be seen in Figure 10–3, if B were offered subsidized medical care, the efficient amount of medical care would be utilized. In this case, a charge of $30 per unit of medical care to B would lead to B's consumption of the optimal of three units. The rest of society must now pick up the remainder of the tab; since the total cost to all members of society of medical care consumed by B is $120 and since B will pay $90 of this, some arrangements must be made to collect the remaining $30 from the rest of society. This can be done in the form of taxes. Various arrangements are discussed in the next paragraphs.

We can conclude from our analysis that some form of cost-sharing arrangement can lead to an optimal or efficient amount of the product being achieved. However, other arrangements can also be efficient, for example, zero prices paid by B and some form of rationing. In practice, this type of arrangement requires that the rationing method used must produce the efficient outcome, and such methods are difficult to design and operate. Our analysis can also be extended to a case in which there are several Bs, each with a different level of income. If their demands differ because of these income levels, a system of variable subsidies tailored to the income level could be designed to have each member consume the right level of output (Pauly, 1972).

What is critical in translating the preceding analysis into a policy prescription to answer the questions posed about the desired nature of the scheme is a clear conception of what the externality might look like in actuality (see Section 4.3). Assuming that external demands for the medical care of some groups do exist and are significant, it is essential that we pin down exactly what services these external demands are for. If the externality is for good health, for example, then the external demanders (the As in our analysis) may have a demand for preventive care consumed by the potential recipients of aid (the Bs). The externality may be much more specific than that, however. It may be that the As are concerned only with those Bs who have catastrophic illnesses requiring large financial outlays. In this case they will not want to pay for the medical care of Bs who have sore throats, ingrown toenails, or acne. We know very little about the nature of the medical care externality; from an efficiency point of view, however, it is necessary to know what the As are concerned about before we design a delivery system that will incorporate these externalities.

Assuming that we have identified the nature of the externality, we can then use the preceding analysis to answer our questions, as long as we have the goal of efficiency in mind. Once the externality has been pinpointed, the types of health care that might improve the situation can be identified, and the potential recipients can be identified as being those who might otherwise not consume a sufficient amount of output. The consumer's portion of cost sharing will be designed to ensure that there is no overuse, which is defined as any quantity beyond which marginal social benefits are less than marginal social costs. The reimbursement mechanism chosen will lead to the least cost output.

Concerning the payments made by the rest of society, we can say nothing about what a fair share would amount to, for this is related to equity considerations. However, another aspect of cost sharing can be illuminated by efficiency analysis, and that concerns the incentive effects of taxes. The rate of any tax may have an effect on the economic behavior of the taxpayer. A high marginal tax rate on income (meaning that additional increments of income earned will be taxed at a high rate) may lead the income earner to work less because the net proceeds will not be worth the effort. Output would be reduced. A high marginal tax on payrolls will increase the price an employer must pay for labor services and will lead the employer to cut back on these services and perhaps substitute cheaper services of capital inputs (payments to which are not taxed on a payroll tax). These are examples of how the tax rate may influence the size and composition of total output produced. Therefore, the cost of a program to society is not merely the amount of taxes transferred. If, in the process of being levied, these taxes cause less output to be produced or fewer workers to be hired, these effects must be counted in the total social cost of any program financed by taxes (Mitchell and Phelps, 1976).

10.4 GOALS OF HEALTH POLICY

Based on the analysis of Section 10.3, we can identify a series of specific goals that must be met for an optimal health policy to be enacted. These goals are no unreasonable demand barriers, technical efficiency, and adequacy of supply. A fourth goal presents itself when government provision or finance enters into the picture, and that is the size of the budget (Stoddart and Labelle, 1985). A fifth goal, although not covered in the preceding analysis, is adequate quality of care.

Demand barriers

Demand barriers refer to the impediments, or lack of them, to an individual receiving care. Within the context of our present model, price is the prime impediment. One can encourage additional care demanded by lowering the direct price through the purchase of insurance, public programs, or charity. To the degree that medical care consumption is thought to be desirable, the absence of demand barriers can be measured by the availability of insurance, or the direct price faced by the individual.

However, money price is not the only factor related to demand barriers. As seen in Section 4.9, time costs and travel costs can also impede individuals from accessing medical care. If certain individuals' medical care consumption is to be encouraged, these costs must also be addressed, either through subsidies, relocating facilities to lower travel time and expenses, or expanding facilities and increasing operating hours to decrease waiting time.

Technical efficiency

Technical efficiency refers to the production at minimum cost of whatever level and quality of output is supplied. Technical efficiency is usually measured by money costs, but, as seen in Section 5.7, great care must be taken when comparing costs between facilities to be sure that all factors other than inefficiency (e.g., quality, input prices, case mix) have been factored out.

Adequacy of supply

Adequacy of supply refers to the availability of sufficient resources to provide care at the efficient level (given quality). As seen in Section 6.7, adequacy of supply depends on the incentive (reimbursement) system developed, the level of reimbursement, and the adequacy of funds.

Public expenditure control

Strictly speaking, the situation of the government budget does not fall out of our model. Of course, a transfer of funds from A to B is consistent with a tax on A by a government body and subsequent expenditures on medical care for B. But the model says nothing about the size of the tax, the expenditure, or the difference (the contribution to the deficit). In recent years, however, the budget deficit and public spending have come under a great deal of scrutiny, and cutbacks in government programs have been widespread. Often the rationale for these cutbacks has not been the worthiness of the program, but rather the contribution to the overall budget. To the extent that cutbacks come out of lower costs because of greater technical efficiency, true savings are provided to society, and there are gains in social efficiency. However, cutbacks may also result in reduced supply. This is not necessarily bad if output was greater than the socially optimum level to begin with. However, if the initial output was at the socially optimum level or below it, cutbacks will lead to reductions in social efficiency because the value of the output that is lost is greater than the savings made by the cutbacks.

Quality of care

Although quality is an elusive concept, the preservation of quality of care is a matter of public concern and therefore should be a consideration in any social evaluation.

10.5 ALTERNATIVE VALUE SYSTEMS

As stated in Section 10.3, acceptance of a Paretean participatory value system means rejecting any allocational change that would not be to the benefit of everyone. Any nonvoluntary confiscatory policy, however well meaning, is simply ruled out. On the other hand, many writers prescribe changes in the allocation that are compulsory and that also may harm some individuals (i.e., leave them at a lower level of well-being after the change). These writers feel that these prescribed changes are fully justified. An example of such an allocational change would be the levying of a compulsory tax, the proceeds of which would be used to pay for medical care for groups who otherwise might not obtain it. While such an allocational change might be acceptable to all parties, one who proposed it on delegatory grounds would do so even if it were not universally acceptable. Some of the grounds on which these nonvoluntary allocations might be justified are inquired into next.

One such basis involves a belief on the part of the value interpreter that he or she is indeed expressing the will of the majority or the entire group when proposing a certain set of values be followed in making allocational decisions. Frequently, those affected have not been consulted for their voluntary consent. Their "wills" are being interpreted (Fein, 1972; Mechanic, 1976). A second basis for positing a set of values is to place the individuals in a hypothetical setting and ask, if faced with a certain problem in this setting, on what values would they agree? An example of such reasoning places 14 men and women in a lifeboat (the game can be played with any number, however) with the necessity of choosing 4 to go overboard in order to save the other 10. Under these conditions, all might ultimately agree to a sweepstake so that each has the same chance of being saved (Beauchamp, 1976). Such exercises led their inventors to conclude that, in a health care context, a widely accepted principle might emerge positing that all should have a fair chance at using any health care resource; that is, there should be a right to health care. A third line of justifying a right to health care is by appeal to a higher authority. This has been discussed in Section 10.2 (Outka, 1974).

It was pointed out in Section 10.2 that the justification of a right or entitlement to health care does not, by itself, give concrete guidance to anyone making pre-scribed changes in the allocation of resources. To translate values into specific prescriptions, a ranking system must be developed. There are a number of such systems in terms of which one might gauge whether the right to health care was achieved. Most of these indicators are really indicators of the degree of fairness or equity. Alternate allocations are ranked according to how access or use of medical care is distributed among potential or actual users. Perhaps the most extreme goal in terms of fairness would be the affirmation that a fair distribution of the product would be achieved when everyone's right to health was recognized and granted. This would mean that, starting from initial health levels, the resources of the community should be employed to ultimately bring about an equal health status for all. Such a proposition is made without regard for the realities of what health care can do to achieve health and for what resources might be available to achieve this goal. Because it is widely believed that pursuing such a goal would involve a strain on resources, it is seldom posited (Hemenway, 1982).

More seriously posited goals relate to equality of access to or use of medical care. One such goal would be that everyone have access to the best medical care. Presuming that the "best" might be measured unambiguously, the resource-use implications of such a measure would be enormous. Achieving such a goal, presumably on a regional basis, would mean a very large investment in health care facilities and personnel, as well as a means of ensuring that they locate in accordance with the equality indicator. Because of the cost implications of this goal, it is seldom posited.

Another indicator that might be accepted would be one of strict equality of health care accessibility for everyone. Such a policy would involve a leveling off of those who have more access and a raising of the level of those who have less. Developing such an indicator and using it as a guide would involve deciding on a level that at least the value interpreter (if no one else) could accept. A third indicator that might be chosen would give everyone a right of access to at least a minimum acceptable level of care. Choosing such an indicator would involve specifying exactly what this minimum might be and deciding to what extent others might exceed this minimum. In addition, it might lead to a two-tier system of care, one for the poor and one for the insured.

No doubt we have only skimmed the surface of possible ranking schemes that might be constructed in order to offer a fair guide to the allocation of resources. Indeed, once we move into the realm of delegatory value making, everybody is entitled to his or her own view about what is best for society, that is, on what course society's resources should be set.

This need not deter one from searching for a system of values for a social welfare indicator with which one can guide the use of medical care resources. The search for a set of values that might prove appealing to a majority of people has been a major preoccupation of philosophers, and a role for such a set of values exists in the health care sector. Even if a unanimous set of values does not emerge, someone may yet design a health care system that satisfies a somewhat less appealing set of goals in a very effective way. While waiting for the perfect system to come along, many would settle for a second best.

REFERENCES

Efficiency Criteria

Arrow, K.J. (1963). Uncertainty and the welfare economics of medical care. *American Economic Review, 53,* 941–973.

Buchanan, J.M. (1965). *The inconsistencies of the National Health Service.* London: Institute of Economic Affairs.

Culyer, A.J. (1971). The nature of the commodity "health care" and its efficient allocation. *Oxford Economic Papers, 23,* 189–211.

——— (1972). On the relative efficiency of the national health service. *Kyklos, 25,* 266–287.

Detsky, A.S. (1978). *The economic foundations of national health policy.* Cambridge, MA: Ballinger Publishing Co.

Pauly, M.V. (1968). The economics of moral hazard. *American Economic Review, 58,* 531–537.

——— (1972). *Medical care at public expense.* New York: Praeger Publishers.

Weisbrod, B.A. (1964). Collective consumption services of individual consumption goods. *Quarterly Journal of Economics, 78,* 471–477.

Equity and Other Social Goals

Beauchamp, D.E. (1976). Public health as social justice. *Inquiry, 13,* 3–14.

Daniels, N. (1982). Equity of access to health care. *Milbank Memorial Fund Quarterly, 60,* 51–81.

Fein, R. (1972). On achieving access and equity in health care. In J.B. McKinlay (Ed.), *Economic aspects of health care* (pp. 23–56). New York: Watson Publishing International.

Friedman, L.M. (1971). The idea of right as a social and legal concept. *Journal of Social Issues, 27,* 189–198.

Goldfarb, R., Havrylshyn, O., & Mangum, S. (1984). Can remittances compensate for manpower outflows. *Journal of Development Economics, 15*(1), 1–17.

Hemenway, D. (1982). The optimal location of doctors. *New England Journal of Medicine, 306,* 397–401.

Lewis, C.F., Fein, R., & Mechanic, D. (1976). *A right to health.* New York: Wiley–Interscience.

Mechanic, D. (1976). Rationing health care. *Hastings Center Report, 6*(1), 34–37.

Mitchell, B.M., & Phelps, C.E. (1976). National health insurance: Some costs and effects of mandated employee coverage. *Journal of Political Economy, 84,* 553–571.

Outka, G. (1974). Social justice and equal access to health care. *Journal of Religious Ethics, 2,* 11–32.

Schwartz, W.B., & Joskow, P.L. (1978). Medical efficacy versus economic efficiency: A conflict in values. *New England Journal of Medicine, 299,* 1462–1464.

Stoddart, G.L., & Labelle, R.J. (1985, October). *Privatization in the Canadian health care system.* Ottawa: Health and Welfare Canada.

Thurow, L.C. (1985). Medicine versus economics. *New England Journal of Medicine, 313,* 611–614.

Whipple, D. (1974). Health care as a right. *Inquiry, 11,* 65–68.

Chapter 11

Public and Private Health Insurance

11.1 INTRODUCTION

In Chapter 10 we presented an overview of the concept of economic evaluation. It was shown that, at a very broad level, there are two major areas of concern, economic efficiency and equity. Furthermore, both efficiency and equity have a number of characteristics associated with them. Efficiency criteria for medical care markets can be categorized into a number of separate policy goals, including absence of demand impediments, technical efficiency, adequacy of supply, quality of care, and overall levels of cost (including the impact on public expenditures). Also, spillover effects and incentive effects of taxes must be considered in any public policy. It was also shown that efficiency does not imply that equity has been achieved, and that equity criteria are important components of any health policy measures.

In this chapter, our welfare framework will be used to analyze selected aspects of private and public health insurance coverage. As has long been recognized, health insurance lies at the heart of the health care system, and public policies related to insurance influence the functioning of the health care market. Indeed, much of our emphasis in Part II of this book has been on models of consumer, provider, and market behavior that explain how these entities function under alternative insurance arrangements (reimbursement, copayments, etc.). Our goal in this chapter is to illustrate how the explanatory economic analysis of Part II can be employed to increase our understanding of how specific policy choices (e.g., reimbursement, cost sharing by consumers, taxes and premiums) can influence the attainment of policy goals identified in Chapter 10.

In Section 11.2 we present an overview of public health insurance in the United States, focusing on Medicare, Medicaid, indigent care, and the role of each of these components in the overall health insurance picture. In Section 11.3 we briefly discuss some of the problems that public policy faces in this area. In

227

Section 11.4 we discuss some of the solutions proposed in recent years and how each solution can be analyzed using our framework of policy goals and the models developed in Part II.

11.2 PUBLIC HEALTH INSURANCE

Public health insurance in the United States involves a number of programs aimed at target populations. In addition, a major aspect of the issue of public health insurance is the large number of individuals who have no coverage and, as a result, frequently have low levels of access to care. In this section we discuss the two major public health insurance programs, Medicare and Medicaid, and major gaps in coverage for indigents.

11.2.1 Medicare

The Medicare program was instituted with the passage of Title XVIII of the Social Security Act, entitled, "Health Insurance for the Aged." It began operation on July 1, 1966. Presently covered under Medicare are individuals over 65 who are eligible for Social Security benefits, disabled individuals, and individuals who have end-stage renal disease. We will focus mainly on the coverage of individuals over 65.

Coverage for these individuals is in two parts. Under Part A, known as hospital insurance (HI), hospitalization and some skilled nursing facility (SNF) coverage are provided. The conditions for coverage by SNF benefits are quite restrictive and must be related to a prior hospitalization. If these conditions are met, Medicare coverage is for 100 SNF days of care. Medicare Part A covers 90 days of hospitalization per benefit period (benefit periods are identified as being preceded by a specified time during which the enrollee is not a bed patient in a hospital or an SNF); in addition, each enrollee has a lifetime reserve of 60 days. Under Part B, supplementary medical insurance (SMI) is provided; coverage includes physician services, drugs, x-ray, lab, and medical supplies.

Because much of the aged population is covered by Medicare *and* Medicaid, a better understanding of the overall financing of public programs in the United States can be obtained with a unified picture. This overall picture will be developed with reference to Figure 11–1.

With regard to Medicare hospital insurance, program enrollees pay no premiums; however, there is a deductible tied to the per diem cost of care, which has been rising steeply in recent years. In 1986 it was $492. After the deductible is met, there are no copayments for the first 60 days, and a copayment of 25 percent of the deductible for days 61 through 90. The public share of HI (exclusive of the deductibles and copayments) is financed primarily through a Social Security tax on

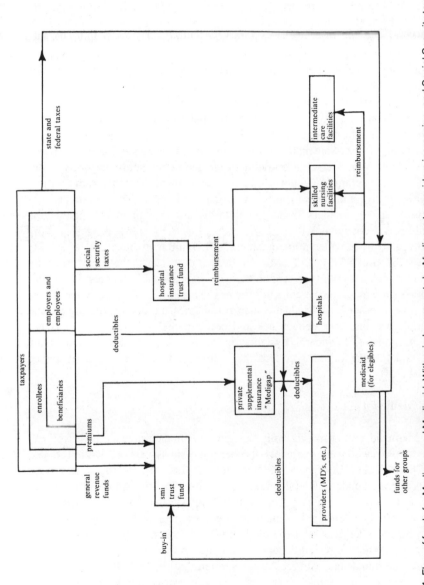

Figure 11-1 Flow of funds for Medicare and Medicaid. With reimbursements by Medicare to providers increasing, and Social Security taxes and Medicare Part B premiums limited, additional pressure is being placed on general revenue funds. Nursing home reimbursements have been taking a larger portion of Medicaid dollars, which has led to stricter policies for the nonaged population.

worker payrolls (see Figure 11–1). Funds from this tax go into the hospital insurance trust fund out of which hospitals and nursing homes are reimbursed.

The SMI program is voluntary, with enrollees buying in with a premium. An enrollee in the SMI program receives benefits subject to a deductible (first $75 of reasonable charges in 1986) and a copayment of 20 percent of reasonable charges. The SMI premium was initially set so that the premium covered one-half of the expenditures of the SMI trust fund (which reimburses providers). Premium increases ($16.80 per month in 1986) are tied to Social Security cash benefits. Recently, because of the restrictions on premium increases, the premium portion has fallen below 30 percent; the remainder of the SMI fund's income comes from general revenues (i.e., public expenditures).

There is an active private market for supplementary insurance to cover the beneficiaries' (those who use services) deductibles and copayments. In terms of our flow of funds diagram in Figure 11–1, enrollees in the SMI program can pay premiums to private insurers for this "Medigap" coverage. The private insurers then reimburse the providers for the beneficiaries' shares of their costs (that is, the deductibles and copayments).

With regard to provider reimbursement, HI reimburses hospitals on a DRG basis (see Section 6.7.3), and SMI reimburses physicians, the major provider group in this category of insurance, on the basis of reasonable charges. If a doctor accepts assignment of the patient's bill, he or she accepts the Medicare reasonable charge for the procedure; Medicare then reimburses the doctor directly for the appropriate amount (less deductibles and copayments). If the doctor does not accept assignment, Medicare pays the reimbursed (reasonable) amount to the patient and the doctor must collect the entire amount from the patient (see Section 8.2.4).

11.2.2 Medicaid

The Medicaid program, originally designed to finance medical care for low-income families who were recipients of other financial assistance, was introduced in 1966 under Title XIX of the Social Security Act. Unlike the Medicare program, which is operated under guidelines set by the Social Security Administration, the Medicaid program is a state–federal partnership. Although the form of the program was initially determined by the federal government, state governments individually decide whether or not to participate in the program, as well as the extent of the program. Who is covered depends to a considerable extent on criteria established by individual states. In recent years federal guidelines have become more flexible, in part to allow states to impose coverage restrictions. Except for a short period in the early 1980s, states have not restricted coverage.

Those individuals covered under the joint federal–state program fall into three groups: (1) cash recipients of the Aid to Families with Dependent Children

(AFDC) program (dependent children, adults in AFDC families, blind, disabled); (2) cash recipients of Supplemental Security Income (SSI) (aged, blind, disabled); and (3) the "medically needy," many of whom would not qualify on an income basis, but who have spent a sufficient amount on medical care ("spend down") such that their incomes net of medical care expenses fall below specific levels. In this exposition we will concentrate primarily on the covered population over 65.

Federally required benefits under Medicaid include physician services, inpatient and outpatient hospital services, lab services, and nursing home services in skilled nursing homes. States can put limitations on benefits, such as on the number of inpatient days covered, authorization requirements for specific medical procedures, and so on. In addition, states can provide optional services such as intermediate care facility (ICF) stays, dental care, and physiotherapy.

The financing of Medicaid is based on a formula that incorporates state income levels. The minimum federal contribution is 50 percent. The state receiving the highest federal share (Mississippi) receives about 77 percent of its approved program costs from federal funds. Medicaid funds come out of general taxation revenues. Medicaid was originally designed as an open-ended program; that is, the federal share would follow the state share with no explicit limitations. In recent years a number of alterations have been proposed that would, in effect, cap the federal contribution (Wyckoff, 1985).

For eligible enrollees who are also Medicare eligible, Medicaid can "buy in" to SMI, paying the SMI premium as well as deductibles and copayments (see Figure 11–1). These enrollees will then be covered by Medicare for SMI and HI and by Medicaid for other benefits such as SNF and ICF care.

Medicaid reimburses physicians on the basis of *reasonable charges* for fees. Medicaid traditionally followed Medicare in reimbursing hospitals on the basis of retrospective costs, but recent reforms have allowed medical programs to develop prospective forms of reimbursement. New regulations have also allowed for reimbursement changes for physicians, nursing homes, and HMOs (U.S. Department of Health and Human Services, 1983, pp. 140–142).

11.2.3 Uncovered Care

Despite the existence of Medicare and Medicaid, many individuals either have no health insurance coverage at all or have large gaps in coverage. According to estimates by the National Center for Health Services Research (Kasper, Walden, and Wilensky, 1979) 12.6 percent of all individuals (about 25 million) had no insurance coverage in 1977. A substantial number of this group were young and/or healthy, but this still left uncovered approximately 4.2 million who were in fair or poor health (as reported by themselves).

In addition to those with no coverage, a substantial number of individuals have gaps in coverage. Catastrophic coverage (expenses per episode of illness in excess of $5,000) is particularly sparse (Birnbaum, et al., 1979), with much of this lack of coverage being in the area of long-term care (Meiners, 1983).

The issue of lack of coverage has surfaced as a major policy issue in the area of inpatient hospital care. The admission of indigent patients has not fallen evenly among hospitals. Teaching hospitals, public hospitals, and hospitals supplying a large proportion of their output in certain product lines (e.g., obstetrics) are all associated with larger portions of charity care and bad debts (Mulstein, 1984).

11.3 SOME PROBLEMS IN COVERAGE ISSUES

In recent years several issues relating to public insurance have dominated the public policy scene. In this section we will briefly review these. In the following section, we discuss specific solutions and show how economic analysis can help us to develop a relation between the solutions and the goals of health policy. Keep in mind that each problem discussed is really part of a larger, overall problem, and so in discussing solutions we must be aware of spillover effects to other markets and groups.

Depletion of the HI trust fund

Medicare's HI funding is tied to the growth of the portion of the Social Security tax that is earmarked for the HI trust fund. However, there is no automatic link between the growth of revenues into the trust fund and the growth of expenditures of the fund, which primarily go to reimburse hospitals (Wolkstein, 1984). The tax is a percent of payrolls and so cannot be increased by more than the increase in payrolls, unless the Social Security tax rate is increased. In the absence of such a tax increase, large deficits have been predicted for the HI trust fund by the mid-1990s. This is because expenditures out of the fund have been growing at a more rapid rate than the receipts of the fund. Let us call total reimbursements from the fund to providers, (R). We can express R as the product of three variables, reimbursement per beneficiary (someone who uses services, termed r/b), the proportion of program enrollees who use services (i.e., who are beneficiaries, termed b/e), and the number of enrollees (termed e). In notational terms:

$$R = \frac{r}{b} \times \frac{b}{e} \times e$$

In Section 2.2.8 it was shown that, when we have a variable that can be expressed as being equal to the product of more than one variable, the growth rate of the first variable (termed Gr) can be approximated by the sum of the growth rates of the products; that is,

$$\frac{Gr}{b} + \frac{Gb}{e} + Ge,$$

where Gr/b, and so on, refer to growth rates of r/b, and so on.

The expenditures for hospital care by Medicare for selected years are shown in Table 11–1. A decomposition of the growth rates, as calculated by the Health Care Financing Administration (U.S. Department of Health and Human Services, Medicare and Medicaid Data Book, 1983, Tables 2–1, 2–7, and 2–10), show that $Gr = 16.4$ percent from 1966 to 1979, while $Gr/b = 1.4$ percent and $Ge = 2.8$ percent. The residual, largely attributable to Gr/b, or expenses per beneficiary, was 12 percent, or about 75 percent of the total growth in expenditures. Now Gr/b includes the growth of service intensity *and* price, and it is difficult to disentangle the two (see Section 2.2.8). Nevertheless, for policy purposes one can see that the problem lies in the higher costs per beneficiary, not in more beneficiaries served. Any solution would have to recognize this issue.

Medicare's SMI revenues and expenditures

SMI funds come from two main sources: premiums paid directly by the enrollees (or by Medicaid for those qualifying) and general revenue funds. Originally, the premium rate was set so that premium revenues of the SMI trust fund were one-half of all revenues. From 1973 the growth of premiums was limited to be no greater than the growth of Social Security cash benefits. As a result, since then the premium share of total fund revenues has fallen to about 30 percent.

Table 11–1 Summary Expense Statistics for Medicare and Medicaid Programs for Selected Years (billions of dollars)

	Medicare			Medicaid	
Year	Hospital Expenses	Physician Expenses	Total Medicare Expenses	Nursing Home Expenses	Total Medicaid Expenses
1970[1]	4.9	1.7	7.0	5.0	1.3
1975[1]	11.6	3.3	15.5	13.2	4.8
1980[2]	2.6	7.8	36.8	26.8	10.2
1981[2]	31.3	9.7	44.8	30.5	11.6
1982[3]	36.8	11.4	51.1	31.3	12.3
1983[3]	40.5	13.4	57.4	34	13
1984[3]	44.4	14.6	63.1	36.7	13.9

Sources: [1]*Health Care Financing Review* 2(1), pp. 1–36, U.S. Department of Health and Human Services, 1980; [2]*Health Care Financing Review* 5(1), pp. 1–31, U.S. Department of Health and Human Services, 1983; [3]*Health Care Financing Review* 7(1), pp. 1–35, U.S. Department of Health and Human Services, 1985.

The growth of reimbursements from the fund has grown by about 17.5 percent annually during the 1970s (U.S. Department of Health and Human Services, Medicare and Medicaid Data Book, 1983, Table 12–1). Since the number of enrollees grew by only 3.2 percent during this period, most of this growth has been in terms of expenditures per enrollee. As in the case of the HI trust fund, this growth in expenditures has been a major cause of concern. In this case, however, increases in tax revenues could be automatically transferred to the SMI trust to meet shortfalls of premium revenues over expenses. Nevertheless, these transfers are a drain on public funds and have been a source of concern.

Medicaid expenditures

Medicaid expenditures have not grown nearly as fast as Medicare expenditures, as can be seen in Table 11–1. A major problem lies in the distribution of expenditures between groups. In 1970, nursing home expenditures were 26 percent of all Medicaid expenditures; in 1984 these expenditures were about 36 percent of the total. This changed composition suggests a displacement of other expenditures by nursing home (long-term care) expenditures.

Beneficiaries over 65 receive the bulk of long-term care, and so the preceding statistics suggest that there has been some type of redistribution of benefits in favor of the over-65 group. Indeed HCFA statistics (U.S. Department of Health and Human Services, Medicare and Medicaid Data Book, 1983, Tables 2–4 and 2–9) show that from 1973 to 1980 the *number* of total Medicaid beneficiaries who were over 65 fell from 22 percent of all beneficiaries to 15 percent. During the same period, the share in dollar benefits of the over-65 group fell from 38 percent of all benefits to 36 percent. These statistics, in conjunction with those in the previous paragraph, suggest that one particular group of old people, those requiring long-term care, has been consuming a substantially larger share of resources. A considerable portion of the growth in total expenditures for SNF and ICF nursing home care has been in reimbursement per beneficiary: with a growth rate for ICF reimbursements of 17.7 percent from 1975 to 1980, the number of beneficiaries increased by 3.9 percent, leaving the difference (almost 14 percent annually) as an approximation of the growth in reimbursement per beneficiary (i.e., of the growth of prices and service intensity).

Uncompensated care

The major problem with uncompensated care is who will ultimately pay for the care. A number of options exist, and they can be broken down into private-sector and public-sector solutions (although some compromise is possible). With a private-sector solution, the burden is shared by fellow patients or by insured individuals part of whose hospital bill or premium would go toward uncompensated care. Public-sector solutions involve taxes, and these can be at any level of government and on almost any conceivable type of tax base (e.g., on health insurance premiums, income, or tobacco and alcohol purchases). The solution must have some broad appeal to equity.

11.4 POLICY ALTERNATIVES

11.4.1 Economic Analysis and Alternative Solutions

A number of policies have been proposed to deal with the problems identified. In this section we will discuss some of these policies in a manner that illustrates the use of economic analysis in health policy evaluation. The evaluations for each market will be conducted in the light of the goals identified in Chapter 10: barriers to demand, technical efficiency, adequacy of supply, quality, and public expenditure control. In addition, we will note any side effects on related markets that might influence our overall assessment of the policy and any equity considerations.

In our evaluation of policies, trade-offs frequently occur. That is, a policy may enhance one goal, say barriers to demand, but at the expense of another goal, say public expenditure control. Indeed, if such were not the case, we would hardly be faced with economic choices. Given these trade-offs, we must make an assessment as to whether the negative consequences are worth the positive benefits. Being able to categorize the consequences of policies is a very useful beginning in the evaluative process. However, economic analysis cannot make clear-cut predictions about all the consequences of every policy. In many cases there are gray areas, such as in some cases our inability to predict how quality will be affected. In these instances we will simply mark our effect with a question mark, ?.

In Table 11-2 we present the expected impact of a number of policies on each goal. Impacts are listed as +, indicating a positive effect *on the goal*; as −, indicating that the policy detracts from the policy goal; and as n.a., indicating that the policy has no expected effect. If our theory is not general enough to make specific predictions about the effect of a policy on a goal, we insert a ?.

There are several bases on which we can make these predictions. First, we can use economic theories, such as those presented in Part II of this book. Indeed, this is the basis on which we will proceed. Alternatively, we could take a more empirical approach; that is, we could study the policies using statistical analysis to determine the effect that these policies have actually had (Stoddart and Labelle, 1985).

In Table 11-2 we also identify the appropriate theory by referring to the section in Part II where it is presented. That is, if a policy is expected to influence supply, we will use supply analysis to determine its effect and will therefore refer to the relevant section in Chapter 6.

Table 11–2 Effects of Policies Related to Public Insurance

Policy (and Related Section in Text)	Barriers to Demand	Technical Efficiency	Adequacy of Supply	Quality	Public Expenditure Control	Side Effects and Equity Considerations
Medicare						
Prospective payment system (PPS): DRGs (6.7.2)	n.a.	+	?	−	?	Early discharges may lead to greater nursing home demand
Medigap premium taxes (4.3)	−	n.a.	n.a.	n.a.	+	
Lower physician fees (8.2.4)	−	n.a.	−	?	+	
Raise SMI premiums (4.3)	−	n.a.	n.a.	n.a.	+	More poor uninsured; pressure on indigent, Medicaid programs
Raise HI/SMI copayment/ deductible (3.6, 4.2)	−	n.a.	n.a.	n.a.	+	Possible increases in Medigap coverage; should be accompanied with catastrophic coverage; possible longer-term adverse effects
Medicaid						
Reduction in benefits: program limits	−	n.a.	n.a.	n.a.	+	Shifts burden to indigent care
Copayments for ambulatory care (3.6, 4.2)	−	n.a.	n.a.	n.a.	+	
Competitive bidding (8.2.1)	n.a.	+	+	−	+	
Prospective reimbursement for nursing homes (6.7.2)	n.a.	+	?	−	?	Depends on per diem level
Indigent Care						
Higher hospital charges: cost shifting (8.2.4)	+/−	n.a.	n.a.	n.a.	+	Redistributive effects; burden on payors of medical care

11.4.2 POLICIES FOR MEDICARE

Prospective Payment (DRGs)

The first Medicare policy we will examine is the implementation of prospective payment of hospitals on a DRG basis. Such a system was implemented to contain costs. If we base our predictions on either the profit-maximization or output-maximization models of Sections 6.2 and 6.4, the predicted effect (see Section 6.7.2) is to increase technical efficiency, that is, encourage hospitals to lower costs, since the extra profits resulting from these cost savings will accrue to the hospital. Hospitals also have incentives to lower quality since these reductions will also yield cost savings. Unless we have some idea about the actual DRG rate levels, we cannot say anything about the supply response and the overall effect on public expenditures: the higher the rates, the greater will be the supply response of providers, and the greater the impact on public expenditures.

The PPS system may also have side effects, which will be felt on the other parts of the health care system. Per case reimbursement provides hospitals with the incentives to shorten length of stay. In some cases, early discharge may result in sending patients to nursing homes (in these cases hospital days and nursing home days are substitutes), thus increasing nursing home demand. In addition, lower rates to hospitals may result in higher charges to other patients (see Section 8.2.4) as a result of cost shifting.

In sum, with the output- and profit-maximizing models, some effects are quite predictable, but we cannot predict the effect of PPS on all the goals. If we change the supplier's behavioral goals to incorporate quality elements (Section 8.5), we no longer have a clear-cut prediction about how quality of care will be affected by PPS: the agency will seek to preserve quality, but we cannot predict how far it will go.

Medigap premiums tax

The purpose of a tax on Medigap premiums is to make insurance coverage for the Medicare copayments and deductibles more expensive, thus discouraging the practice by Medicare enrollees of obtaining first dollar coverage on medical expenses. Such a tax would raise the direct price to consumers of Medigap coverage and would reduce the demand for this coverage (see Section 4.3).

One policy effect is to increase barriers to demand. This is listed as having a negative effect in Table 11–2, although some might argue otherwise: first dollar coverage may encourage the overuse of services and thus contribute to higher system costs. The predicted effect on public deficits is to reduce them (1) by the amount of the tax and (2) by the additional amount of lower government reimbursements because of the reduction in the demand for medical care (Section 3.6).

Lower physician fees

A lowering of Medicare's reasonable charge for physicians who accept assignment will result in fewer assignments and a reduced supply of care to Medicare patients (see Section 8.2.4). At the same time, because of the reduction in assignments, those patients whose physicians would have accepted assignment before face higher direct prices. The effect on public expenditures is favorable. However, the analysis does not predict what will happen to the patients whose access is reduced by the reduced availability of care. They may seek assignment care (possibly of a lower quality) elsewhere or else go without care.

Increase in the SMI premium

An increase in the SMI premium would cause a reduction in those who would be willing to purchase SMI coverage. This would raise barriers to demand (the uninsured would have to pay full price for medical care) and reduce public expenditures. Unlike the case of Medigap premiums, however, the reduction in medical care demand resulting from reduced coverage will more likely include many necessary cases, because in this case the options are no coverage versus coverage limited by copayments and deductibles.

Raising the SMI copayments and deductibles

The effect of this policy would be very similar to that of raising the SMI premium. In this case, demand could be directly choked off. Because the population affected is elderly, there are more likely to be adverse ill-health effects resulting from reduced demand.

11.4.3 Policies for Medicaid

Limitations on benefits

Limitations on benefits, such as maximum number of days of hospital care per beneficiary, would create a barrier to demand and reduce the public program's expenditures. However, some needs simply will not go away, and some other outlet will be necessary for these patients. For these cases, the policy simply shifts the costs from one source of funds to another.

Copayments for ambulatory care

Choking off the demand of the poor, who are more likely to be needy cases, is more likely to have adverse health effects in subsequent periods (see Section 4.2). In addition, it is likely that such a policy merely shifts costs between programs or levels of government.

Competitive bidding of suppliers

Such a policy, which has been implemented by the California and Arizona Medicaid programs, has the objective of providing cost-effective care for indigents. If the buyer has a considerable degree of market power, it can extract a lower price from competitive sellers (see Section 8.2.1), and if there was any room for cost reductions, either through increasing efficiency or lower quality, these will be incorporated into the providers' responses. However, the bidding process is a complex one and may not automatically lead to savings (see Section 9.5).

Prospective payment for nursing homes

The effect of prospective payment for nursing homes is similar to that of PPS on hospitals (Section 6.7.2) with the exception that, because the lengths of stay in nursing homes are so variable, the rates must be on a per diem (daily) basis. If the nursing home is an output maximizer, we can expect lower costs because of greater efficiency and lower quality. The actual supply will depend on the level of rates that are set. With a per diem basis of payment, we can also expect longer stays per patient (Section 6.7).

11.4.4 Indigent-Care Policies

With indigent-care policies, we reach the bottom of the pile of public policies. If this group is to be treated at all, the choices amount to either raising some tax at some level of government or else allowing the costs to be shifted on to some unsuspecting group.

Hospital cost shifting

If hospitals are to provide free care to charity patients, their costs for these patients must be covered from profits obtained in serving paying patients. To be able to shift costs in this way (Section 8.2), a provider must have some degree of market power. The $+/-$ in Table 11-2 refers to the reduced barriers of the charity care patients coupled with the higher prices paid by the paying patients. As the market increases in competitiveness, an individual hospital has less ability to increase profits by raising prices, and thus less ability to subsidize charity patients in this way.

Such a solution to finance indigent care involves distributional considerations. It shifts the responsibility for the charity patients onto the other patients. If the other patients have insurance coverage, the shifting is ultimately to the individuals who pay their insurance premiums. Even *this* burden is hidden, however, because of tax subsidies for employer-provided health insurance. Nevertheless, the avoidance of political action in the area of indigent care does not mean that no one bears the burden.

11.5 PRIVATE HEALTH INSURANCE

In the United States the issue of overinsurance because of tax subsidies to employment-provided insurance has surfaced (Feldstein and Friedman, 1977). Current tax law treats employer health insurance premiums as a nontaxable benefit. That is, if total employee compensation of $20,000 is composed of

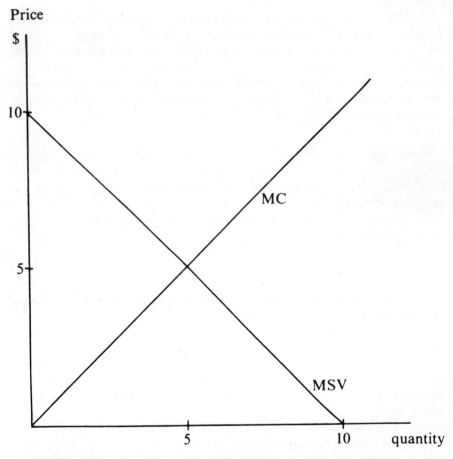

Figure 11–2 Representation of efficient allocation of resources. Efficient allocation occurs where marginal social value equals marginal social cost; in this diagram, this occurs at an output of 5.

$18,000 in wages and $2,000 in health insurance premiums, the employee will pay income tax on the $18,000. If the income tax rate is 20 percent, the employee would have had to earn $2,400 to buy this health insurance in the absence of the subsidy. With marginal income tax rates of 20 percent, for example, the subsidy can be considerable.

The effect of this subsidy has been to encourage the demand for more complete insurance coverage. Let us say that such insurance arrangements lead to full-service coverage (zero deductibles and copayments). Then, in terms of the efficiency model of Chapter 10 (see Figure 11–2), output will expand to a level of 10. At this level, *MC* is well above *MSV*, and so output is greater than the optimal amount.

As shown in Section 4.3, there are utility gains from shifting the risk of uncertain expenditures by insuring. These gains must figure into the overall net benefit picture, and they offset to some degree the losses from overinsurance. Nevertheless, the overall situation, even incorporating these benefits from insurance, may be one of an oversupply of health insurance.

REFERENCES

Medicare

Congressional Budget Office. (1983, March). *Changing the structure of Medicare benefits*. Washington, DC: Congressional Budget Office.

Davis, K., & Rowland, D. (1984). Medicare financing reform: A new Medicare premium. *Milbank Memorial Fund Quarterly, 62*, 300–316.

Ginsburg, P.B., & Moon, M. (1984). An introduction to the Medicare financing problem. *Milbank Memorial Fund Quarterly, 62*, 167–182.

Hsiao, W.C., & Kelly, N.L. (1984). Medicare benefits: A reassessment. *Milbank Memorial Fund Quarterly, 62*, 207–229.

Long, S.H., & Smeeding, T.M. (1984). Alternative Medicare financing sources. *Milbank Memorial Fund Quarterly, 62*, 325–348.

Luft, H.S. (1984). On the use of vouchers for Medicare. *Milbank Memorial Fund Quarterly, 62*, 237–250.

Rice, T., & McCall, N. (1985). The extent of ownership and the characteristics of Medicare supplemental policies. *Inquiry, 22*, 188–200.

Smits, H.L., Feder, J., & Scanlon, W. (1982). Medicare's nursing home benefit: Variations in interpretation. *New England Journal of Medicine, 307*, 855–862.

U.S. Department of Health and Human Services. (1983). *The Medicare and Medicaid data book*, (HCFA Publication No. 03156). Baltimore, MD: Health Care Financing Administration.

Wolkstein, I. (1984). Medicare's financial status: How did we get here? *Milbank Memorial Fund Quarterly, 62*, 183–206.

Medicaid

Brecher, C., & Knickman, J. (1985). A reconsideration of long-term-care policy. *Journal of Health Politics, Policy, and Law, 10*, 245–272.

Buchanan, R.J. (1983). Medicaid cost containment: Prospective reimbursement for long term care. *Inquiry, 20*, 334–342.

Congressional Budget Office. (1981, June). *Medicaid: Choices for 1982 and beyond*. Washington, DC: Congressional Budget Office.

Davis, K., & Schoen, C. (1978). *Health and the war on poverty*. Washington, DC: Brookings Institute.

Harrington, C., & Swan, J.H. (1984). Medicaid nursing home reimbursement policies, rates and expenditures. *Health Care Financing Review, 6*, 39–49.

Holahan, J. (1975) *Financing health care for the poor*. Lexington, MA: Lexington Books.

Meiners, M.R. (1983). The case for long-term care insurance. *Health Affairs, 2*, 55–79.

Stuart, B. (1972). Equity and Medicaid. *Journal of Human Resources, 7*, 152–178.

Wyckoff, P.G. (1985, August 15). *Medicaid: Federalism and the Reagan budget proposals*. Economic commentary of the Federal Reserve Bank of Cleveland.

Indigent Care, Catastrophic Coverage, Cost Shifting

Birnbaum, H., Naierman, N., Schwartz, M., et al. (1979). Focusing the catastrophic illness debate. *Quarterly Review of Economics and Business, 19*, 17–33.

Hadley, J., & Feder, J. (1985). Hospital cost shifting and care for the uninsured. *Health Affairs, 4*, 67–81.

Kasper, J.A., Walden, D.C., & Wilensky, G.R. (1979). *Who are the uninsured?* National health care expenditures study, data preview 1. Hyattsville, MD: National Center for Health Services Research.

Mulstein, S. (1984). The uninsured and financing of uncompensated care. *Inquiry, 21*, 214–229.

Stoddart, G.L., & Labelle, R.L. (1985). *Privatization in the Canadian health care system*. Ottawa: Health and Welfare Canada.

Taxes and Private Health Insurance

Brandon, W.P. (1982). Health-related tax subsidies. *New England Journal of Medicine, 307*, 947–950.

Congressional Budget Office. (1980, January). *Tax subsidies for medical care*. Washington, DC: Congressional Budget Office.

Feldstein, M., & Friedman, B. (1977). Tax subsidies, the rational demand for insurance and the health care crisis. *Journal of Public Economics, 7*, 155–178.

Ginsburg, P.B. (1981). Altering the tax treatment of employment-based health plans. *Milbank Memorial Fund Quarterly, 59*, 224–255.

Mitchell, B.M., & Vogel, R.J. (1975). Health and taxes: An assessment of the medical deduction. *Southern Economic Journal, 41*(4), 660–672.

Wilensky, G.R., & Taylor, A.K. (1982). Tax expenditures and health insurance. *Public Health Reports, 97*(5), 438–444.

Chapter 12

The Political Economy of Regulation

12.1 INTRODUCTION

The commodity medical care possesses several characteristics that have led many observers to ask whether a freely operating market for such a commodity will adequately serve consumer interests. First, there is the potential importance of the commodity on whose receipt good health and life may frequently depend (Section 4.2). This characteristic by itself could be the basis of an external demand for the commodity (Section 4.3) or could be the basis for one positing that individuals have a right to health care (Section 10.5). Second, there is the potential for ignorance on the part of the patient both as to his or her health status and the likely effectiveness of medical care in restoring health (or preventing illness) (Section 4.11). Coupled with the potential importance of the commodity, such a characteristic could place the consumer in a submissive position in relation to the practitioner and lead to excessive supplier-induced demand (Section 9.2). Third, the consumer frequently does not know when illness will strike, a characteristic leading to the demand for insurance (Sections 4.4 and 4.5) and reduced incentives for consumers to conserve in the consumption of medical care.

In the light of these arguments, it has been questioned whether a truly free market is likely to operate in the interests of the consumers. One outcome attributed to a totally free medical care market is the possibility of harmful services being administered by unqualified practitioners (Avellone and Moore, 1978). A method of redressing such market inadequacies is to legitimize the role of the qualified physician as the consumer's agent. Indeed, in this century institutions have grown up that have offered recognition to physicians as the legitimate agents of their patients. As a result, physicians have been allowed a considerable degree of self-regulation in the form of licensing and immunity from procompetition laws.

In the 1970s a growing concern developed that physician (as well as other) self-regulation had a considerable degree of physician self-interest built into it and did not automatically lead to economic efficiency. In addition, there was growing concern that the insurance mechanism was resulting in excessive hospital inflation (Section 9.4). An obvious answer to these problems was to appeal to the political mechanism, since it is through this mechanism that the rules of the marketplace are set. One general approach to rule setting is to impose politically mandated regulations on the providers of the market. These regulations are introduced to restrict the opportunities of the producers and ensure that they behave more in the interests of the public. Such a general approach assumes that the regulations and regulators will automatically act in the interest of the public; it is thus termed the *public-interest* approach to regulation. This approach is discussed in Section 12.2.

The public-interest approach to regulation does have a touch of faith attached to it. It assumes that the right forces will bring pressure to bear on the political system to change the rules of the game and that the changes will somehow improve matters. If matters do not then improve, the public-interest approach calls for still more regulation. This entire approach has been called into question primarily because there has been a good deal of criticism of the market as it has operated *under* regulation. It has been contended that the facts show that regulations have not unequivocally aided in the achievement of social goals. Indeed, it has been suggested that regulation usually will work in favor of special-interest groups; these groups are often the regulated rather than the consumers.

To explain this bias in regulation, another explanation of the role of the political process in influencing the market has been developed. This explanation regards the political process as a series of exchanges between consumers, producers, politicians, bureaucrats, and regulators. Out of this complex web of exchanges, policies are formulated and implemented that change the rules under which the market (especially providers) operate, but these rules do not necessarily favor consumers. Providers in a particular market may have enough to offer politicians so that they receive favorable regulations in exchange. Section 12.4 examines this approach.

12.2 MARKET REGULATION

12.2.1 The Market and Professional Dominance

Because of the potential importance of medical care and of potential ignorance regarding health and the impact of health care on health, it has been contended that a truly free market may operate in the interests of (often unethical or incompetent) providers. In addition, because of possible large losses due to uncertain illness, patients will insure and the lower postinsurance (direct) price will create a disincentive for the consumer to economize on medical care. Even *if* providers were fully qualified, insurance would create the incentive toward more use.

Let us examine these contentions in light of the flows in the hospital care market. In Figure 12–1, inside the circle we present the flows of money and services in the hospital market. To simplify matters, the government as a financing body is left out of the picture. In such a market, patients receive hospital services

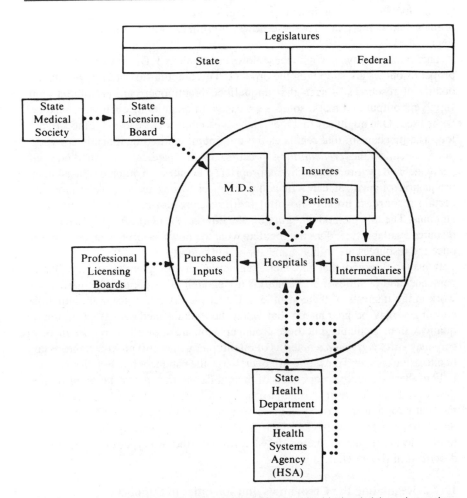

Figure 12–1 Jurisdictions of credentialing bodies. Suppliers (inside the circle) receive credentials certifying or licensing them to provide services from credentialing bodies (shown outside circle). The solid line represents money flow, and the dotted line represents service flow (inside) and regulatory control (outside).

prescribed by their doctors. These services are reimbursed for either by their insurance companies or jointly between the patients and the third parties when there are copayments. The contentions regarding the operations of a free market are as follows. First, the providers, both doctors and hospitals, may not be well qualified and may provide an inferior flow of services to the patient. In the extreme, these services may even be harmful to the patients. Second, the flows of services from even well-qualified doctors and facilities may be excessive, in the sense that they contribute little to the maintenance of health. The public-interest approach to regulation stipulates that, on appeal to the legislatures, regulations and laws can be brought into being that alter these flows, presumably to the interests of the patients.

There are two ways in which these flows can be altered. One is to ensure that the proper resources are supplying the product. This amounts to determining that the quality of resources is such that unqualified practitioners are prohibited from supplying output and that resources excessive in quantity or quality are also not being used. One might say that the ''right'' resources will be used for the ''right'' job. The mechanism that regulates the minimum required qualifications of suppliers is called the *credentialing* process. In the medical care market, both personnel and facilities must have appropriate credentials in order to be used in the production of medical care. In addition, mechanisms exist to determine that certain resources, notably hospital facilities, are not produced in excessive amounts. The first method of regulating the flows in the market merely determines resource availability; it does not regulate what the flows of services and money are once the resources are in place and supplying output.

It may be argued that the mere regulation of the quantity and quality of personnel and facilities (i.e., capital) is not enough to ensure that the market will work in the interests of the consumers. Under facility and personnel regulation, consumers may be guaranteed that when they obtain medical care a minimum quality will be available; but those producers who are allowed to produce medical care may still *overproduce* in terms of quality; they may still provide unnecessary or excessive care; and they may still overcharge the patient or the third party. In the light of these excesses, proponents of the public-interest interpretation of regulation would call for further regulations, controlling the quality and quantity of medical care and the prices of these services. This type of regulation is more direct, bearing on the behavior of the providers. In the process of such regulation, market flows are further altered. In what follows, the two types of regulation are described in more detail.

12.2.2 Regulating the Credentials and Facilities of Suppliers

Our description of the regulation of the necessary credentials and number of facilities of suppliers will be made with regard to Figure 12–1. Outside the circle we draw the regulating or credentialing bodies of the various suppliers; dotted arrows are drawn from these regulating bodies to the regulated market participants. The regulating body has received its authority from a legislature, either federal or state. In our description we focus on a few examples of the many forms of regulation.

We begin with a description of the method of credentialing the primary practitioners of medical care, the physicians. The prime method of determining the credentials of those who practice medicine is through state licensure, a process by which those who meet specific criteria are granted licenses to practice medicine. The criteria are determined by state licensing boards and include graduation from an accepted (by the physician's association) medical school and completion of one year of internship in an acceptable institution, usually a hospital. The composition of state licensing boards is of particular interest. These boards are given the power to legally determine who can and cannot practice medicine and what the practice of medicine constitutes. The members of the boards are frequently recommended to the state legislatures by the state medical associations. Since these state medical associations are bodies made up of member practicing physicians in the state, the licensing boards in effect are organizations that represent the suppliers of medical care in the state. To put the matter another way, the credentialing of physicians amounts to *self-regulation* on the part of the suppliers.

Other types of health personnel are also licensed by state bodies. For example, registered nurses, physician assistants, physical and occupational therapists, and optometrists all require licensure through a professional board to practice their trade. As in the practice of medicine, the licensing boards determine what credentials are required for the practice of the various professions and exactly what constitutes a professional practice: that is, what tasks the various professionals can and cannot perform. These determinations are made in the context of state licensure laws for the practice of medicine and cannot supersede them. For example, nurses cannot prescribe treatments of prescription drugs; optometrists can neither use certain drugs nor perform eye surgery. The main difference between the boards of other-than-physician health professionals and those of physicians is that nonphysician boards are usually not autonomous, and the laws and regulations they administer are legislated in the context of medical licensure laws. Physicians will have representation on these nonphysician state boards or will serve as advisors and thus will be in a position to influence what acts can and cannot be performed by these various groups.

Nonpersonnel resources are also subject to credentialing processes. Hospitals must be licensed by state licensing agencies, usually the state health department. These licenses require that a minimum level of facilities and personnel be present.

A second type of regulation for hospitals is more concerned with excess quantities of facilities, rather than with the attaining of minimum quality levels. This type of regulation attempts to limit investment (capital expansion) to those types of facilities that are "necessary," avoiding duplication or simply unneeded resources. Perhaps the best known of these regulating agencies is the Health Systems Agency (HSA), which was legitimized by the U.S. National Health Planning and Resources Development Act (Public Law 93-641) of 1974. According to this law, investment in institutional facilities exceeding a certain sum (usually $100,000) must be approved by the HSA for the area in which the HSA operates; these approvals are called *certificates of need* (CON). If the institution does not obtain a CON before expanding, it can have its license to operate withheld or a fine imposed.

The membership composition of the HSA's managing board is stipulated by the enacting legislation to include a specified number of consumers and a specified number of providers in the area. These individuals act as voting members of a voluntary board. The HSA also hires a full-time staff to study regional requirements and prepare files. The granting (or not) of a certificate of need lies with the board rather than with the staff of the HSA. The HSA board's vote is not final; in some cases it may be overturned by a state planning agency, which is often located in the state health department. It should be pointed out that at the time of writing, local planning agencies faced the prospect of losing federal funding. This would jeopardize the operation of many HSAs.

The role of the HSA can be contrasted with that of credentialing and licensing activities. The HSA is concerned with "too much" of either quantity or quality. Its initial concern was with restricting investment that would lead to increased institution costs. The state licensing activities are concerned with the setting of a floor below which quality will not fall. Both types of activities are carried out under the auspices of legislatures, either federal or state. A doctor cannot practice medicine without a license from the state licensing board and a nurse cannot practice medicine at all. In either case, if individuals violate laws, they are subject to legal sanctions. Similarly, an institution that expands without a certificate of need may be subject to legal sanctions. In addition to these legally authorized processes, certain professionally authorized processes influence the credentials of those who operate in the market.

One type of professional qualification involves the certification by a professional board of a physician in a specific specialty. For example, physicians who complete a specified time in a hospital-based residency program and subsequently pass the exams of a board that is linked to a specialty association (e.g., the examining board of the American Association of Internal Medicine) can become *board-certified* specialists. This form of certification does not grant them any *legal* privileges over and above those granted to them by the state licensing board. However, such certification is frequently a requirement, set down by members of a hospital staff, for a part- or full-time position in a hospital. The effect of extralegal certification is similar to that of licensing. It has the effect of setting the standards of those who practice in certain settings, mostly in hospitals.

12.2.3 Regulation of Suppliers' Behavior

In addition to determining the quantities and qualities of personnel and facilities of suppliers, regulations exist to influence the behavior of these suppliers. The reasons given for these types of regulations are that the mere regulation of credentials and quantities of resources is not enough; suppliers may still behave in manners detrimental to the public interest. As with the preceding types of regulations, behavior can be regulated at the legal and nonlegal levels. We will look at examples of each. The relation of these regulating bodies to actual participants in the marketplace is shown in Figure 12–2.

Peer review organizations (PROs) are set up under the legitimation of the Social Security amendments; they review providers' activities to determine whether they

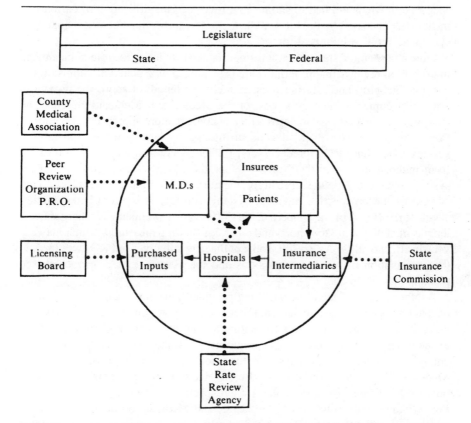

Figure 12–2 Jurisdictions of behavior-regulating bodies. Suppliers (inside the circle) have their supply behavior controlled legally and professionally by regulatory and professional bodies (outside the circle).

are reasonable, necessary, and appropriate and assess the quality of these activities. These agencies are selected by the U.S. Department of Health and Human Services on a competitive basis. Preference is given to organizations that are associated with area physicians (e.g., state medical associations), as this assures some degree of local provider representation. The prime responsibility of PROs is to conduct reviews of potential or ongoing utilization of Medicare and Medicaid reimbursed hospitalizations. All hospitals receiving Medicare and Medicaid reimbursement must contract with the area PRO to conduct reviews of patient utilization. PRO staff consist primarily of nurses and part-time area physicians. Any admissions that do not meet review criteria are subject to claims denial.

PROs are continuations of professional standards review organizations (PSROs), which were set up under Public Law 92-603. Under these amendments, all health care institutions that received reimbursement from federal funds under Medicare or Medicaid had to submit to a review of the utilization of care in the institution conducted by the PRO of the area. Any utilization deemed inappropriate would not be reimbursed for.

From an economic standpoint, it is important to categorize the role of incentives in utilization review. Inappropriate care is penalized by a denial of claims; in the event of inappropriate care (such as an excessive length of stay), the providing hospital becomes liable for the cost of the Medicare or Medicaid patient. The review and the penalties associated with it encourage more appropriate utilization. Peer review cannot be regarded as occurring in a vacuum, however. Indeed, the very excesses that PROs' predecessors, PSROs, were designed to curb resulted from inducements *to overutilization* under the old cost-based reimbursement system (Section 6.7). Not surprisingly, the more recent orientation of PROs in the context of the prospective payment system with DRGs is toward maintaining adequate *quality*. A prime concern under DRGs is with premature discharges (i.e., lengths of stay that are too short) and other cost-cutting measures, which may adversely affect quality. As a result, some of the new initiatives of PROs will include the examination of quick readmissions and the assurance of proper discharge planning.

Another means of legally controlling provider behavior comes in the form of hospital prospective reimbursement (Section 6.7.3). A number of states have set up agencies that are responsible for setting or controlling hospital charges. There are considerable variations in these programs. First, the programs can control the charges or set rates for all payors or for a selected group of payors. Under the Medicare PPS system, rates are set by the Health Care Financing Commission only for Medicare cases; and under the prospective payment system in Western Pennsylvania, only Blue Cross, Medicare, and Medicaid reimbursements were covered (Worthington and Piro, 1982). Only a few prospective reimbursement systems cover all payors: these include the Maryland system, the New Jersey system, and the Rochester and Finger Lakes systems in upstate New York.

Second, the base of payment has varied widely: New York has chosen a daily rate and New Jersey and Medicare a per case (DRG) rate, and the upstate New York programs have placed the hospitals on a total budget system. Third, actual rates can vary from being extremely stringent (as in the case of the New York per diem rates) to reasonable or generous. In addition, the rates can exclude certain items from payment. At the inception of the PPS system, Medicare's DRG rate excluded costs for depreciation and interest; such reimbursement was passed through to the hospitals on the basis of actual costs incurred, although there has been consider- able discussion of building the capital component of costs into the prospective rates (Anderson and Ginsburg, 1983).

In addition to legal forms of behavior control, there are also informal forms of control. Perhaps the most significant of these have been attempts by the medical profession to curb "unprofessional" behavior on the part of its members. Two examples are advertising to gain business from a colleague and practicing medi- cine in a prepayment setting. These so-called unprofessional activities have been policed at the local level by the county medical society. Membership in county societies was frequently required for a physician to have a full- or part-time position in a hospital (Kessell, 1958). Not having a hospital position could be financially damaging to a physician who practiced in any of a large number of specialties. Recently, the legality of such sanctions has been called into question as being violations of antitrust law. However, while formal anticompetitive practices can be dealt with by law, informal ones are more difficult to curb.

Since it is the existing staff who determine who is to have hospital privileges, physicians who behave "unprofessionally" can be excluded from having hospital positions by very informal means, not requiring any legal sanctions. In addition, they can be denied referrals by their colleagues. Since referrals constitute a large portion of business for specialists, their denial can be very damaging. As a result, physicians have generally refrained from such competitive behavior and may continue to do so despite the absence of any formal mechanisms to deter them.

12.2.4 Evaluating Regulation

Legally sanctioned regulations have been instituted to ensure that the market operates in the consumers' and taxpayers' interests. Recently, a number of evaluations have been conducted, and the results of these have formed the general impression that the regulations studied have not unequivocally been beneficial to consumers and taxpayers. In this section we will summarize the economic impact of four such sets of regulations: (1) prohibition of professional advertising, (2) capital expenditure review, (3) rate review or prospective reimbursement, and (4) utilization review. Our summary will be conducted in the light of the social goals outlined in Chapter 10: the reduction of demand barriers, technical effi- ciency of suppliers, adequacy of supply, quality of care provided, and public expenditure control. Rather than basing our reviews of these policies on theoretical grounds (as we did in Chapter 11), we will base them on the results of empirical studies. Note, however, that empirical studies might conflict with one another and so results are not always clear-cut. The results are summarized in Table 12–1.

Prior to having been curbed on antitrust grounds (see Section 12.3), many states had laws prohibiting competitive advertising in certain professions (medicine, optometry, and pharmacy); the bans included the advertising of prices for specific products or services. The rationale given for these laws was that such advertising frequently accompanied unprofessional practices, including the provision of low-quality services and products. Whether or not this is true, advertising also has another effect. It increases the flow of information to an individual about the supply opportunities available and permits him or her to choose a source of supply on the basis of price and other supply characteristics. Advertising also encourages suppliers to actively seek out consumers by offering prices and product characteristics that are favorable relative to those of other suppliers. In essence, it encourages a bidding down of prices. Restrictions on advertising, on the other hand, permit suppliers to behave more like monopolists, because they restrict the flow of information to consumers about alternative sources of supply.

An analysis was conducted of the effects of state laws on advertising for eyeglasses. The restrictions placed on advertising according to state laws varied considerably from state to state: they ranged from a total ban on advertising to permitting advertising. Most states fell in between, having a greater or lesser degree of restrictiveness. The analysis conducted a statistical study of the degree of state restrictiveness on the price of eyeglasses, controlling for other factors that might cause demand to increase and thus cause prices to be higher (Benham, 1972). The data on price and consumer characteristics (which might influence demand) were obtained from a nationwide survey on consumer expenditures on

---

Table 12–1 Effects of Alternative Regulations

Regulation	Barriers to Demand	Technical Efficiency	Adequacy of Supply	Quality	Public Expenditure Control
Capital expenditure review (Certificate of Need)	n.a.	−	+	+	?
Peer review	n.a.	n.a.	n.a.	+	?
Prospective reimbursement	n.a.	+	−	−	+
Prohibiting advertising	−	n.a.	n.a.	?	?

Note: + refers to conformity of program with policy goals (not to the direction of the effect).

health services. Since consumers were identified by state, the data permitted a comparison of the prices paid for eyeglasses according to that state. The results of the study showed a net positive relation between restrictiveness of advertising and price. States with complete advertising restrictions had an average price paid for eyeglasses of about $33, while in those with no restrictions the average price paid was about $26. The study did not adjust for all factors (both on the demand and supply side) that might influence differences in price; such data were not available. Nevertheless, the study provided a good first indication of one of the effects of advertising, notably that it is associated with lower prices and presumably lower provider profits.

Capital expenditure reviews were instituted to curb spending on excessive capital equipment so that the expensive procedures performed with the equipment would not proliferate. A study of the actual effects of certificate of need laws (Salkever and Bice, 1976) questioned whether these effects were achieved. Between 1968 and 1972, considerable numbers of states either did or did not require HSA approval of capital expenditure projects. This permitted a comparison of the effects on supplier behavior between the states that had capital expenditure review mechanisms and those that did not. The main purpose of certificate of need requirements was to restrict capital expansion to those projects that were "needed"; presumably all excessive expenditures would be stopped, and the net increase in new capital stock would decline. As a result, in terms of our cost curve analysis (Section 5.4), the upward shift in cost curves (i.e., for care with excessively high technology) would be slowed, and unit costs would not increase at as high a rate as when no capital review was performed.

The study examined two categories of investment: the increase in the number of beds and the dollar amount of investment per bed. The method of analysis was to separate those states that did have certificate of need requirements for new investment from those that did not; to control for other factors that might influence the volume of investment in these states, such as the volume of investment and the availability of funds; and then to determine the net influence of these laws on differences in investment among states. The results of the study showed that the existence of capital review procedures had a deterrent effect on the number of new beds created (bed capacity). Given that bed overcapacity has been a problem in recent years, the associated public goal with regard to supply is the elimination of unneeded beds, and so the plus sign in Table 12–1 refers to the conformity of the laws in achieving a more appropriate (smaller) supply. In addition, the existence of capital expenditure review was *positively* associated with the amount of new investment per bed. More investment per bed means more equipment of presumably a higher level of technology, and so quality (interpreted as being more technology-oriented care) was enhanced. Some of this additional capital investment may well be excessive; and so at the same time that quality is enhanced, technical efficiency may be adversely affected. The net effect on public expenditure control is in doubt:

fewer beds create a favorable outcome while more investment per bed will create a negative one. On average, the results of this analysis did not create a great deal of public confidence in capital expenditure review.

A large number of studies have been undertaken to analyze the impact of rate review and prospective reimbursement on many different aspects of hospital activities and on some nonhospital activities (e.g., nursing homes and physicians). As pointed out in Section 6.7.2, a hospital's response will differ greatly between an all-payor system and a system where some payors are under regulated rates while others are not. We will center our analysis on that of an all-payor system, where payment is on a per case basis. New Jersey's DRG system best fits this description.

Prior to 1980, New Jersey hospitals were reimbursed on the traditional multi-payor system, with Medicare reimbursing on a cost-based system, Medicaid and Blue Cross on a budget-based cost system with interim payments made on a per diem basis, and the commercial insurers reimbursing on the basis of charges. Beginning in 1980 the New Jersey Health Department began regulating all-payor rates for some hospitals on a DRG basis. During 1980 and 1981, some hospitals were being reimbursed on each basis, permitting a comparison to be made among hospitals under each payment system.

One study (Rosko and Broyles, 1986) conducted a comparison of the hospitals under each system with regard to cost per admission, cost per patient day, length of stay of admissions, and the number of admissions. Controlling variables related to demand and hospital characteristics. The study results indicated lower costs per admission and higher admissions for the group under DRGs. With regard to policy objectives (Table 12–1), it seems likely that under such a scheme (and based on the study results) technical efficiency improved. Some of the cost reduction may also result in lower quality, although few studies have addressed this directly. Supply increased, but this may not be a positive factor because some of the increased admissions may be unnecessary; certainly the incentives were in that direction. While technical efficiency and perhaps lower quality lead to lower costs, increased admissions lead to higher costs, and the net effect on total costs and public expenditures is uncertain. In sum, the overall effect of prospective reimbursement is therefore unclear.

There is no general agreement in the health services literature regarding the policy-related impact of prospective reimbursement. Perhaps some of this uncertainty results from the fact that programs vary considerably and it is difficult to generalize. In many ways, however, the New Jersey results are typical of what one can expect from an evaluation study. Given the difficulties in pinning down quality variables and the offsetting impacts of variables on total costs, it is not surprising that there has been much disagreement over how well prospective reimbursement works.

Analyses of PSRO activities have indicated that there have been some resulting reductions in inappropriate care (Schwartz, 1981). Quality is likely to have gone up. The effect of the program on hospital expenditures is uncertain, however; a Congressional Budget Office review (United States Congress, 1979) concluded that there were no net savings from the program. As a result, the overall picture, as shown in Table 12–1, does not indicate a very positive evaluation.

In sum, reviews of the major types of regulation discussed have raised substantial doubt as to whether or not the programs attained the social goals they were intended to achieve. An explanation for these observations might be that the regulation was done incompetently, and that if it were done competently, it might yield advantageous results.

While this is a plausible explanation, it does not explain why regulation so frequently and, indeed, almost systematically failed to serve the public interest. Incompetent regulators would at least be unsystematic in their efforts. Another explanation for the disappointing results is that regulation takes place in an environment in which it might be expected to operate systematically, at least at times, in the interests of the *suppliers*. This explanation regards regulation as an integral part of the marketplace rather than being the activity of independent, impassive regulators who are enforcing consumer-oriented "rules of the game." From this vantage point, regulations can be bought and sold just like medical care and pharmaceuticals. Thus, by changing the "rules of the game" the governance of the market can be changed, but this is not automatically done in the interests of the consumer. It is the buyer of favorable regulation in whose interests these rules will be altered. This approach to regulation might be regarded as the political economy view of regulation. This interpretation is explained next.

12.3 POLITICAL ECONOMY OF THE HEALTH CARE MARKETPLACE

In this section we examine the alternative explanation of regulatory activity: that this activity is the outcome of a complex series of exchanges between producers, consumers, politicians, and regulators. In a sense, this type of explanation regards the political process as a type of market process in which participants, if the terms of exchange are right, can "purchase" from politicians laws or regulations that have a favorable impact on the purchasers' incomes. The vantage point of this theory is one of examining *exchanges* between the various participants in the political marketplace and identifying the conditions under which specific exchanges favoring a particular group will arise.

12.3.1 Flows in the Political Marketplace

Figure 12–3 presents a simplified picture of the participants in a political marketplace. Incorporated in this diagram are the consumers and producers in a commodity market and the exchanges between them of money and services. This representation would be the equivalent of the inside of the circle shown in Figures 12–1 and 12–2. In this instance, there is no group outside the circle because the political system, rather than acting as a watchdog to guard the consumers' interests, is regarded as an integral part of the mechanism by which prices, quantities, and qualities are set. In Figure 12–3 the legislators are drawn inside the circle and the regulators (to some extent employees of the politicians) are also included inside the circle; the commodity marketplace has become politicized.

We can now look at the dimensions of self-interest of each of the four groups in our simplified system, that is, what they can gain from the system and what they can offer other participants of this expanded marketplace in return. The first group, the *politicians*, maintain their positions in office by obtaining a sufficient number

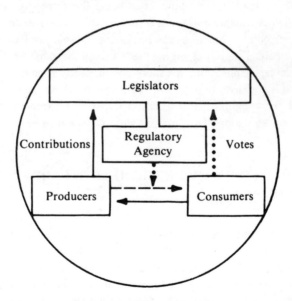

Figure 12–3 Picture of the expanded, politicized marketplace. Producers and consumers both may "purchase" credentialing and regulatory benefits from legislatures via the political process. The process, viewed as an integral part of the market mechanism, leads to an expanded picture of the medical care marketplace. The dotted line represents service flow, and the solid line represents money flow. The dotted line from the regulatory agency represents regulatory influence.

of votes. Their efforts at election and reelection are aided by campaign contributions from consumer and producer groups. In return for this support, politicians can supply sympathetic legislation and regulation favoring the interests of the supporting groups. Politicians can also supply publicly provided goods, such as fire protection services; public health services; subsidized services, such as medical care; and money payments, such as welfare payments and subsidies to producers.

 ̄ Consumers can obtain benefits through the political system from the consumption of publicly provided or subsidized commodities and services, from money transfers, and from low prices caused by strict (consumer oriented) regulation. Their participation in the political system includes bearing some of the costs of operating the public system; this takes the form of taxes. The main form of payments that consumers can offer politicians for beneficial packages of politically provided services and regulations is votes and campaign contributions.

Providers or suppliers of commodities gain from the system through subsidies (e.g., government scholarships and subsidized loans for medical students), contracts for work provided for the public sector (e.g., Medicare and Medicaid payments), and favorable regulations and laws that enable prices and profits to be maintained at high levels and that restrict competition. Providers are also, like consumers, subject to taxes that help to finance the activities of the political system. The main form of support that providers can offer to politicians in exchange for a favorable mix of political services and regulations is made in terms of campaign contributions. (Though they are voters, providers usually do not form large voting blocs.)

Regulators are appointed, full-time employees of regulatory commissions. Their appointments are usually for fixed terms, for example three to five years. The main benefits regulators can obtain are expanded budgets and wider mandates for their agencies and good future job prospects for themselves. The former types of benefits can be obtained from the political system. Since the budgets for regulatory commissions come from legislative appropriations, regulators can offer satisfactory performance to satisfy their employers, the legislators. Job prospects for regulators may come from the civil service or from the industry being regulated. It is not uncommon for regulators to work for regulated industries once their terms of office have been completed.

12.3.2 Political Exchanges

Given the potential benefits and costs each group can incur from participating in the system, we now seek to explain what exchanges will likely occur in the political marketplace. We assume that all participants will follow the *net benefit* or *profit* principle; that is, in participating in political exchanges they pursue their own self-interests and attempt to obtain the maximum net benefits possible from the system. Even though all participants would like to obtain favorable bundles of commodities and taxes and favorable regulations, conditions are such that some groups will be in a better position than others to obtain favorable bundles. Let us make the assumption that it is costly for an individual to participate actively in the political marketplace because of the resources (including time) needed to make his or her preferences known to the politicians, to organize blocs of voters to obtain some bargaining advantages, to make contributions, and so on. This costliness varies across groups such that for some it is more costly to bargain for political exchanges. These variations mean that some individuals or groups are more likely to bargain and strike exchanges with politicians than are others.

With this perspective, we can identify two pertinent factors that influence exchanges between beneficiaries and politicians. The first is the cost of organizing a group that will bargain with the politicians of one of the political parties. The second is the incidence of the costs resulting from the exchanges made. Regarding the first factor, the costs of organizing involve identifying those individuals with similar interests, organizing these individuals into a group, bargaining for benefits with politicians, paying campaign contributions, and sharing the benefits from the system. It has frequently been asserted that the costs of organizing are substantially lower for producers than for consumers because it is very easy for producers to recognize common areas of interest (in part, because there are fewer of them and it is less costly for them to reach an agreement). To the extent that this is true, producers will be more successful in obtaining favorable regulations and laws than will consumers, and the regulations enacted will be in the producers', rather than the consumers', interests.

The second factor deals with who bears the burden of providing these benefits and in what manner these costs are borne. If one group, say a producer group, obtains favorable regulations such that competition is reduced and prices are increased, the consumers of the industry's output will bear the cost of this regulation in that they must pay higher prices. If these higher prices are not clearly traceable to the regulations that cause them, that is, to the exchanges struck between politicians and producers, the politicians clearly have more leeway to offer the producers regulations that lead to higher prices and profits. This is certainly true in the case of licensing, where the influence of licensing on lower quantities supplied and ultimately, but indirectly, on higher prices and producer profits is not direct and clear to the consumers of the service. The profits obtained from licensing may be considerable because of the high prices caused by restrictions on supply. However, the consumers may not draw the link between high prices and licensing (and they may even applaud the protection from low quality that they obtain).

The role of the consumer in the political system provides a check on how far many types of political exchanges can go. Since many of these exchanges do affect the consumers, they will feel these effects in terms of higher prices or taxes. When the consumer pays higher taxes, he or she can more directly trace the effects to the political exchanges than when paying higher prices for regulated services. The recent interest in health care role of cost containment shown by the federal government with regard to the health care sector is associated with the major role that the federal government now plays in financing medical care. The large increases in health care costs that have occurred in recent years have a direct impact on federal taxpayers and are a source of concern to federal lawmakers. The ability of taxpayers to transfer their votes to more cost-conscious politicians (witness the Gramm-Rudman–Hollings bill) has certainly placed a brake on a number of federal programs.

12.3.3 Explaining Regulatory Patterns

The failures of regulation discussed in Section 12.2.4 are not mysterious when viewed in a self-interest rather than a public-interest light. For example, we noted the failure of capital expenditure review to reduce the quantity of investment per bed. At the same time, these reviews did curb new bed capacity. An explanation for these phenomena has been offered in terms of the *political-marketplace* concept. Capital expenditure review is conducted by local review agencies with voluntary boards; some of the members of these boards represent existing suppliers. If these agencies did become captives of supplier groups (i.e., hospitals), they might be expected to restrict new competition from potentially new suppliers; this restriction would show up in terms of the number of beds in a region. However, if such agencies were captives of the existing industry, they would not be expected to curtail the investment of existing suppliers. If desired investment by existing suppliers is largely in terms of higher-quality facilities rather than more bed capacity, investment per bed would not be restricted. This explanation would provide a rationalization of observed findings in terms of the political-economy theory.

The preceding analysis is merely an extension of the self-interest assumption extended to *all* participants of the marketplace. What the political-economy approach does is extend the concept of what the marketplace is. Still in the picture are providers and consumers, of course. But beyond that the picture includes all participants whose efforts affect indirectly the demand and supply positions of the commodity in question. This includes those lawmakers and regulators who are in positions to impose (at a price) better terms for demanders or suppliers. Which group will be favored will depend on a number of factors, including the political benefits from using the political system and the costs of doing so. What is clear is that the outcome in the wider market system, in terms of quantity, cost, distribution of outputs, and so on, cannot automatically be assumed to meet the social goals of the system.

REFERENCES

Regulation: General

Avellone, J.C., & Moore, F.D. (1978). The Federal Trade Commission enters a new era. *New England Journal of Medicine, 299*, 478–483.

Dittman, D., & Peters, J.A. (1977). A foundation for health care regulation. *Inquiry, 14*, 32–41.

Posner, R.A. (1971). Regulatory aspects of national health insurance plans. *University of Chicago Law Review, 39*, 1–29.

Schwartz, W.B. (1981). The regulation strategy for controlling hospital costs. *New England Journal of Medicine, 305*(21), 1249–1255.

Regulation: Prospective Reimbursement

Anderson, G., & Ginsburg, P.B. (1983). Prospective capital payments to hospitals. *Health Affairs, 2*, 52–63.

————, & Lave, J.R. (1984). State rate setting programs: Do they reward efficiency in hospitals? *Medical Care, 22*, 494–498.

Biles, B., Schramm, C.J., & Atkinson, J.G. (1980). Hospital cost inflation under state rate-setting programs. *New England Journal of Medicine, 303*, 664–668.

Coelen, C., & Sullivan, D. (1981). An analysis of the effects of prospective reimbursement programs on hospital expenditures. *Health Care Financing Review, 2*, 1–40.

Cromwell, J., & Kanak, J. (1982). The effects of prospective reimbursement programs on hospital adoption and service sharing. *Health Care Financing Review, 4*, 67–88.

Detsky, A.S., Stacey, S.R., & Bombardier, C. (1983). The effectiveness of a regulatory strategy in containing hospital costs. *New England Journal of Medicine, 309*, 151–159.

Farnand, L.J., Jacobs, P., & Dickson, W.M. (1986). An evaluation of a program to regulate rural hospital costs: The Finger Lakes Hospital experimental payment program. *Inquiry, 23*, 200–208.

Guterman, S., & Dobson, A. (1986). Impact of the Medicare prospective payment system for hospitals. *Health Care Financing Review, 7*(3), 97–114.

Hellinger, F.J. (1981). Recent evidence on case-based systems for setting hospital rates. *Inquiry, 22*, 78–91.

Rosko, M.D., & Broyles, R.W. (1986). The impact of the New Jersey all-payer DRG system. *Inquiry, 23*, 67–75.

Salkever, D.S., Steinwachs, D.M., & Rupp, A. (1986). Hospital cost and efficiency under per service and per case payment in Maryland. *Inquiry, 23*, 55–66.

Warner, K.E. (1978). Effects of hospital cost containment on the development and use of medical technology. *Milbank Memorial Fund Quarterly, 56*, 187–211.

Worthington, N., & Piro, P. (1982). The effects of hospital rate setting programs on volumes of hospital services. *Health Care Financing Review, 4*, 47–66.

Regulations: Other

Benham, L. (1972). The effect of advertising on the price of eyeglasses. *Journal of Law and Economics, 4*, 337–352.

Christianson, J.B. (1979). Long-term care standards: Enforcement and compliance. *Journal of Health Politics, Policy, and Law, 4*(3), 414.

Cohen, H.S. (1973). Professional licensure, organizational behavior, and the public interest. *Milbank Memorial Fund Quarterly 51*, 73–88.

Feldstein, P.J. (1977). *Health associations and the demand for legislation*. Cambridge, MA: Ballinger Publishing Co.

Joskow, P.L. (1981). *Controlling hospital costs*. Cambridge, MA: MIT Press.

Havighurst, C.C. (1978). Professional restraints on innovation in health care. *Duke Law Journal*, 1978, 304–385.

Hellinger, F.J. (1976). The effect of certificate of need legislation on hospital investment. *Inquiry, 13*, 187–193.

Kessell, R. (1958). Price discrimination in medicine. *Journal of Law and Economics, 1*, 20–35.

Lave, J.R., & Leinhardt, S. (1976). An evaluation of a hospital stay regulatory mechanism. *American Journal of Public Health 66*, 959–967.

Salkever, D., & Bice, T. (1976). The impact of certificate of need controls on hospital investment. *Milbank Memorial Fund Quarterly, 54*, 185–214.

Shepard, L. (1978). Licensing restrictions and the cost of dental care. *Journal of Law and Economics, 21*, 187–201.

United States Congress. (1979, June). *The effects of PSRO's on health care costs*. Washington, DC: Congressional Budget Office.

United States Department of Health and Human Services. (1980). *Professional standards review organization 1979 program evaluation*. Baltimore, MD: Health Care Financing Administration.

White, W.D. (1979). Why is regulation introduced in the health sector? A look at occupational licensure. *Journal of Health Politics, Policy, and Law, 4*, 536.

Chapter 13

Competition Policy

13.1 INTRODUCTION

In the late 1970s a growing dissatisfaction with regulatory solutions to resource-allocation problems in general carried over to the health care field. Several authors, spurred by the apparent success of (primarily inter-HMO) competition in a few local markets (Christianson and McClure, 1979), began to suggest that the medical care marketplace could indeed be successfully transformed into a competitive mold.

Based on the analysis in previous chapters, it is possible to develop a checklist of preconditions that must be met for a medical market to successfully fit a competitive mold (i.e., to yield an efficient outcome). Such a list is presented in Table 13–1, along with the section in the text where the precondition is discussed. First, demanders must know their health levels and any appropriate medical treatments (Section 4.11). Second, demanders must have an incentive to economize on insurance (Section 4.3). Third, demanders must have an incentive to economize on medical care (Section 3.6). Fourth, suppliers must have an incentive to minimize production costs (Section 6.2). Fifth, suppliers cannot collude to engage in anticompetitive practices, and there must be free entry of suppliers (Section 8.3.2). These preconditions, if met, will facilitate the attainment of a competitive solution, but not necessarily an equitable one. A competitive solution is fully consistent with insurance problems of self-selection, where potentially heavy users of medical care are priced out of the insurance market or where the poor cannot obtain any insurance coverage. For these reasons, equity must be considered in any discussion of preconditions to a *viable* market solution.

In the traditional, professionally dominated medical care marketplace in the United States, virtually all the above mentioned preconditions were violated. Consumer ignorance has precluded the market from meeting the first precondition, and advertising bans contributed to this barrier. Tax subsidies for employer-

Table 13–1 Preconditioning for a Viable Competitive Market

Preconditions	How Traditional Markets Violate Preconditions	Suggested Competitive Policies
Demanders know health levels, appropriate medical treatments, and their impact (4.11)	Consumer ignorance Advertising bans (8.3.2)	Antitrust policies
Demanders price conscious with regard to purchase of health insurance (4.3)	Tax subsidies for insurance (11.5)	Cap employer health insurance benefits
Demanders price conscious with regard to medical care (3.6)	Overinsurance (4.3)	Copayments/deductibles
Supplier incentives to minimize costs	Cost-based reimbursement for hospitals (6.7.2) Fee for service reimbursement for physicians (6.7.1)	Hospital DRGs; HMOs
Suppliers cannot collude to engage in anticompetitive practices (8.3.2)	Professional organization boycott of HMOs, insurer cost containment (8.3.2)	Antitrust
Free entry of suppliers (Ch. 8)	Professional licensure, capital expenditure review (8.3.2)	Antitrust
No cream skimming	Self-selection, uninsurable, high-cost cases (4.4)	Health plan regulations

provided health insurance detracted from price consciousness in the purchase decision of health insurance (Section 11.5). As a result, first dollar coverage prevailed in the medical care (especially hospital care) marketplace (Section 4.3), reducing the incentive for consumers of medical care to be price conscious. Hospitals were reimbursed on a retrospective cost-based system (Section 6.7.2), and physicians were reimbursed on a fee-for-service system (Section 6.7.1), neither of which provided inducements for technical efficiency. Professional organizations prevented entry into the market by HMOs and impeded third-party cost-containment activities (Section 8.3.2). Professional licensure and certificate of need laws restricted the free entry of suppliers (Section 8.3.2). In short, the traditional medical care marketplace was a conglomeration of practices that virtually assured inefficiency and inflationary growth (see Section 9.4), and even the most well-intentioned regulations would be hard pressed to forge an efficient outcome out of such a situation.

In response to this market structure and to the failures of regulation to ensure efficiency and curb inflation, proponents of competition have proposed reforms along two major lines: (1) the curbing of anticompetitive practices by resorting to the antitrust laws, which have traditionally not been applied to the professions, and

(2) the altering of tax laws and public medical care insurance programs to create a more competitive environment. In Section 13.2 we discuss antitrust laws and the role they have attempted to play in restricting noncompetitive practices. And in Section 13.3 we discuss proposals to alter tax laws with regard to health insurance benefits, creating inducements for consumers to economize on health insurance coverage.

13.2 ANTITRUST POLICY

Antitrust laws attempt to combat anticompetitive practices such as boycotts and price fixing. Their purpose is to set basic rules for the marketplace, thus attempting to ensure that competition is conducted on a fair basis. A major concern of these laws is to ensure that suppliers do not gain or use market power, jointly or individually, to extract an unfair price from consumers.

Until 1975 there was a presumption that antitrust laws did not apply to the professions, including medicine. The prevailing belief in the health care field was that professional ethics would regulate providers and ensure that they behaved in a manner so as to promote the consumers' interests. In 1975, however, a landmark court decision, *Goldfarb* v. *the Virginia Bar*, stated that the antitrust laws did apply to price fixing in the legal profession. Prior to 1975, there had been a longstanding concern with many practices of professional organizations in the health care field, and after the *Goldfarb* decision, attention rapidly turned to the examination of the applicability of antitrust laws in curbing these practices. Among the issues examined were boycotts by physicians of HMOs, organized physician opposition to insurers' cost-control techniques, bans on advertising, and price fixing.

The main federal antitrust laws that are potentially applicable to the health care field are the Sherman Act, the Federal Trade Commission Act, and the Clayton Act. The Sherman Act was passed in 1890 in response to monopoly practices by railroads. The relevant portions are Section 1, which bans collusion between parties (including boycotts) in restraint of trade, and Section 2, which bans attempts to monopolize trade. The Federal Trade Commission Act (1914) set up the Federal Trade Commission (FTC), which can investigate potential anticompetitive practices and issue injunctions to violators. Of particular relevance to the health care field is Section 5 of the FTC Act, which declares illegal unfair methods of competition affecting commerce or unfair competitive practices. Section 7 of the Clayton Act (1914) has also been used to arrest the growth of hospital mergers.

Antitrust laws can be enforced in criminal or civil suits. Criminal suits are enforced at the federal level by the Antitrust Division of the Department of Justice. Civil suits can be instituted by private parties (who may have been damaged) or by the FTC. For civil suits, remedies might include the issuance of cease and desist orders (by the FTC), divestiture of some lines of business by the violators, or the payment of triple damages (three times the value of the damages incurred by the injured parties) by the violators.

Among the initial actions by the FTC in the health field was the filing of a complaint against the American Medical Association (AMA) in 1975, referring specifically to the legality of several codes in the AMA's Principles of Medical Ethics (Avellone and Moore, 1978). The AMA codes cited were those prohibiting advertising by physicians and prohibiting physicians from bidding for contracts with lay organizations, from billing jointly with lay organizations, and from entering into partnerships with nonphysician health professionals (e.g., psychiatrists with psychologists). Such codes, it was contended, set up barriers to the implementation of more effective business practices. Since the initial complaint, a number of other practices have been questioned, including situations where dentists refused to provide insurers with patients' x-rays to permit utilization review, and where a hospital and local physicians excluded HMO-based physicians from hospital appointments. Successful suits such as these have resulted in a challenge to the dominant role that physicians traditionally have had in shaping the rules of the medical marketplace. The way has been opened for more innovative forms of medical care practice (such as HMOs and PPOs), which do not necessarily meet the general approval of the medical profession.

13.3 TAXATION AND INCENTIVE PLANS

While antitrust laws have created a general environment in which competition can work, a number of other characteristics of the medical care market have created barriers to the formation of a more competitive market. In response to these barriers, several proposals have been made to alter the income tax laws so that economizing behavior at the consumer level is rewarded (see especially Enthoven, 1980). While many different arrangements are possible, we will briefly outline one proposal that allows the medical care market to meet many of the preconditions for a competitive market (see Table 13–1).

The first step in setting up such a plan would be to introduce incentives and penalties into the system such that consumers would be rewarded for seeking out and choosing economical forms of medical care. Limiting tax credits on employee benefits would begin to move the system in such a direction. Several steps would have to be undertaken to implement such a proposal. First, a basic minimum bundle of services would have to be selected. Second, an average reasonable cost (called A) for this bundle would have to be determined. Thus one might determine that the annual average cost might be $200 for individuals aged 0 to 19, $400 for individuals aged 20 to 64, $800 for individuals aged 65 to 74, and $1,200 for individuals over 74. The basic cost for a family of two adults and two children would be $1,200 (2 × $200 + 2 × $400).

Based on the value of the bundle, a tax credit could be established for those families who purchased health insurance. The credit would be the same whatever the amount of insurance covered. The credit would not equal A because that would discourage individuals from seeking out less costly plans whose value was less than A. One suggested figure for the credit was 60 percent of A (Enthoven, 1978) because this would encourage price consciousness (by rewarding those who accept cheaper plans), but would not be so low that it would not be worthwhile to adopt *some* plan. For the family of four and a value of A of $1,200, if an employer provided health insurance worth $2,000 the family would receive a tax credit of 60 percent of $1,200, but the remaining $800 would be considered as additional taxable income. On the other hand, if a family chose a low-cost insurer who provided the basic benefits for $300, the tax credit would still be 60 percent of $1,200, or $720, and the family would benefit financially.

Certain regulations would have to be enforced to avoid abuse of such a scheme as well as encourage choice. Health plans would have to qualify as acceptable plans by offering at least the basic minimum level of services. Otherwise, some insurers might offer less than this in order to enroll only the healthy, who could then take undue advantage of the tax credit. Also, employers of a certain size would be required to offer employees a choice of (say three) different health plans. Furthermore, each plan would have to have open enrollment to ensure access. Finally, for each category of insurees, each plan would have to charge all individuals the same rate (*community rating*). Thus, if the premium for those aged 20 to 64 was $330, this rate would have to be the same for everyone purchasing insurance. This requirement would be necessary to curb some insurers from skimming the market of the low-cost cases, creating possible problems associated with adverse selection and resulting in the uninsurability of high-risk individuals.

The organizational form that a health plan might take is deliberately left unspecified in such a scheme to encourage diversity. A plan might be of the traditional variety (with choice of physician, and the like) or of an HMO variety. Specific plans may be operated on a for-profit or a nonprofit basis. Different plans might experiment with a variety of constraints, such as limitations on choice of physician and hospital or differing levels of copayments and deductibles.

If some plans decided to use deductibles and copayments, they would have to have a limit on insuree out-of-pocket payments (say $1,500 per family). This stipulation would be necessary to avoid problems associated with cream skimming (some plans might otherwise deliberately set a high deductible to capture the low-cost end of the market).

A scheme such as this would move a considerable way toward rationalizing the health care marketplace. Health plans would have an incentive to produce efficiently (or to contract economically with physicians and hospitals) in order to offer coverage at low prices. Consumers would have an incentive to seek out low-cost packages of coverage because they would pay the direct extra cost of any higher quality of coverage. This is not to say that high-cost and high-quality plans would not be chosen; after all, firms compete on both nonprice and price bases, and quality of care might be attractive to some. It simply says that, if high-quality care were chosen by some consumers, they would have to bear the burden of the excess costs of these plans.

Such a plan as outlined is largely employment related, but would be fully consistent with public programs as well. Public programs such as Medicare and Medicaid could offer enrollees vouchers equal to a specified amount. A voucher equal to the value of A should permit the enrollee to have access to the basic amount of care at no personal cost. The amount of the voucher would be decided by public-policy considerations.

13.4 COMPETITION AND SOCIAL GOALS

The growth of competition in the medical care marketplace should permit the policy goals of technical efficiency and adequacy of supply. Competitive bidding would go some way toward weeding out some inefficient providers. The effect on other goals, notably absence of demand barriers, quality, and public expenditures, is less clear.

The effect on demand barriers would depend on the specific provisions for encouraging the purchase of insurance. Under limitations placed on tax subsidies, insurance coverage will fall for some groups; but it is a matter of judgment as to whether this reduction would constitute a movement from overinsurance to a more adequate level of coverage or to an inadequate low level.

The effect on the public budget cannot be specified before the facts relating to Medicare and Medicaid coverage and the size of the cap on subsidies are known. A competitive marketplace is consistent with very generous government allowances and subsidies or very stringent ones (Caper, 1982).

Great concern has been expressed over the impact of such a scheme on quality of care. Competition, in the present sense, would encourage a growing role for health plans in cost-containment activities. These activities might be in the form of review of doctors' and hospitals' supply behavior or in the form of competitive bidding. The external review of physicians' supply behavior constitutes a growing area of regulation and could result in a loss of physician autonomy. This concern has been stressed particularly because the regulating groups may be nonphysicians, a circumstance that may herald a considerable loss of professional control (Saward and Sorensen, 1982). It is an open question as to how such imposed regulations will affect the quality of medical care.

In health care, wide variations can exist in patients' medical conditions and in the nature of the product. This leaves much opportunity for cream skimming (of healthier individuals) and cost cutting (perhaps at the expense of quality). How-

ever, regulations can be built in to ensure plans do not skim off the healthiest patients; but the interpretation of such regulations could become ambiguous, leading
to further regulations, and finally back to a more heavily regulated system.

One type of organization that would be most vulnerable in a competitive
environment is the teaching hospital. Teaching requires additional resources, and
a hospital that has both teaching and patient care functions will be more expensive
to operate than one with only patient care functions. Teaching hospitals would
therefore lose out in competitive bids. One solution might be to separate funding
sources for the teaching hospitals' teaching functions. In theory, it would be
possible to subsidize a teaching hospital for the additional costs that it would incur
because of the teaching function.

Despite these shortcomings, which are admittedly serious concerns, the competitive view of the medical marketplace has provided an alternative against which
the traditional system can be compared. Many shortcomings of the traditional
system—the incentives that were counterproductive in many ways and the regulations that may have acted as barriers to the achievement of policy goals—are more
clear now than before the competitive strategy was mapped out. Any changes in
the health care system henceforth will have to be forged with these new insights in
mind.

REFERENCES

Incentives and Competitive Health Plans

Caper, P. (1981). Competition and health care. *New England Journal of Medicine, 304*, 1296–1299.

———— (1982). Competition and health care. *New England Journal of Medicine, 306*, 928–929.

Enthoven, A.C. (1978). Consumer-choice health plan. *New England Journal of Medicine, 298*, 650–658 & 709–720.

———— (1980). *Health plan*. Reading, MA: Addison-Wesley Publishing Co.

———— (1981). The competition strategy. *New England Journal of Medicine, 304*, 1109–1112.

Fein, R. (1985). Choosing the arbiter: The market or the government. *New England Journal of Medicine, 313*, 113–115.

Ginzberg, E. (1980). Competition and cost containment. *New England Journal of Medicine, 303*, 1112–1115.

———— (1984). The monetarization of medical care. *New England Journal of Medicine, 310*, 1162–1165.

Luft, H.S. (1985). Competition and regulation. *Medical Care, 23*, 383–400.

Rossiter, L. (1984). Prospects for medical group practice under competition. *Medical Care, 22*, 84–92.

Saward, E., & Sorensen, A. (1982). Competition, profit, and the HMO. *New England Journal of Medicine, 306*, 929–931.

Stano, M. (1981). Individual health accounts: An alternative health care financing approach. *Health Care Financing Review, 2*, 117–120.

Vladeck, B. (1981). The market vs. regulation: The case for regulation. *Milbank Memorial Fund Quarterly, 59*, 209–223.

───── (1985). The dilemma between competition and community service. *Inquiry, 22*, 115–121.

Competition and Antitrust Regulations

Alpert, G., & McCarthy, T.R. (1984). Beyond Goldfarb: Applying traditional antitrust analysis to changing health markets. *Antitrust Bulletin, 29*, 165–204.

Avellone, J.C., & Moore, F.D. (1978). The Federal Trade Commission enters a new era. *New England Journal of Medicine, 299*, 478–483.

Blair, R.D., & Fesmire, J.M. (1986). Antitrust treatment of nonprofit and for-profit hospital mergers. In *Advances in Health Economics, 7*.

Castilo, L.B. (1983). Antitrust enforcement in health care. *New England Journal of Medicine, 313*, 901–904.

Dolan, A.K. (1980). Antitrust law and physician dominance of other health practitioners. *Journal of Health Politics, Policy, and Law, 4*, 675.

Havighurst, C.C. (1978). Professional restraints on innovation in health care financing. *Duke Law Journal, 1978*(2), 303–388.

───── (1980). Antitrust enforcement in the medical services industry. *Milbank Memorial Fund Quarterly, 58*, 89–124.

───── (1983). The doctors' trust: Self-regulation and the law. *Health Affairs, 2*, 64–76.

Pollard, M.R. (1981). The essential role of antitrust in a competitive market for health services. *Milbank Memorial Fund Quarterly, 59*, 256–268.

Chapter 14

Cost–Benefit Analysis

14.1 INTRODUCTION

In Chapters 11 and 12 we saw that market forces, left to themselves, do not necessarily lead to the right amount (an admittedly vague term) of medical care being utilized. Whether the amount actually produced is greater or less than the right amount depends on two things: (1) on how the market is operating, and (2) on our choice of criteria by which we measure the right amount. As shown in Chapter 12, the special characteristics of the commodity medical care, coupled with widespread third-party financing, make this market ripe for an overproduction of quality of care. On the other hand, as seen in Chapter 11, the care received by some individuals may be judged as too little. Whether, in fact, too much or too little care is produced will depend on the yardstick chosen to evaluate the market, as well as on the market outcome.

It was also shown in Chapter 12 that we can hardly presume that health policy will automatically correct matters. When viewed as the outcomes of transactions in an expanded marketplace, there is no presumption that health policy will ensure that the right amount of care is provided. In some cases, for example with licensure, the policy-influenced market will probably unduly restrict output.

In this chapter we examine one tool that measures the "right amount" in light of one specific set of values, the goal of economic efficiency. This tool, termed cost–benefit analysis, provides separate measures of the economic costs and benefits of various programs and projects and permits one to determine whether, at any level of output, further expansion or contraction of services will yield additional net benefits or losses. It should be stressed that, in making a recommendation based on cost–benefit analysis, one is accepting the efficiency goal. If some other goal, for example, an equitable distribution, overrides efficiency goals, the cost–benefit measure will not allow one to determine the "right amount."

As seen in Sections 4.11 and 9.2, the value that people place on medical services varies depending on their circumstances and also on the physicians' abilities to stimulate consumer wants. In the latter case, individual valuations of medical care may be subject to physician-induced shifts; the question, What value does one place on medical care?, may well be unanswerable in such circumstances. If this is the case, the value of benefits placed on medical care may not have a stable measure, and our cost–benefit ratio will itself shift whenever the value of medical care shifts. Because there is no unique measure of benefits, cost–benefit measures would be unreliable even if we accepted the efficiency goal.

There may be a way out of this quandary, however. Medical services are required for the restoration and maintenance of life and health. Doctors can influence a patient's valuation of medical services by convincing the patient that these services are required to maintain health. It is less likely that doctors can influence consumer attitudes toward life and health. If this is the case and if these more basic sources of benefit have some degree of stability in their own right, perhaps we can find the measure of constancy we are seeking in terms of the more basic entity, health. Perhaps we can measure the outcome of medical and health care activities in terms of the costs and benefits of obtaining health.

This chapter proceeds along these lines. We begin in Section 14.2 with a brief example of a cost–benefit analysis. In cost–benefit evaluations there are a number of rather knotty measurement problems that, while not always accommodated in a study, should certainly be acknowledged. These problems are discussed in Section 14.3. In Section 14.4 we discuss cost-effectiveness analysis.

14.2 A SIMPLE COST–BENEFIT ANALYSIS

Our simple example is presented in the context of a government program designed to immunize the individuals in a certain region. The background of this program is as follows. With a zero level of immunizations, there are 500 illnesses annually. Each illness is assumed to impose a cost of $30 on the patient as viewed by the patient. These costs can be measured in terms of direct costs (medical care) and indirect cost (pay lost from missed work); pain and suffering costs are assumed to be negligible. Immunizations have an illness-reducing effect as shown in Table 14–1. The first 1,000 people immunized reduces total illness by 100, bringing it to a level of 400. The next 1,000 people immunized reduces the level of illness by 75, bringing it to a level of 325. The next 1,000 immunizations further reduce the number of illnesses by 50, and so forth. Note that we are assuming a diminishing marginal effect from immunizations in terms of reducing illness. In Table 14–1 the total number of illnesses is shown in column 3; the additional reduction in illness associated with each extra 1,000 immunizations is shown in column 5; and the money value of this reduced illness, our "benefits," is shown in

Table 14–1 Data for Cost–Benefit Analysis of Community Immunizations

(1) Number of Immunizations	(2) Total Cost	(3) Total Number of Illnesses	(4) Marginal Additional Cost of Immunizations	(5) Net Reduction in Illnesses	(6) Money Value of (5)	(7) Benefit : Cost Ratio (6) (4)
0	$ 1,000	500				
1,000	3,000	400	$2,000	100	$3,000	3 : 2
2,000	5,000	375	2,000	75	2,250	2.25 : 2
3,000	7,000	275	2,000	50	1,500	1.5 : 2
4,000	9,000	250	2,000	25	750	0.75 : 2
5,000	11,000	235	2,000	15	450	0.45 : 2

column 6. Column 6 values are obtained by multipying column 5 by $30, which is the money value of losses per episode of illness.

The resources used in the provision of immunizations include a building owned by the government, a nurse whose hourly wage translates into $1 per shot, and drugs and supplies that cost an additional $1 per shot. The additional cost per shot is thus $2. Variable costs for 1,000 shots are $2,000; for 2,000 shots, $4,000; and so on. The total cost measures the total resource commitment made by the government in providing the services; it should include a value of the services provided by the building. We will assume that the government could have rented out the building space for $1,000; this will be used as a measure of the economic cost of the building space.

The total cost of immunizations includes the building space cost, assumed to be a fixed cost once the decision to use the space for this purpose has been made, and the variable costs comprising nursing services and supplies. Total costs are shown in column 2, and additional or incremental costs of each extra 1,000 shots are shown in column 4.

Given these figures, two benefit–cost ratios can be calculated: a total benefit–cost ratio for each level of output and a marginal benefit–cost ratio calculated for any movement from one level to the next. Let us look, for example, at these ratios when 1,000 immunizations have been given. In this case, the *total* benefit–cost ratio is shown by total benefits created divided by total costs incurred: this is $3,000/$3,000 or 1 : 1. The project breaks even at this level of output using the total criteria. Using marginal valuations, the project can be shown to be profitable at a level of output of 1,000 immunizations. This ratio shows the ratio of additional benefits to additional costs from producing 1,000 immunizations rather than producing none. Given that the building costs are already committed and thus fixed, then the marginal costs are $2,000, and the marginal benefit–cost ratio (column 7) is 3 : 2. An additional 1,000 immunizations beyond this would yield a marginal benefit–cost ratio of 2.25 : 2.00. This is still in excess of a ratio of 1 : 1; such a ratio would indicate that additional benefits were just equal to additional costs. The third 1,000 immunizations have a marginal benefit–cost ratio of under 1 : 1. This would indicate a net social loss from expanding to a level of 3,000 from 2,000. The right number of immunizations is 2,000. Any expansion beyond this, say to 3,000, would yield greater additional costs than benefits; in terms of our efficiency goal, we should not move to a level of 3,000 immunizations.

In identifying 2,000 immunizations as the right quantity of output, we are identifying an ideal or optimal quantity, rather than an actual one. In fact, the actual quantity produced may be greater or less than the ideal or efficient quantity. For example, if the reimbursement of physicians is such that they have no incentives to offer immunizations, then, in the absence of a public health effort, very few immunizations will be made. The actual quantity will be less than the optimal one. On the other hand, if the immunizations are made by a public health department that has encouraged the legislature to make immunization mandatory, 5,000 or more immunizations will be made. From an efficiency standpoint, this is too many and would show up in the marginal benefit–cost ratio, which would be less than 1.

14.3 INFORMATION REQUIREMENTS AND MEASUREMENT PROBLEMS

The previous example presents a picture of some overall elements of a cost–benefit analysis. The next step in our exposition is to examine in more detail the overall informational requirements and some of the major measurement problems in conducting such an analysis.

14.3.1 Information Requirements

Figure 14–1 summarizes the data requirements for a cost–benefit analysis in the health field. To begin with, we have the scarce resources (medical personnel and equipment) that can produce medical care or health care, such as hospital treatment. The relation between the inputs and the throughputs (medical care) is called the *production relation*. It measures how productive resource inputs are producing medical care. Medical care is referred to as a *throughput* rather than an output because it is not regarded as the end in the system. The second relation is between medical care activity and the level of health. This relation measures how effective medical care is and is referred to as the *effectiveness relation*. The measure of this relation is beyond the scope of the economist and is usually done by medical researchers.

The two relations together form the link between resource use and health. This link measures how effective resources are in producing health. Note that resources can be ineffective in this task because either they are not used productively or the treatments produced have no influence on health, or because of both.

With these two relations determined, we have established the relation between inputs and outputs of the project or system. Recall that generally it is the incremental or marginal relation that is of concern to us, that is, how much more health can be produced with an extra unit of resources. We move next to the valuation process, that is, determining the worth to society of an extra unit of health. When this is done, we have a measure of the social benefits attributable to changes in the health status of the community members.

These benefits must be compared with the opportunity costs of the project to obtain a benefit–cost ratio. Strictly speaking, the opportunity cost is the benefits given up by *not* using the resources in the highest-valued alternative use. This is

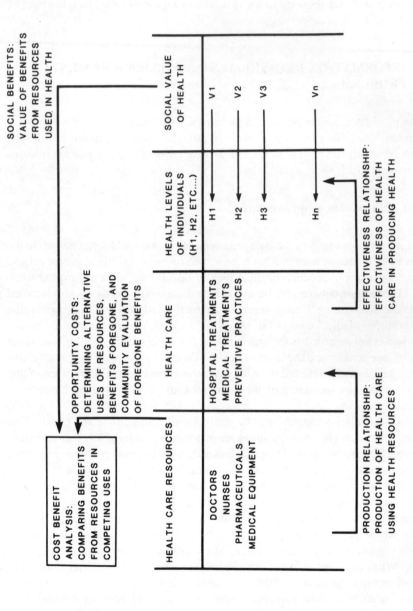

Figure 14–1 Outline of information requirements for a cost–benefit analysis. The complete cost–benefit analysis requires tracing through the effectiveness of resources in producing health, evaluating health output, and determining opportunity cost of resources used.

frequently measured by the money cost of the paid resources and by the imputed cost of unpaid resources (see Section 14.3.4).

A complete cost–benefit analysis requires that all the preceding information be available, which is seldom the case. Because of this, a less demanding sort of analysis, a cost-effectiveness analysis, has become popular. Cost-effectiveness studies examine the cost–output relation between alternative methods of achieving the same goal, for example, of treating kidney failure or of preventing heart attacks. Such an analysis stops short of comparing alternative objectives by the placing of money values on these objectives. Only a cost–benefit analysis will allow one to compare the net social values of alternative goals. However, a number of evaluational problems must be surmounted before obtaining true cost–benefit calculations. The remainder of Section 14.3 discusses some of the major problems.

14.3.2 Production Relation

The production relation represents how productive inputs are in producing medical care. As seen in Section 5.7, the measure of physician care or hospital care can have certain ambiguities; in particular, they can vary considerably in quality, which is difficult to measure. The production relation must take this quality variance into account so as not to have intensive medical care appear unproductive, when it is, by its nature, more resource intensive.

14.3.3 Effectiveness Relation

To determine the relation between one variable and another, clear definitions and measures are required for both variables. As shown in Chapter 1, there is neither an unambiguous definition nor a standard measure of health. Also, numerous potential factors might influence the health of a patient in addition to medical treatment. These include, among others, the predisposition of the patient to recover on his or her own and the environment in which the care is administered. In the absence of a well-defined effectiveness relation, a key piece of information in a cost–benefit relationship will be missing (Cochrane, 1972).

14.3.4 Opportunity Cost and Money Cost

As discussed in Sections 2.2.3 and 5.3.1, the *money cost* is the actual payout to a resource, while the *opportunity cost* is the money measure of the resource's commitment (whether or not the resource was paid). The opportunity cost is measured in terms of what the resource could earn in its highest-valued alternative use (the market value). Under the presumption that what consumers would have paid the resource in this alternative use is a reflection of what the resource would be worth *to them*, using the opportunity cost allows us to obtain a measure of what the resource would be worth in its next highest-valued use. Under many circumstances the money cost is a good approximation of the opportunity cost; that is, what resources earn are roughly the same in their present use and in their next highest-valued use.

To identify a resource's opportunity cost, we must first identify what that resource's highest-valued *alternative* use is. This is by no means an easy task. Take, as an example, a radiologist in Green Bay, Wisconsin, emergency clinic who earns $60 an hour. If she were not practicing radiology, what would her highest-valued alternative be? Would it still be in medicine, but in some other specialty or community? Would it be as a dentist or lawyer? There are no easy answers to these questions. Indeed, one of the most difficult tasks of evaluation economics is to identify what the resources *could* be doing in an alternative use. One of the main determining factors of a resource's alternative use is the time allowed for the resource to adjust to the alternative use. If our time horizon is 3 years, the radiologist might well retrain and become a pathologist. Her opportunity cost in such a case might be what she could earn as a pathologist. On the other hand, if we are speaking about a horizon of several months, the radiologist's highest-valued alternative may be a position as a radiologist somewhere else.

Let us assume that we are talking about the short run and that the radiologist's highest-valued alternative is a position as a radiologist in a Chicago hospital, at $60 an hour. This is the radiologist's opportunity cost, and in this case it equals her money cost.

There are instances when money costs will not equal opportunity cost. Money costs may be an *underestimate* of economic or opportunity costs when the resources are underpaid or are unpaid. If the radiologist donated her time for free, money costs are zero; if we valued her resource input at zero, we would be underestimating the value of resources used. In this case we would use the opportunity cost as the measure of the resource commitment. Other instances when money costs underestimate opportunity costs occur when buildings or equipment are donated or used but not costed.

Sometimes resources may be *overvalued* when measured by their money costs. One example might be if Wisconsin radiologists were successful in having a law passed that placed strict limitations on the number of radiologists who could practice radiology in the state. This might drive their prices up; such a law may create a price of $80 in Wisconsin as compared with one of $60 in Chicago. In these circumstances the money price would be too high a measure of the resource's opportunity cost.

14.3.5 Benefits and Cost Accruing in the Future Periods

Until now, our analysis has considered only current period costs and benefits. In fact, many types of health program benefits continue to occur in future years. An individual saved by an intensive-care program for heart attack victims may obtain benefits that last a number of years.

To evaluate these benefits and costs, two things must be recognized: (1) we are evaluating these as of the current period, and (2) future benefits and costs, valued as of the current period, must be discounted to account for individual's valuations of these benefits and costs.

The first observation is that, when a program for 1979 is proposed, the valuations to be considered are made as if they were all occurring in 1979. If the beneficiaries of a heart attack program are told that benefits will occur through 1990, the benefits for 1980, 1981, 1982, and so on, are valued as of 1979. That is, if $10,000 in benefits will accrue from the program in 1985, they will be valued at what the individual thinks they are worth to her or him in 1979.

It is generally assumed that $1,000 in benefits accruing now will be worth more to an individual than $1,000 accruing one year from now. The value of these preferences of earlier over later periods can be expressed in terms of the discount rate, called r. If an individual is asked how much money he or she would accept in 1980 in order to be worth as much to him or her as $1,000 in 1979, the person might say $1,100. In other words, $1,000 in the current period 1979 would be worth as much as $1,100 one year later. The discount rate is 0.10, and the equivalency of values it brings about can be expressed as $1,000 $(1 + 0.10) =$ $1,100, or symbolically as $1,000 $(1 + r) = $1,100$. This may be rewritten as $1,000 $= $1,100/(1 + r)$. This equation says that, in the individual's eyes, $1,100 next year will be equivalent to $1,100/(1 + r)$ or $1,000 this year. The existence of discounting on the part of individuals is an assumption derived largely from introspection. It is based on the idea that there is some discount rate an individual is willing to make to equate present and future benefits.

The same principle holds for comparisons between 1980 and 1981. That is, $1,000 in 1980 is equivalent to $1,100 in 1981, if the individual's discount rate is 0.10. By inference, then, $1,000 in 1981 will be worth $[\$1,000/(1 + r) (1 + r)]$ in 1979; this can be expressed as $\$1,000/(1 + r)^2$. Similarly, $1,000 in 1982 can be expressed as the equivalent of $\$1,000/(1 + r)^3$ in 1979, and so on. Generally, improved health or added life yields a stream of benefits; that is, a saved life in 1979 will yield benefits in 1980, 1981, 1982, and so on. If such benefits are $2,000 each year, the present value of future benefits can be expressed as

$$\$2,000 + \frac{\$2,000}{(1 + r)} + \frac{\$2,000}{(1 + r)^2} + \frac{\$2,000}{(1 + r)^3}$$

and so on, for as long as benefits last. The letter usually used to symbolize the annual benefits is B, with subscripts 0, 1, 2, and 3 for right now, one year hence, two years hence, and so on. In our present example, $B_0 = B_1 = B_2 = B_3$ and the present value of benefits can be expressed symbolically as

$$B_0 + \frac{B_1}{(1 + r)} + \frac{B_2}{(1 + r)^2} + \frac{B_3}{(1 + r)^3}$$

If the number of years in which benefits will last is quite large and $B_0 = B_1 = B_2$, and so on, the present value of benefits can be expressed as B_0/r. If benefits of $10,000 a year will last forever and if the discount rate is 0.10, the present value of these benefits will be $10,000/0.10 = \$100,000$. Benefits lasting for long periods can be approximated with this formula.

The present-value formula tells us what a discounted stream of benefits is presently worth. The same formula can be applied to value costs. If C_0, C_1, and C_2, are costs of a program applicable to periods 0, 1, and 2, and the discount rate is i, the present value of costs is

$$C_0 + \frac{C_1}{(1 + i)} + \frac{C_2}{(1 + i)^2}$$

Note that i is used as the discount rate for costs and r for benefits. This is merely to bring out the point that the benefits may be accruing to individuals other than those who bore the costs and that these individuals may have different discount rates. In practice, we seldom make this distinction, and so we will use r as the discount rate both for beneficiaries of a program and for those who suffer costs.

The equation used to summarize the cost–benefit ratio of a project, that is, to compare costs and benefits, is the net present value (NPV) equation, which measures the net difference between the present values of costs and of benefits. This is expressed for a three-period evaluation as

$$NPV = B_0 + \frac{B_1}{(1 + r)} = \frac{B_2}{(1 + r)^2} - C_0 - \frac{C_1}{(1 + r)} - \frac{C_2}{(1 + r)^2}$$

Many health programs are financed through general taxes. If we assume the foregone benefits would all have occurred in the present period, that is, they would have occurred at the expense of current consumption, then the opportunity costs of these programs can be represented as C_0, and our equation is

$$NPV = B_0 + \frac{B_1}{(1 + r)} + \frac{B_2}{(1 + r)^2} - C_0$$

Given the extension of benefits and costs of a program into future periods, the analyst is faced with the problem of assigning an appropriate discount rate to the net present-value equation. Controversy exists over which rate to employ. If we believe that market interest rates clearly reflect supply and demand forces for saving and investment, it can be argued that at current levels of savings (e.g., transforming present into future wealth through bonds and mortgages) the market interest rate is an expression of the marginal consumer's discount rate. On the basis of this reasoning, the interest rate in the market for riskless bonds (e.g., bonds of most governments) expresses the discount rate of consumers and can be used as a discount rate for the evaluation of riskless projects, that is, those whose return is certain. For more risky projects, a higher discount rate, one incorporating a risk premium, should be used based on this reasoning.

There is a complication, however. The market interest rate reflects the discount rates of present consumers at present saving levels. The preferences of future generations are not incorporated into the picture. A generation of high-living, heavy-spending people may discount future benefits at a very high discount rate and may not care to preserve the environment for future generations or, in general, to undertake projects that benefit future generations. If future generations' benefits are to be taken into account, this will call for a lower discount rate than that which the present generation would choose in the absence of such consideration.

An advocate of this viewpont might place the discount rate choice in the hand of the government, which presumably would act as arbiter between resource demands of present and future generations. However, the government can hardly be considered an impartial party. If the bureaucrats and technicians who heavily influence government decisions act to any degree in their own self-interests, they would choose a rate that is as low as possible! The reason for this is that at low discount rates future benefits will be valued higher relative to present consumption than at high rates. By using a low rate more long-lasting projects will be justified on a cost–benefit basis, and hence an expansion of the bureaucracy will be better justified.

In the wake of such conflicting views, analysts have established the practice of taking a neutral view to the issue of discounting by calculating the net present value using several rates and letting the policymaker choose the appropriate one. The sensitivity of the *NPV* to alternative discount rates can be illustrated in the context of an example. Assume that a health program costing \$43,000 (all resources used are taken from current consumption) yields benefits equal to \$10,000 a year for 5 years, beginning with the current year. To determine if the program will yield greater benefits than costs, we must find an expression for the present-value equation. With $B_0 = B_1 = B_2 = B_3 = B_4 = \$10,000$, we can apply a discounting factor to find the present value of this benefit stream. The present-value (*PV*) equation is

$$PV = B_0 + \frac{B_1}{(1 + r)} + \frac{B_2}{(1 + r)^2} + \frac{B_3}{(1 + r)^3} + \frac{B_4}{(1 + r)^4}$$

The values of $(1 + r)$, $(1 + r)^2$, and so on, are shown in Part A of Table 14–2 for three alternative discount rates: a low rate of 4 percent, a middle rate of 8 percent, and a high rate of 12 percent. Applying these rates to B_1, B_2, B_3, and so on, yields the values shown in Part B of Table 14–2. The present value of the income stream is \$46,298 using the low rate, \$43,232 using the middle rate, and \$40,839 using the high rate. Notice how the total present value of the stream falls as future benefits are given less importance (higher rates of discount). To determine whether the program would yield positive net benefits, we must calculate the *NVP*. Given that C_0 equals \$43,000, the *NVP* is positive at a 0.04 discount rate, just barely positive at a 0.08 rate, and negative at a 0.12 rate. An individual's prescription of whether or not to undertake the program will depend on the discount rate used.

14.3.6 Measuring the Benefits from Survival and Better Health

By far the most widely espoused benefit to be obtained from increased survival and better health has been the increase in working time that this health affords. A very convenient money measure of these benefits is the earnings made by the worker during this added healthy time. If the benefits from reduced illness or reduced death last longer than 1 year, the future benefits can be discounted with an appropriate discount rate.

Turning this measure around, one can use it to measure the indirect cost of illness or death. In this case, the economic cost of illness or death can be estimated as the discounted money value of work time lost. Since illness also results in medical treatment, we must add the direct costs of medical care to obtain a more complete measure of the burden of illness (Rice, Hodgson, and Kopstein, 1985). This approach to the measurement of illness costs has been called the *human capital* approach.

The human capital approach is really a lower bound to the total economic burden of illness, even if we were only counting the *private* costs of illness (i.e., those borne by the afflicted or foregone by the deceased). Since illness or death is accompanied by pain and suffering, the avoidance of illness and death is accompanied by the avoidance of pain and suffering. The patient presumably would place a value on avoidance over and above the value of earnings gained and medical costs avoided. Furthermore, these measures ignore the value of avoided death and illness as valued by others (i.e., *external* valuations placed on better health). Individuals (family members and others) do value health and the survival of others. Difficult as it may be to estimate them, these valuations must be added to private values to equal the *social* value of health and survival.

Recently, a more unified approach has been developed to obtain a measure of the *private* benefits of increased survival. Such an approach examines the value people place on the probability of increased survival. It approaches the problem in terms of saving a "statistical life" rather than a specific, identified life. One virtue of this approach is that it frames individual decisions in the terms of which many

Table 14–2 Calculation of Present Value of Benefits under Alternative Discount Rates

Part A: Discounting Factor

Discount Rate	$(1 + r)$	$(1 + r)^2$	$(1 + r)^3$	$(1 + r)^4$
0.04	1.04	1.08	1.12	1.17
0.08	1.08	1.16	1.25	1.36
0.12	1.12	1.25	1.41	1.57

Part B: Discounted Present Value of Benefits

Discount Rate	B_0	$\dfrac{B_1}{(1 + r)}$	$\dfrac{B_2}{(1 + r)^2}$	$\dfrac{B_3}{(1 + r)^3}$	$\dfrac{B_4}{(1 + r)^4}$	Present value (row sum)
0.04	10,000	9,615	9,233	8,896	8,554	46,298
0.08	10,000	9,259	8,620	8,000	7,353	43,232
0.12	10,000	8,928	8,000	7,029	6,369	40,839

decisions are made in reality. A large number of resource-allocation decisions in the health field take place in risky and impersonal rather than certain and personal contexts. When attempting to place a value on life and health, analysts originally conceived of the problem in terms of questioning how much someone's life would be worth to him or her. This places the question in rather dramatic, gunpoint terms. Undoubtedly, there have been instances when life or certain decisions have been placed in the hands of society or the medical profession. The case of kidney dialysis treatments in the early 1950s for which "life and death committees" were established to ration life-saving dialysis treatments to known victims of kidney failure, leaving the nonrecipients to die, created a great public stir. Not all, or even most, life or death decisions are made in such certain contexts. Individuals who would offer their souls to avoid a certain death will, in less certain circumstances, behave to *increase* their chances of dying or becoming ill. People willingly smoke, eat potentially hazardous foods, and accept dangerous jobs despite the fact that the likelihood of illness or death will increase. One can only conclude that, while facing certain death may be intolerable, activities that increase the *risk* of death may be acceptable. They are acceptable because the gains in income or satisfaction that accompany them exceed their costs.

The willingness-to-pay approach, placed in a risky context, has been used to derive estimates of the money value of increased or reduced risks of illness or death. For example, assume that a perfectly riskless occupation, folding paper airplanes and packaging them, pays a wage of $400. A second occupation that is somewhat more risky, cleaning asbestos pipes, becomes available. We assume that the riskier occupation requires exactly the same skills as the riskless one, and furthermore, that 3 in every 1,000 asbestos workers eventually contract lung cancer, whereas none of the airplane folders do. If the workers in the asbestos industry were aware of these risks and were still willing to accept them, provided that they were suitably compensated for doing so, the additional compensation they would accept, called a *risk premium*, would be a measure of the value of this extra risk. If the asbestos workers were willing to accept a wage of $450 a month, then, if all other factors were held constant, the wage differential would be a measure of the value they placed on this extra risk. This value will depend on several factors; these include the degree to which the workers are risk averse and the size of the risk (see Section 4.4 for a discussion of decision making under conditions of uncertainty). For example, the greater the adversity of the worker to risk is, the more utility will be gained from the safe alternative. The risk premium required to compensate the individual who is more risk averse would be greater.

Recent investigations have been undertaken to estimate the risk premiums in risky occupations, as well as the amounts consumers are willing to pay for goods that reduce the probability of death, such as seat belts and fire alarms (Blomquist, 1981). The results, when extrapolated to calculate a value per statistical life, show a wide variation in such values, ranging from $300,000 to $2.5 million. Despite these wide variations, there is a considerable usefulness in such studies. The value of benefits from many health-related projects and programs can be expressed in terms of reducing the likelihood of illness and death. Heart attack prevention programs, early disease detection programs, water and air purification programs, and work safety measures, among others, can all have their benefits measured in terms of the reduced likelihood of illness and death. In these instances the measures obtained of the value of these programs in reducing the probability of illness and death can be used as measures of the benefits of the programs (Muller and Reutzel, 1984; Thompson, 1986).

14.4 COST-EFFECTIVENESS ANALYSIS

Frequently, situations arise where we want to evaluate the economic consequences of alternative courses of action, but where we do not wish to place values on life. For example, if we are treating a 70-year-old woman with no financial assets for a peptic ulcer, according to both the human capital and willingness-to-pay approaches, our results may come up short on the benefit side if we conducted a cost–benefit analysis using increased earnings as a measure of benefits. It may well be that on equity grounds we have decided to go ahead and treat her. If alternative courses of treatment exist, we are still faced with an economic problem, that of choosing the lowest-cost alternative. The task of a *cost-effectiveness* analysis is to rank alternative treatments on the basis of cost per unit of output.

As seen in Section 1.3, there is no unique measure of health output. The output "life years saved" refers only to those treatments that save lives. But one can save a life (or a statistical life) and have the recipient end up in a wheelchair. In such a case the outcome will not be the same, qualitatively, as if the recipient were perfectly healthy during the years saved. Additionally, many treatments do not save lives but they change the quality of life (i.e., improve health status).

For these reasons, physical measures of health status have been developed that rank individuals according to health status for certain dimensions such as mobility and pain. As seen in Section 1.3, a scale can be developed for each dimension; mobility, for example, can be ranked from 0 (for totally immobile) to 10 (for completely mobile). Additional dimensions can be ranked, and a "superindex" can be developed that aggregates the indexes for each dimension. (The development of these indexes requires the insertion of values on the part of somebody with regard to developing values for each unit on the scale; see Williams, 1974b.)

With the development of a *physical* measure of output, this index can be applied to each treatment. For example, the 70-year-old woman might move from 6 to 7 when treated with drugs and from 6 to 8 when treated with surgery for her peptic ulcer. But which is "better"?

From an economic standpoint, if we accept the values embedded in the physical output scale, the better treatment will be the one with the lower cost per unit of

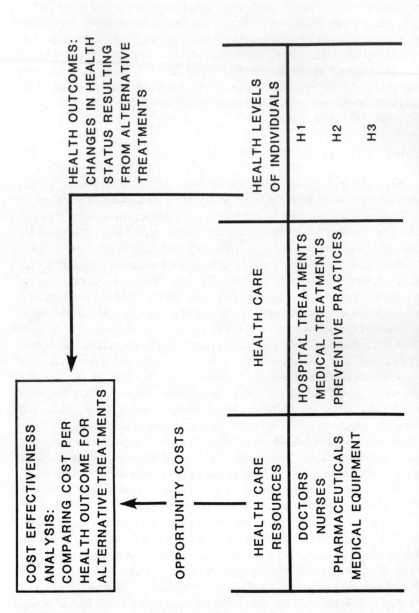

Figure 14–2 Outline of information requirements for a cost-effectiveness analysis. The complete cost–benefit analysis requires tracing through the effectiveness of resources in producing health, evaluating health output, and comparing cost per unit of health output for alternatives.

physical output. If the drug treatment cost $800 and the surgery costs $2,000, then *per unit of physical output*, the drug treatment is more cost effective.

The elements of a cost-effectiveness analysis are shown in Figure 14–2. As can be seen in comparison with Figure 14–1, values are not placed on improved health outcomes. Rather the costs for each alternative are related to the physical measures of health outcomes themselves. Because dollar values are not placed on health outcomes, cost-effectiveness analysis cannot tell us whether something is worth doing. However, when dollar measures of output are either unavailable or unacceptable, we still have a tool to gauge the economic desirability of alternative courses of action.

REFERENCES

Cost of Illness

Hodgson, T.A., & Meiners, M.R. (1982). Cost-of-illness methodology: A guide to current practices and procedures. *Milbank Memorial Fund Quarterly, 60*(3), 429–462.

Rice, D.P., Hodgson, T.A., & Kopstein, A.N. (1985). The economic cost of illness: A replication and update. *Health Care Financing Review, 7*(1), 61–80.

Zook, C.J., Savackis, S.F., & Moore, F.D. (1980). Repeated hospitalization for the same disease. *Milbank Memorial Fund Quarterly, 58*, 454–471.

Cost–Benefit and Cost-effectiveness Analysis: General

Carr-Hill, R.A. (1985). The evaluation of health care. *Social Science & Medicine, 21*, 367–375.

Cochrane, A. (1972). *Effectiveness and efficiency.* New York: Oxford University Press.

Doubilet, P., Weinstein, M.C., & McNeil, B.J. (1986). Use and misuse of the term "cost effective" in medicine. *New England Journal of Medicine, 314*(4), 253–256.

Drummond, M.F. (1980). *Principles of economic appraisal in health care.* New York: Oxford University Press.

——— (1981). *Studies in economic appraisal in health care.* New York: Oxford University Press.

Hellinger, F.J. (1980). Cost–benefit analysis of health care: Past applications and future prospects. *Inquiry, 17*, 204–215.

Stoddart, G.L., & Drummond, M.F. (1984). How to read clinical journals: VII. To understand an economic evaluation (Parts A and B). *Canadian Medical Association Journal, 130*, 1428–1433 and 1542–1549.

Warner, K.E., & Hutton, R.C. (1980). Cost–benefit and cost-effectiveness analysis in health care. *Medical Care, 18*, 1069–1084.

——— (1982). *Cost–benefit and cost-effectiveness analysis in health care.* Ann Arbor, MI: Health Administration Press.

Weinstein, M.C., & Stason, W.B. (1977). Foundations of cost-effectiveness analysis for health and medical practices. *New England Journal of Medicine, 296*, 716–721.

Williams, A. (1974). The cost benefit approach. *British Medical Bulletin, 20*, 252–256.

——— (1974). Measuring the effectiveness of health care systems. *British Journal of The Preventive Medicine Society, 28*, 196–202.

Value of Health and Life

Avorn, J. (1984). Benefit and cost analysis in geriatric care. *New England Journal of Medicine, 310*, 1294–1301.

Blomquist, G. (1981). The value of human life: An empirical perspective. *Economic Inquiry, 19*(1), 157–164.

Landefeld, J.S., & Seskin, E.P. (1982). The economic value of life: Linking theory to practice. *American Journal of Public Health, 72*(6), 555–566.

Mooney, G. (1977). *The valuation of human life.* New York: Macmillan.

Muller, A., & Reutzel, T.J. (1984). Willingness to pay for a reduction in fatality risk. *American Journal of Public Health, 74*(8), 808–812.

Rice, D.P., & Hodgson, T.A. (1982). The value of human life revisited. *American Journal of Public Health, 72*(6), 536–538.

Schelling, T.C. (1968). The life you save may be your own. In S.B. Chase (Ed.), *Problems in public expenditure analysis* (pp. 127–157). Washington, DC: Brookings Institute.

Thaler, R., & Rosen, S. (1975). The value of saving a life. In M.E. Terleckyj (Ed.), *Household production and consumption* (pp. 265–302). New York: National Bureau of Economic Research.

Thompson, M.S. (1986). Willingness to pay and accept risks to cure chronic disease. *American Journal of Public Health, 76*, 392–397.

Viscusi, W.K. (1978). Labor market valuations of life and limb. *Public Policy, 26*, 359–385.

Zeckhauser, R. (1975). Procedures for valuing lives. *Public Policy, 23*, 419–464.

Specific Cost–Benefit and Cost-effectiveness Analysis

Berwick, D.M., & Komaroff, A.L. (1982). Cost effectiveness of lead screening. *New England Journal of Medicine, 306*, 1392–1398.

Bloom, B.S., & Jacobs, J. (1985). Cost effects of restricting cost-effective therapy. *Medical Care, 23*, 872–880.

Detsky, A.S., & Jeejeebhoy, K.J. (1984). Cost-effectiveness of postoperative parenteral nutrition in patients undergoing major gastrointestinal surgery. *Journal of Parenteral and Enteral Nutrition, 8*, 632–637.

Doherty, N., & Hicks, B.C. (1975). The use of cost-effectiveness analysis in geriatric day care. *Gerontologist, 15*, 412–417.

Evans, R.G., & Robinson, G.C. (1980). Surgical day care: Measurements of the economic payoff. *Canadian Medical Association Journal, 123*, 873–880.

———— (1983). An economic study of cost savings on a care by parent ward. *Medical Care, 21*, 768–782.

Hammond, J. (1979). Home health care cost effectiveness: An overview of the literature. *Public Health Reports, 94*, 305–311.

Lave, L.B. (1980). Economic evaluation of public health programs. *Annual Review of Public Health, 1*, 255–276.

Russell, L.B. (1986). *Is prevention better than cure?* Washington, DC: Brookings Institute.

Scheffler, R.M., & Paringer, L. (1980). A review of the economic evaluation of prevention. *Medical Care, 18*, 473–484.

Stern, R.S., Pass, T.M., & Komaroff, A.L. (1984). Topical v. systemic agent treatment for papulo-pustular acne. *Archives of Dermatology, 120,* 1571–1578.

Weinstein, M.C. (1983). Cost-effectiveness priorities for cancer prevention. *Science, 221,* 17–23.

Weisbrod, B.A. (1971). Costs and benefits of medical research. *Journal of Political Economy, 79,* 527–544.

_____ , Test, M.A., & Stein, L.I. (1980). Alternative to mental hospital treatment. *Archives of General Psychiatry, 37,* 400–405.

Economic Evaluation and Technology Assessment

Detsky, A.S. (1985). Using economic analysis to determine the resource consequences of choices made in planning clinical trials. *Journal of Chronic Diseases, 38,* 753–765.

Drummond, M.F., & Stoddart, G.L. (1984). Economic analysis and clinical trials. *Controlled Clinical Trials, 5,* 115–128.

Weinstein, M.C. (1981). Economic assessments of medical practices and technologies. *Medical Decision Making, 1,* 309–330.

Index